Praise for Jax Peters Lowell
and *The Gluten-Free Bible*

"With her trademark cheekiness and deep-hearted wisdom, Jax Lowell serves up another celiac classic."

—Diane Eve Paley, president, Celiac Society of America

"I have never read an allergy book that I could say had a heart, but this one does."

—Jim Burns, food editor, *Los Angeles Times* syndicate

"Aren't we lucky this talented writer is one of us!"
—Alice Bast, executive director, National Foundation for Celiac Awareness

"Jax Lowell proves it's possible to live *and* eat happily ever after."
—Connie Sarros, *The Wheat-Free, Gluten-Free Cookbooks*

"Lowell has succeeded in creating a work that will inspire the patient, dietician, and doctor—RUN, don't walk, to pick up your copy!"
—A. Myron Falchuk, M.D., associate professor of medicine at Harvard Medical School

". . . Just what the doctor ordered."
—Alessio Fasano, M.D., Center for Celiac Research

"A lot of attitude and a terrific sense of humor."

—*New York Daily News*

"A book that nurtures as it advises."
—*Better Homes & Gardens*'s Cooks' Catalog

Also by Jax Peters Lowell

No More Cupcakes & Tummy Aches:
A Story for Parents and Their Celiac Children to Share,
illustrations by Jane Kirkwood

Against the Grain: The Slightly Eccentric Guide
to Living Well without Gluten or Wheat

Mothers: A Novel

the gluten-free bible

➤ JAX PETERS LOWELL

the
gluten-free
bible

The Thoroughly
Indispensable Guide
to Negotiating Life
without Wheat

Foreword by Anthony J. DiMarino Jr., M.D.

An Owl Book

HENRY HOLT AND COMPANY · NEW YORK

Owl Books
Henry Holt and Company, LLC
Publishers since 1866
175 Fifth Avenue
New York, New York 10010
www.henryholt.com

An Owl Book® and ® are registered trademarks of
Henry Holt and Company, LLC.

Owing to limitations of space, all acknowledgments of
permission to reprint previously published material
will be found with the recipe acknowledgments.

Library of Congress Cataloging-in-Publication Data
Lowell, Jax Peters.
    The gluten-free bible : the thoroughly indispensable
guide to negotiating life without wheat / Jax Peters Lowell ;
foreword by Anthony J. DiMarino.
      p. cm.
    "An Owl book."
    Includes bibliographical references and index.
    ISBN-13: 978-0-8050-7746-9
    ISBN-10: 0-8050-7746-4
    1. Wheat-free diet. 2. Gluten-free diet. I. Title.

RM237.87.L683 2005
613.2'6—dc22   2004059709

Henry Holt books are available for special promotions and
premiums. For details contact: Director, Special Markets.

First edition published in hardcover in 1995 as
Against the Grain by Henry Holt and Company

First Owl Books Edition 1996
Revised Edition 2005

Printed in the United States of America

10 9 8 7 6 5 4 3

In memory of Kay and Jack Peters
and Catherine Petitpain, the angels at my table
And, always, for John

When one door of happiness closes, another opens;
but often we look so long at the closed door
that we do not see the one
which has been opened for us.

—HELEN KELLER

contents

foreword: the well-informed celiac . . .

Just as patients should and do "size up" their doctors as people and communicators, so, too, the judicious physician takes careful note of how patients present themselves in order to decide how much information, support, and guidance each person needs. It was clear to me when I first met Jax Lowell in September of 1996 that I was in the presence of one of the most highly motivated patients I'd met in my many years of practice. Here was someone possessed of enormous energy and who had great respect for knowledge. She was willing and able to do her homework, assessing treatment options so that her decisions were always well informed. It was apparent to me from the start that we would be colleagues in our joint effort to understand and to overcome the medical obstacles and complications presented by long-standing celiac disease.

But that is only half the story. The other side of this highly motivated, smart, and courageous woman is that of a skilled communicator, first-rate writer, and gifted speaker. Add to this her great humor and a powerful desire to use her talent to help others, and it's no surprise that her first book, *Against the Grain*, became a landmark resource. I have asked Jax to apply her quietly persuasive humor to more than one recalcitrant celiac patient and she has done so with tact, charm, and her trademark resourcefulness.

Much has been learned about celiac disease since *Against the Grain* first made its debut in 1995. Once thought to be present in approximately 1 in

10,000 North Americans, we now recognize that this immune response to the gluten in common grains was merely the tip of the iceberg. Work by Dr. Alessio Fasano and others at the Center for Celiac Disease at the University of Maryland would suggest that the condition may occur in a quiescent but insidious form as frequently as 1 in 132 individuals in the United States. Whatever the prevalence, what we do know is that the symptoms of frequent diarrhea, malodorous/fatty stools, extreme weight loss, and subsequent malnutrition occur only in the minority of celiac patients.

The more subtle presentations of this genetic disease include unexplained bone loss, anemia—especially iron deficiency anemia—or any number of autoimmune or allergic-like disorders, including a blistering itchy rash called dermatitis herpetiformis, headaches, dental enamel defects, fatigue, and aphthous ulcers, among other wide-ranging symptoms. For a few young women, the inability to become pregnant or miscarriage exposes the underlying celiac disease. These atypical presentations make up the majority of celiacs, many of whom report having vague symptoms for many years prior to diagnosis. Others pick up an incorrect diagnosis of irritable bowel disease along the way.

Physicians can establish a diagnosis simply and easily by testing for antibodies to CD. Subsequent biopsy of the small intestine or duodenum showing atrophy, or damage to the intestinal villi, confirms it. Subsequent serological screening of the immediate family is important as well, with as many as 10 percent of first-and second-degree relatives testing positively.

It has been said that "if life is theater, physicians have a front row seat"— and I do! The majority of patients, especially those with classic presentations, are vigilant about their diets and often fearful of ingesting hidden gluten. But more and more celiacs, especially those with few symptoms or who have been diagnosed through family screening, completely deny the existence of this condition, tolerating abdominal bloating and gaseousness out of a belief that it is impossible to enjoy life without gluten. Many deny even the increased risk of malignancy that can be associated with failing to strictly observe the gluten-free diet, as well as autoimmune problems such as diabetes millitus, rheumatoid arthritis, and Sjögren's syndrome. While most are relieved to know they do not have a life-threatening disease, they are despondent over the fact that they have to religiously observe a diet that eliminates their favorite foods.

While physicians must rigorously pursue follow-up care for their celiac patients—identifying and treating nutritional deficiencies, monitoring bone density, calcium absorption, assessing vitamin and mineral levels, offering dietetic education, and using periodic serological screenings and/or repeat biopsies to check for compliance and healing—there are no magic pills, no prescriptions to write for this condition. This is one case where food *is* the medicine and lifelong adherence to the gluten-free diet is the path to good health.

Education and confidence is paramount, as is the physician's attitude toward the diet. If a physician delivers the news with gloom and doom, the patient will respond accordingly. It is incumbent on all of us to communicate the accessibility and rewards of truly satisfying gluten-free foods. Congratulations are in order, not condolences. For surviving years of uncertainty, for enduring missed diagnoses and debilitating malaise, and for sticking with it.

Inspiring this kind of educated optimism is where Jax Lowell is at her best and where *The Gluten-Free Bible* offers the greatest reward to the reader. This comprehensive follow-up to her best-selling *Against the Grain* is as much literary gift as it is invaluable resource. That she is an incredibly talented writer is apparent in every paragraph. The chapter headings alone make one laugh out loud, but there is real insight behind the author's humor. You know you are in the hands of someone who's been there and doesn't take no for an answer. Lowell's witty and wise advice on the doctor-patient relationship can make visits with willing and cooperative physicians much more pleasant and informative. Other chapters offering commonsense tips on general health, sexual matters, and tough situations like college, dating, and family holidays exude optimism, creativity, gratitude, and grace. From nitty-gritty label reading to shopping and traveling tours, to negotiating a safe restaurant meal, this truly is "the bible" for the newly diagnosed and veterans alike.

Everywhere in this book is wonderful gluten-free food, the best of what's available today, and recipes that prove there is life after diagnosis, a good and full one. But lest you think you are in store for nonstop laughs, Lowell offers the full range of human response to a diagnosis of celiac disease. Moments of deep personal insight are written with poignancy and emotional truth.

The Gluten-Free Bible is indispensable reading, not only for patients who have celiac disease, but also for the physicians who care for them. I have recommended *Against the Grain* to my patients for many years, along with my encouragement to join local and national support groups in order to learn more about the gluten-free life. Now we have, in my opinion, one of the most valuable, comprehensive, and well-written of the numerous "self-help" books I have ever read. It is no accident that Jax Lowell's incredible energy, enthusiasm, and wonderful outlook have enabled her to overcome her diagnosis. That she continues to guide others to do the same is an extraordinary gift to an entire generation of American celiacs and their families.

Thank you, Jax Peters Lowell.

Anthony J. DiMarino Jr., M.D.
William Rorer Professor of Medicine
Chief, Division of Gastroenterology and Hepatology
Thomas Jefferson University Hospital, Philadelphia

introduction: the fork in the road

I am descended from a long line of Cassards and Petitpains, the latter name belonging to my maternal grandfather and French for "little bread." My mother's people included a statesman, bishops, naval officers, farmers, merchants, housewives, lamplighters, and one pirate by marriage, Jean Lafitte. Originally from Nantes, they scattered to Paris, Marseilles, Venezuela, and to Saint Domingue, which would one day become Haiti. It was here that Madame Marguerite Cassard, a young widow, was trying to figure out how to get her bakery out of debt even as the uprising cut a bloody machete swath to her door. Faced with the prospect of certain death, she fled to France with barely a sou and the shirt on her back while her sons Jean, Gilbert, and Louis made for America and New Orleans. According to the family historian, cousin Jean prospered in a series of businesses, one of which was a bakery on a par with Fauchon.

At the age of eighty-three, my mother demonstrated all the classic signs and symptoms of celiac disease. Stubborn as her forebears for whom good French food was a matter of honor and already ill with something far worse, she ignored my pleas and dunked her morning brioche into a bowl of café au lait right up to the day she died.

And so the baker's children come home to roost. After years of puzzling and increasingly dramatic symptoms, my own celiac disease was diagnosed in 1983, and among the first and second cousins in my generation, there are five more cases, as well as a persistent family rumor that Aunt A. is showing symptoms at the age of eighty-nine. Cousin Patricia, too, is beginning to see her lifelong plumbing problems in the light of her heritage. It wasn't until I published *Against the Grain* that my own more than slightly eccentric clan took seriously the idea that gluten intolerance is not something you outgrow. Add to this, dear reader, the fact that the undersigned descendant of "little breads" and master bakers now makes her home in a former bread factory and you have the irony of all ironies. A better case for genes as destiny, I challenge you to find.

❧

Thanks to a landmark study funded by the National Institutes of Health and spearheaded by the best minds in the international celiac community, we now know what many of us knew only in our gut—celiac disease does indeed run in families and at the staggering rate of 1 in 132 people and even more in some groups. The NIH estimates that we are 1 percent of the U.S. population, roughly 3 million strong. As more and more doctors are learning to recognize CD's protean symptoms, we are getting diagnosed faster and better every day. Major articles are being published in mainstream consumer magazines, as well as in important medical journals. Television reporters, talk show hosts, actors, and football players are going public and gluten-free jokes are finding their way into the lexicon of late-night comedy. Some of these jokes ruffle our feathers, but as an old PR hack once said, "It doesn't matter what they say, as long as they spell your name right." In America, awareness and incorporation into the national culture is everything. Celiac disease is gaining what marketers like to call "critical mass."

Today doctors and patients know a great deal about celiac disease, who gets it and why. We are organized to the hilt and we have become a powerful consumer voice. We are learning, down to a microscopic fraction, what amount of gluten can keep us sick and what can't hurt. There is new thinking about what foods are safe, which ones are not, and healthy arguments about it. There are walks for awareness and walks for the cure. There are foundations, celiac disease centers, and a task force has taken the first successful steps toward gluten-free labeling legislation. There are rumors of pills, patches, and patents pending. There has never been a better time to be gluten-free.

❧

When *Against the Grain* first appeared in 1995, getting a good and safe gluten-free meal was about as easy as finding an oat in a sack of buckwheat. The Internet was an idea Al Gore hadn't yet taken credit for and writing a book about a condition nobody had ever heard of was considered professional suicide. As many of you already know, pigheadedness is woven into my DNA. I persisted, believing CD wasn't rare at all, just grossly underdiagnosed.

No one could have predicted the sensation the book caused among my fellow celiacs who had been handed a bag of rice cakes, a mimeographed diet, and thereafter ignored. Readers laughed out loud, many for the first time. Tears were shed, cleansing the spirit like a good rain. Letters poured in praising the book and thanking me for addressing the emotional and social issues the medical community had no time for. Support groups prepared their members for the cruel, glutenous world by role-playing a chapter called "Restaurant Assertiveness Training" and people faced up to friends, family members, spouses, and in-laws who could not and would not honor their special needs. The book inspired many new gluten-free businesses and, rumor has it, was even the inspiration for one celiac tour company. Suddenly it was okay to carry gluten-free bread in your purse, march into a restaurant kitchen, travel with foreign language dining cards in one's luggage, and expect answers from a food company. No more eating the middle of a sandwich, picking the crust off a pie, taking second place. Going "against the grain" and being slightly eccentric about it was in. Sitting in the corner and suffering was out. It still is.

To my everlasting surprise, *Against the Grain* was quoted in a *Newsweek* article entitled *The Perils of Pasta* and was featured on the Food Network program, *In Food Today,* National Public Radio, and the *New York Times.* A certain New York rabbi wrote to tell me I had saved his life and that, according to Jewish tradition, my life was forever bound up with his. I never called him on it, but the idea that a kind stranger might someday pluck me from the brink is an indescribable comfort in an increasingly dangerous world.

No one expected *Against the Grain* to become the beloved classic it is, least of all me. Nor did I expect the outpouring of friendship and gratitude from gluten-challenged friends and fans in every city and town in America and Canada. I have looked into your eyes and seen my own fears mirrored there and I have been privileged to share your amazing stories of survival, of courage, of transcendent optimism. I have answered your questions to the best of my ability, my healthy and well-fed presence proof that you, too, will live to eat another day. In times of sadness and personal challenge, I have been buoyed and blessed by my extended family of celiacs. One letter I cherish thanks me for helping the correspondent find a sense of self-assertion that has

xxiv   Introduction: The Fork in the Road

affected her life well beyond the dinner table. Satisfaction doesn't get much better than that.

My mother taught me never to make reciprocation a term for giving. She always said "a gift will come back to you on its own." *Against the Grain* has come back to me a hundredfold and with it, a joy beyond measure.

———

Today's celiac lives in a universe that is vastly larger than the narrow world of inedible food I was thrust into. Mail-order businesses and specialty stores have bloomed, offering high-quality products that, to my mind, taste as good or even better than the foods we must forgo. Gluten-free chefs have stirred, concocted, sizzled, and tempted us with delights that are downright delicious. Gluten-free inns and sleepaway camps are flourishing. Caterers, personal chefs, cooking teachers, dieticians, au pairs, and nannies are specializing in the gluten-free diet, as well as a growing number of restaurants that offer gluten-free menus. Our very own magazine, *Living Without*, arrives every season on our doorsteps, full of great articles and mouthwatering food and photography the likes of which we are used to seeing in mainstream magazines like *Gourmet* and *Bon Appetit*. It is no longer necessary to hunt down every product that is gluten-free just to have something to eat. With so many choices, we can shop for only the ones that are worth our time and the extra expense.

———

An edition big enough to capture this brave new world had to be called *The Gluten-Free Bible*, its name a fitting tribute to the nickname many of you gave its predecessor. At twice the size of the original (like a favorite candy bar that got bigger), this was no small undertaking—it is, as the subtitle says, "The Thoroughly Indispensable Guide to Negotiating Life without Wheat." With all-new and totally comprehensive resources, all-new recipes for kids and adults, and some new foreign delights that will get you cooking in ways you never imagined, this edition captures the complexity of the choices and information facing the celiac today.

Food will always be paramount to anyone on the gluten-free diet, and chapter 5, "And the Winner Is . . . ," will guide you to the best of the best gluten-free companies. Chapter 9, "A Map of the Gluten-Free World," is just that, a guide to celiac-friendly restaurants, hotels, airlines, countries, tour companies, camps, hotels, and bed-and-breakfasts, far and near. Brand-new and updated foreign dining cards now total seventeen, including Arabic, Thai,

Dutch, and Swahiili. Chapter 6, "Separating the Wheat from the Chef," with all new recipes, proves America's favorite chefs are still the most generous.

I've tackled the tough issues, too, ones that that go well beyond the problem of what's for dinner. I have consulted with the experts, and answers to important questions, like what other autoimmune problems may be associated with celiac disease and how to get them diagnosed, can be found in "The Seven-Year Itch & Other Associated Conditions," chapter 16. The tricky business of getting something to eat during a hospital stay and managing your doctor and other specialists in the age of managed care is addressed in chapter 15, "The Doctor Will See You Now," along with a guide to America's best celiac-friendly doctors. "Sex and the Celiac," chapter 13, takes on both the lighter and the more serious side of reproduction. You'll find answers to many other questions of concern to newcomers and veterans alike such as, How do you decide which group to join? in chapter 19, "How Many Celiacs Does It Take to Change a Label?" What *is* the latest thinking about what's gluten-free and what's not?

The Gluten-Free Bible is about the whole celiac, not just the one sitting at the dinner table. How do we grow up gluten-free? How do we make sure we remain gluten-free in an emergency, manage our medicine, survive dating, college, a trip to the hospital, organize our kitchens, go trick-or-treating, negotiate all the twists and turns on the gluten-free path?

A cheeky attitude helps, of course, and that is something I will never change. While I have focused on the new, I think I have had the good sense not to fiddle with what many of you now consider classic wisdom. There is comfort, strategy, and take-no-prisoners attitude adjustment for everyone who has ever faced a howling hunger, an empty plate, a noncompliant waiter, or worse, a member of the family who just doesn't get it. It's enough to make you wonder if you'll ever eat again.

All these years later, I know that nothing hurts more than giving up the deep pleasure and satisfaction of one's favorite foods. I still remember in piercing detail the aching sense of loss that accompanied my own diagnosis. How sick I was. How thin I got (contrary to what the Duchess of Windsor may have thought, there *is* such a thing as being too thin); my jutting bones and skin had all the elasticity and appeal of an old handbag. Everywhere I looked I saw evidence of other people's pleasure. Every season was its own form of hell—summer's warm fruit pies, fall's darkly satisfying soups, winter's thick stews, and spring's never-ending *bruschetta*. I wept at the sight of spaghetti, became morose at the mere glimpse of a brownie, and was struck by sudden urges to fondle warm rolls in restaurants, as you will be, too. No longer could I join my friends in sending out for pizza, never again would I dip warm bread in good, herb-scented olive oil.

How could I explain all that to friends who were battling breast cancer and brain injury and hearts that ticked like time bombs, while I had gotten off with a mere dietary restriction? I secretly and guiltily grieved for all the foods I could never taste again and did what most people in total denial do. I cheated. Every chance I got.

I tucked pastries in kitchen drawers, carried croissants in my handbag and nibbled them on the street disguised behind dark glasses. Positive that flying across time zones suspended the problem, I smuggled cupcakes in my carry-on luggage. In the middle of the night, I shaved the sides of a lemon pound cake, convincing myself that the thinner the slice, the safer the serving. Who knows where this dangerous behavior may have led or what further complications my future would have in store, had I not discovered richly satisfying risotto, Thai rice noodles, and the fiery Indian pancake called *papadum*. In a flash of inspiration, I tucked a silver spoon into my evening purse and headed for the caviar. Real pleasure, I learned, does not rest solely on toast points.

Certain foods led me out of danger—the one brand of rice pasta that tasted good, the gluten-free baking mix that enabled me to arrive at a reasonable and safe version of the lemon pound cake I grieved for, the old-fashioned chocolate leaf cookies from a Jewish bakery in Brooklyn, or the muffins made for me by a now shuttered neighborhood café. My readers have similar stories to tell. How little it takes to change one's attitude.

These early victories led me out of my own kitchen and into the world of dinners, brunches, lunches, parties, holidays, vacations, and business trips. Creativity, quirky behavior, emotional directness, and a good bit of chutzpah soon had friends fussing, hostesses adjusting, and chefs rising to the culinary challenge. The UPS person and I became bosom buddies.

When you have celiac disease, half-empty versus half-full is no longer a meaningless cliché; it's the difference between being well-fed and feeling like a victim.

Born on a perfect rose-scented morning in Nantucket where blueberry muffins are as ubiquitous as sand and sea, *Against the Grain* was my personal fork in the road. It was, and still is in this new and exhaustively expanded reincarnation, a gauntlet thrown down to a glutenous world.

My purpose is no different today than it was then. I am convinced nothing is beyond the person who can conquer the loss of something as important, primal, and as basic to one's comfort as food. With *The Gluten-Free Bible* I present my case for choosing joy over sorrow, self-assertion and resourcefulness over fear and negative thinking, pleasure over regret. Whether you are a veteran or a newcomer, have endured a lifetime of being sick, a brief but puzzling illness, or no symptoms at all, my modest hope is that you will find on these pages one of life's most transforming lessons, that imperfection is what makes us interesting, injury the motive that makes us shine.

What follows is the only way I know to live: with a glad heart, a wise head, a healthy sense of self-worth *and* a full stomach. Chapter and verse, *The Gluten-Free Bible* is the story of how I saved my own life and ate happily ever after. It's my proof that living gluten-free has never been easier or more satisfying. You can, too. With all that is available to us today, no celiac should ever have to go hungry, miss a celebration, be ignored, or think he or she is not worth making a fuss over.

Here you stand—at the intersection of what was and what is, about to embark on the journey toward feeling healthy and alive, maybe for the first time in memory. Know that you join a large and boisterous family, all of whom have walked in your gluten-free shoes. Armed with information, a good sense of humor and food you never thought you'd eat again, there's no reason this can't be one of life's excellent adventures.

If I have learned anything on my own twenty-year sojourn on this path, it's that no road is long with good company and no day that includes laughter is ever wasted. Allow me to be your guide. "When you come to a fork in the road," as Yogi Berra so famously advised, it's always a good idea to "take it."

I've Got What?

the brave new celiac

O brave new world,
That has such people in't!

—SHAKESPEARE
The Tempest

Congratulations.

You've just discovered you're the 1 in 132 in the general population of otherwise healthy Americans who have celiac disease or CD, sometimes referred to as gluten-sensitive enteropathy, the quaintly archaic celiac sprue, or, even more remote, nontropical sprue. By now you know that due to an autoimmune response that causes damage to your small intestine you can't digest any grain containing gluten, which includes wheat, rye, barley, and possibly oats. You can eat rice and corn (if you're not allergic to them for a different reason) and a few odd and exotic grains you've never heard of, much less know how to cook. If you've had the classic symptoms related to CD (diarrhea, weight loss, abdominal distention, flatulence, frequent bulky, foul-smelling stools) and if one of your parents, children, or siblings are celiacs, your universe could be as narrow as 1 in 56, or even 1 in 22. If any of your second-degree relatives are celiacs, chances are 1 in 39 that you've got it. If you are African-American, Hispanic, or Asian-American, you could be the 1 in 236 people genetically unable to digest gluten, according to a landmark study published by Dr. Alessio Fasano, in the *Archives of Internal Medicine* in February 2003, which proves once and for all that celiac disease is not and never has been rare, just underdiagnosed.

Even if you think you're the only celiac in the clan, guess again. Subclinical or atypical symptoms include bone pain, anemia, ataxia, dental enamel defects, brain fog, fatigue, irritability, weakness, weight gain, constipation, spontaneous miscarriage, infertility, intensely itchy and burning rash, depression, and peripheral neuropathy. Remember Uncle Max with the delicate stomach, Grandma Reilly who always fell asleep after a spaghetti dinner, the extremely small, fussy baby your nephew was, or your cousin Minnie who couldn't get pregnant if she stood on her head (didn't she try that, too)? And come to think of it, there's poor second cousin Fred who just can't seem to ever get out of the bathroom and Uncle Harry whose foot slapped when he walked. Shake a celiac's family tree and others will fall. It's just a matter of time and testing. More about that later.

Right now, you've got a lot to digest. Your odd little immune system and the pool in which your particular genes are swimming have tricked your body into thinking bread and other foods containing gluten are poison. Foods as basic to human life as breathing, are now verboten. Suddenly the staff of life is life's big stiff. As I'm sure everyone has told you by now, it could have been worse.

Good News, Bad News

The good news is, you're not dead. Not only are you not dead, you don't have anything that could be even remotely construed as fatal or life threatening, unless you cheat constantly, and you're not going to do that, are you? Even better, your condition can be managed quite nicely without drugs, frequent doctor visits, and expensive hospital stays, nor does it require that you suffer any more bad news than you have already gotten. No surgery, no nasty procedures, no worsening symptoms—how many diseases can claim that? All those years of terrible, puzzling, and often conflicting symptoms are over. Gone. History. *Hasta la vista, baby.* This is very good news.

More good news—if you stay on your diet, you will feel good again. Even if you had no symptoms and took the blood test only to humor your grain-challenged sister, you will feel better than you have in years.

Better still, when you know where to look, there is more good gluten-free food than you have time to eat it.

You are not alone. In fact, it is estimated there are upward of 2.2 million of us, either newly diagnosed or about to be, in the United States alone. Although more and more cases are being diagnosed through family screening, the typical celiac knocks around from doctor to doctor for an average of eleven years before somebody figures out what is wrong.

My own celiac disease took years and a huge toll on my health before it was discovered. I suffered mild and seemingly unrelated symptoms all my life without ever getting sick enough to seek help. Then, in my thirties, during a particularly stressful period, I expressed full-blown celiac syndrome, losing as much as five pounds a week and developing bizarre symptoms, from mysterious and gigantic hives to bone pain and a constant mild nausea that seemed to point to serious illness.

My intestinal villi were so scarred from gluten that I had literally stopped absorbing any food at all and had fallen prey to all kinds of nutritional deficiencies. My hair had lost its shine and was falling out in clumps. My muscles had begun to atrophy from a lack of protein. I suffered from anemia. Two bones had fractured from lack of calcium absorption, and I weighed approximately ninety pounds, which at five foot eight gave me the distinct look of a person wearing someone else's skin. My heart had developed a murmur. (What *was* it saying?) I was wobbly from my frequent visits to the bathroom; my condition got so bad I had to nap in order to recover from the exertion of taking a nap.

The smart money was on a diagnosis of lymphoma, a cancer of the lymphatic system that reveals itself in many of the same ways as CD. I was given a bed in a section of the hospital grimly dubbed "the bone yard." Most of my fellow patients were not going home. Happily, the smart money lost.

Once I was diagnosed, all my past health problems suddenly made sense. My long history of painful and overly long periods was due to my inability to absorb vitamin K, which is necessary in the coagulation of blood. This, too, was the reason for my puzzling and worrisome resistance to healing. A lack of vitamin B_{12} was the culprit in the anemia department, and poor calcium absorption, not a forgotten fall, as one X-ray technician had insisted, was the reason for the constant pain in my joints and the onset, years later, of osteoporosis. A bone in my right knee and another in my left wrist had developed small fractures consistent with years of calcium deprivation. All the years spent doubled over with what I repeatedly described as the feeling of "glass in my stomach" were not due to a teenager's panic over the SATs or, later, the adrenaline rush of an advertising career, or a nervous temperament. It wasn't PMS, or the push and shove of a marriage settling in, or because it was Thursday, or because I was "neurotic," as one baffled diagnostician opined, playing a pernicious form of "blame the victim" when her search for the cause stalled.

In the end, I read the entire physician's diagnostic reference, a doorstop of a book called *The Merck Manual*. I cross-referenced my symptoms, slogging through the sequelaes, epithelia, crypts, and unexplained lymphocytic proliferations with a medical dictionary and a legal pad by my side. When I had the problem narrowed down to the field of gastroenterology, I made an appointment with a superb doctor whose job I made vastly easier by virtue of my self-education (something I advocate for everyone, because no one has a better reason to keep trying to find out what's ailing you than you). Together we began the search for the disease that had eluded diagnosis for over thirty years.

There were no simple blood tests to screen for celiac disease then and the inquiry focused on my diminished ability to absorb foods, particularly those with a high fat content. There was an odd and distasteful assortment of tests no longer necessary today, which led to a surgical biopsy or upper endoscopy, still considered the gold standard for a definitive diagnosis. One look through his fiber-optic viewer at my battered and scarred intestinal villi and a careful examination of the snip by the pathology lab told my doctor everything he needed to know. I had celiac disease and was told I could thank my father's Irish roots for this peculiar reaction to the gluten found in most grains (CD is quite common in Ireland and England, as well as in those of northern European ancestry). It would be years before I stopped blaming the folks from Donegal and looked to my mother's French forebears with their bakers and brioche for the real culprit.

No one really knows why CD is so much more prevalent in certain countries (CD is so common in Finland that the local McDonald's serves Mc-Gluten-free.) Legend has it that hundreds and hundreds of years ago invaders poisoned the wheat harvest. Goths, Huns, the Uncle Ben's people? The more scientific explanation is the discovery that nuts and seeds would turn into edible plants ushered in the Paleolithic Age, along with the first food intolerance (maybe the hunter-gatherer Atkins people are on to something after all). No one really knows, but as the myth goes, over the next several generations the locals adapted by reprogramming their bodies to react to gluten as the poison it was for their ancestors. While there is no basis for any of this in scientific fact, I particularly like this theory because it allows me to imagine I have descended from a fierce and courageous tribe that would not be conquered. They adapted instead and became the first humans to discover the ultimate power in passive-aggressive behavior. Whatever gets you through the night.

My doctor said as long as I lived on a gluten-free diet for the rest of my life (thank God I found one who didn't think this was an allergy I would outgrow), I would be healthy and symptom-free. No medication, no medical supervision, save a snip or two every few years to make sure the intestinal wall was healing. He ordered B_{12} shots and lots of vitamins and minerals to help compensate for the anemia and other deficiencies and to speed up my body's badly needed repair.

"Go home, take your supplements, and live a normal life," he said, bursting with pride at having detected what in his misguided, yet professional, opinion was a rare disease. "Just don't eat any bread, pasta, cookies, sandwiches, tarts, croissants, bagels, granola, cereal, cakes, pies, muffins, pastries, sauces, soufflés, stuffing, prepared gravies, crab cakes, pancakes, carrot cakes, birthday cakes, frozen dinners, canned soups—and, in fact, pretty much everything on the supermarket shelf—and oh, by the way, Happy Thanksgiving."

It dawned on me very quickly: life after diagnosis was not going to be a piece of cake. People stared. Waiters glared. Hostesses greeted my presence at their tables with weak smiles. I was the object of rude questions, questionable dinner conversation, and bad jokes, like "Is a celiac anything like a maniac?" After a while I just stayed home, ate tuna fish, and avoided the whole thing. I didn't know what to do, so I did nothing.

I soon fell victim to what I call the-children-are-starving-in-China syndrome, something my grandmother used to tell me to make me eat lunch (she stopped only after I tried to mail a ham-and-cheese sandwich to Beijing). Everyone around me was profoundly relieved that I was not going to die or waste away before their eyes. All I had to do was follow a simple diet (simple for whom?) and I'd be fine. While the doctors congratulated themselves on my difficult diagnosis, my family shed tears of joy and relief. As they celebrated, remembering how as an infant I refused to be weaned and clung to my mother's breast as if my little intestines *knew*, and how the summer I was four, I threw every bit of food I was given against our cottage's knotty pine wall—I suffered an odd form of survivor's guilt, feeling selfish and petty for whining about what seemed like a minor inconvenience in the face of so much real illness in most lives. I secretly wondered what was wrong with me. Why didn't I feel as lucky as everyone said I was?

Once my symptoms began to recede and I could see beyond the physical wreckage, it became clear that I had to make a choice. I could continue to feel sorry for myself. I could see myself as a sick person and go on being the focus of negative attention, which for me was an odd mixture of pity and annoyance. Or I could turn that attention into a positive and teach myself how to enjoy life again. I resolved to see the good news, but it wouldn't be good news until *I* said it was.

We all get to diagnosis via a different route. For some, the path is littered with pain and confusion and frustration and angst. It is a journey marked by challenge and determination and courage. We have listened to our bodies and persisted despite the fact that our complaints did not fit neatly into one diagnostic box or another. We stumped the professionals whose areas of specialty were too narrow to include all of our symptoms or whose detective skills were not as sharply honed, or whose schedules did not accommodate the time for thorough investigation. We faced up to the HMO and demanded to be referred to the right people. For others, the bagel eaten one day is verboten the next. The news is swift and terrible.

The truth is, whether it took years or a few miserable months to figure out the problem, you hung in there. You kept pushing, despite the fact that you may have been told more than once that your only problem was an overactive imagination. Whether it was a hard-won battle or a brief skirmish, your suffering needs to be acknowledged before you move on. This may come as a surprise to some of you, especially those who were taught to keep a stiff upper lip, but you really don't have to feel better because other people say you do.

For those of you with no symptoms or a low-level malaise recognized only in gluten-free retrospect, the suddenness of the gluten-free diet is a shock. In some ways, it's even worse than being sick. Something very important is missing from your life, an entire food group. It deserves its own mourning period.

This really is the first step in healing—being aware of and acknowledging how much it hurts. As I said, with so much real suffering in the world, it is tempting to trivialize a food intolerance, but if you do, you are trivializing yourself and your own loss. You are overlooking the basic first step in getting healthy—acknowledging the importance of what has happened to you. And talking about it.

Tell your story, as I have just told you mine, over and over again, until you no longer need to tell it. Unfortunately, this may take longer than the time usually allotted to you by others, even friends and family. Never mind. Find somebody who hasn't heard it yet.

❧

The bad news? Well, you knew there'd be *some*. If you want to avoid serious long-term complications, you've ordered your last pizza with everything on it. You've eaten your last cheeseburger on a sesame seed bun, buttered your last croissant, and bought your last frozen dinner, ice-cream cone, slice of apple pie.

The bad news is that from now on you have to think about every bit of food you put in your mouth. No more aimless grazing, nibbling, or grabbing something, anything, when you're hungry. You've got to plan meals and snacks and restaurant dinners.

The bad news is that you are on a diet that allows no slack, one that will test your resolve and turn even the meekest among us into a serial killer (which, in your case, is spelled *cereal*).

More bad news.

Not all celiacs agree about what is and what is not gluten-free. Did I say this would be a piece of cake? Let's look at what two well-respected sources have to say on the matter.

The Basics

Before you can elaborate on the theme, you have to know the score. You can't be creative about a problem until you know the extent of it. Let's get down to business.

Here's the basic gluten-free diet as it is described in *The Merck Manual*, and expanded upon by the American Dietetic Association. Look carefully. The foods bearing asterisks, which are explained below, are those that have been reevaluated in light of what we are learning right now.

THE BASIC GLUTEN-FREE DIET

Type of Food	Yes Foods	No Foods
Beverages	Carbonated beverages, pure cocoa powder, tea, pure instant or ground coffee, all milk products, except those on the excluded list, fruit drinks, wines and rums, sake, vermouth, cognac, tequila, vodka derived from grapes or potatoes	Cereal beverages, malted milks, milk with cereal additives, drinks made with malt or other excluded cereals, commercial chocolate, herbal teas with barley or barely malt, alcoholic beverages distilled from cereal grains such as whiskey, vodka, gin, aquavit*, beer, ales, malt liquor
Bread	Bread and muffins made with arrowroot, corn, tapioca, potato, rice, soybean, chickpea, soy flour, potato starch; bean flours, pure corn tortillas, breads and other baked goods prepared with special gluten-free flours, rice cakes, and crackers	Any bread made with wheat, barley, rye, oats**, durum, semolina, graham flour, or wheat starch; commercial mixes for biscuits, muffins, cornbread, wheat germ, bran, bulgur; any bread made with low-gluten flour; crackers, rusk, pretzels

Type of Food	Yes Foods	No Foods
Cereal	Ready-to-eat corn and rice cereals containing malt made from corn; puffed rice, cream of rice, cornmeal; hominy, grits, popcorn, rice noodles, corn and rice pasta, pure buckwheat kasha, millet, teff	Any cereal made with wheat, rye, bran, barley malt, kamut, spelt, wheat germ, oats**, bulgur; couscous, pasta with wheat, semolina, spelt, and other excluded flours
Dessert	Custards and puddings made with allowable flours or starches, gelatin desserts, sherbets, tapioca, homemade or commercial ice cream made without fillers, add-ins, or flavorings.	Any dessert containing wheat, rye, barley, commercial cakes, cookies, ice cream, pastries, pies, puddings, or those made from commercial mixes
Fat	Butter, margarine, pure mayonnaise, cooking oils, shortening, olive oil	Commercial salad dressings containing gluten stabilizers; wheat germ oil
Fruit	Any pure fruit or fruit juice	Any fruit, juice, or fruit pie filling made with gluten thickeners
Meat, Eggs, or Cheese	Any plain meat, fish, or fowl except those excluded, natural aged cheeses, eggs	Meat, fish, or chicken made with bread or bread crumbs, seitan, processed cheese spreads, canned meat dishes, cold cuts unless pure meat, bread stuffings, gravy thickened with flour, any product containing hydrolyzed or texturized vegetable protein (HVP)
Soups	Broth or bouillon; vegetable soup and cream soups made from allowable foods thickened with cornstarch or potato flour only	Any soup containing excluded flours or starches; bouillon cubes made with HVP
Sweets	Any sweets except those prepared with excluded grain products	Candy containing wheat (i.e., licorice and jelly beans), rye, barley malt sweeteners

Type of Food	Yes Foods	No Foods
Vegetable	Any pure vegetables except those prepared with excluded grain products	Any creamed or breaded vegetables
Miscellaneous	Salt, spices, vinegar*, herbs, pickles, baking chocolate, chocolate, olives, nuts, peanut butter	All gravies or sauces thickened with wheat flour, flavoring syrups, rice malt, bottled meat sauces, malt extract, soy sauce, any product containing unidentified starch

So should I photocopy this and stick it on my refrigerator door? Not so fast....

In a perfect world, everyone would agree on what is and what is not gluten-free. In the gluten-free world, however, not all celiac organizations, Internet sources of nutritional information, and medical practitioners offer the same guidelines for safe eating. This needs to change, but in the meantime, a celiac must be prepared to do his or her homework on any given substance and make an informed decision, ideally with his or her doctors. This is especially important for the newly diagnosed whose bodies are still on the mend. To complicate matters, what we know about the presence or absence of gluten in food is evolving as research catches up with our diet.

Let's start with those pesky little asterisks.

Yes, No, Maybe Foods

*GRAIN ALCOHOL

The American Dietetic Association (*Manual of Clinical Dietetics*, 6th edition) now considers distilled alcoholic beverages like gin, whiskey, and vodka (but not beer, which contains malt), and other products that contain distilled alcohol like vinegar and vanilla and other flavored extracts, safe for celiacs to consume. This is because the distilling process itself renders the end result virtually free of gluten.

Some celiacs still prefer to avoid these products. While you're making up your mind what is best for you (discuss it with your doctor, assuming he or she is up on all the new research), there's always wine, potato vodka, and gluten-free cider vinegar, wine, balsamic, or rice vinegar.

**OATS

The oats debate rages. Some consider oats safe for all but the most sensitive celiacs to enjoy in moderation and, in fact, they are consumed by many. Others feel that because of the difficulty in measuring the varying degrees in sensitivity between celiacs, it's hard to know how many oats a celiac can consume without damaging the villi.

The Seattle-based Gluten Intolerance Group (GIG) reports the recent discovery of the specific reactive peptide involved in gluten intolerance. Research conducted by Dr. Don Kasarda, on the amino acid sequencing of oats versus this now-known peptide, put oats in the clear—they don't contain the reactive peptide sequence known to be a problem for gluten intolerance. Based on numerous recent studies like this one, the group clearly states that oats are gluten-free.

But before you grab the nearest oatmeal cookie . . . GIG also says, "Because of the worldwide level of contamination with unacceptable grains, GIG does not recommend oats at this time."

Why? Because it is virtually impossible to find commercial oats that have not been contaminated by wheat or other toxic grains in the milling process or in the manufacturing of the food itself. Again, this is a conversation you need to have with your doctor (my own doctor warns his new patients not to try oats for at least a year after diagnosis and only then with extreme caution). If you do decide to try a bowl of oatmeal, please do so under medical supervision and make sure you buy whole, steel-cut Irish oats like McCann's. No quick cooking or processed domestic brands like Quaker. These are always mixed with wheat or other glutenous grains. And never consume a product that lists oats among the ingredients. You have no idea what form it's in. For you, the expression "feeling one's oats" takes on a whole new meaning.

Proceed with Caution

Buckwheat. Pure buckwheat is gluten-free, but it is almost always contaminated (there's that scary sounding word again) by unsafe grains at the growing, milling, or processing stage. If you love the stuff, find a company like Bob's Red Mill or Pocono that gets it from dedicated fields and mills it in a safe facility.

Millet. This is another grain that is gluten-free, but is often mixed or milled with wheat. Always consider the source and make sure a millet product is not being baked or processed in a facility that handles unsafe flours or grains.

Quinoa, amaranth, manioc or cassava, and teff. These grains are naturally gluten-free as well, but always make sure they have not been mixed with couscous, wheat flour, barley syrup, or other unsafe ingredients as they often are, either in the recipe or in the milling process.

White and brown rice, corn, wild rice, and sorghum. These grains are gluten-free as well as long as they haven't been "enhanced" in any way.

Roots and tubers like tapioca, potato, sweet potato, yams, arrowroot, and manioc or cassava are quite safe.

Legumes like lentils, beans, soy, and peas are a safe choice, as long as you know what else has been cooked with them.

The Bottom Line?

Ask questions first. Eat later. Push for a standardized global gluten-free diet. Even better, lobby for uniform standards for processing all gluten-free food products.

When the guy in the health food store tells you it okay to have spelt because it is a more digestible form of wheat, walk away. It's only more digestible if you're not a celiac. I was once told by a zealous macrobiotic counselor that if I ate seaweed, brown rice, and ground my own *gomasio* (roasted sesame seeds and salt) by hand while facing east and standing on my left foot, my celiac disease would go away. Don't fall for that, either. Eating whole, unre-

---

Travel Advisory

. . . .

While American and Canadian celiacs follow a zero-gluten diet, Europeans allow miniscule amounts of what they consider safe wheat starch in their gluten-free commercial products. According to an article published in April of 2000 in the *Journal of the American Dietetic Association*, "Wheat starch used in European gluten-free foods is specially formulated to comply with the Codex Alimentarius Standard for gluten-free foods. Based on this standard, gluten-free products abroad may contain wheat, rye, barley, oats, and triticale that have been rendered gluten-free. To be rendered gluten-free, the nitrogen content of the gluten-containing grain cannot exceed 0.05 g per 100 g of grain on a dry matter basis."

Don't stay home because of this, but do discuss it with your doctor and have a strategy in place before traveling abroad.

fined, unprocessed, unengineered foods is a great way to get real quality and vitality from what you eat, and it may even hasten the healing process, but it won't "cure" celiac disease.

Forget kamut bread or cereal on the gluten-free diet.

Go nuts with peanuts, almonds, cashews, pecans, and other tree nuts unless you are allergic, in which case, don't you dare.

This brings up an important point. To further confuse the issue, celiacs often have allergies that coexist with CD: lactose intolerance, peanut allergy, carbohydrate intolerance, casein allergy, chemical sensitivities, etc. It's important to sort out where the reaction is coming from before you blame it on gluten.

It's a good idea to avoid processed cheeses and spreads and dips and other flavored, herbed, and otherwise enhanced products, which can contain gluten. Best to buy natural cheeses like cheddar, Swiss, mozzarella, and ricotta and imported cheeses like Brie, Camembert, chèvre, cheddar, and Gouda. It is said that richly veined cheeses like Maytag blue and Stilton are off-limits because the culture that makes them so rich and gorgeous is made with bread mold. Nobody really knows how much, if any, gluten is broken down in the aging process, but most celiac groups advise caution. Better to be safe than sorry.

Many candy bars are not gluten-free even though there is no gluten in the ingredients. Why? It's because wheat flour is often used on the gooey confections to help mold them into shape or to keep them from sticking to each other and gumming up the works on the conveyor belts. Oh Henry, what's a celiac to do? Contact the company that makes a candy bar you really love and ask how it's made. Then give yourself a Hershey's Kiss and a big box of Goobers, they're both gluten-free.

Did you know licorice contains wheat flour? Ditto for many brands of jelly beans and other jelly candy. But take heart, there is a gluten-free licorice, as well as a gluten-free beer.

Strange as this may sound, not all turkeys are gluten-free. It's not because the turkey may have eaten wheat in his or her lifetime, it's because pre-basted turkeys and other poultry products such as Butterball brand may contain gluten in the "butter" mixture injected into the bird.

You'd think you'd be able to find out exactly what's in or on a product just by reading a label. Well, think again. Until such time that Congress and the FDA agrees on standards for a gluten-free label and passes a law making it mandatory for all gluten-containing ingredients to be labeled as such (more about that later), you are on your own.

What's a consumer to do? Memorize these basic rules.

Basic Rule No. 1

Never forget that you are the customer, and, as such, you are entitled to a complete explanation of a food manufacturer's process.

Remember, without you, companies are out of business. They are not doing you a favor by answering your questions and/or complaints. They want you to tell them what you think. That's why they post their Web sites, e-mail, and snail-mail addresses prominently on their packages. It's why they put "cookies" on your tail when you go browsing. It's why they send you free stuff when you get something bad like a piece of gravel in your soup or a pit in a box of pitted prunes. It's why McDonald's finally downsized its portions. Why Coke went away and came back as Coke Classic.

If you really love a product and are not sure how it's made, call or e-mail the manufacturer's customer service department and find out. If they give you a hard time, tell them you and your friends and family, and everyone you've ever met in this life and the next will boycott their products. If what you are told meets with your satisfaction and you get a clear answer regarding the gluten-free status of the product, call back every few months. Manufacturing standards and formulas change. Labels, which are extremely expensive to reprint and apply, often lag behind in this process. If you get trouble, mention you got very sick eating something the company made. All of which leads to . . .

Basic Rule No. 2

Take food company disclaimers with a grain of salt.

We live in litigious times. People sue companies because they get fat eating too many french fries, because they spilled their coffee and got burned (isn't coffee supposed to be hot?), because they ate thirty-seven jelly donuts and went into a diabetic coma. Soon Oreo cookies will be on a government watch list. It's sad, but true. Americans have learned to blame somebody else for every dumb thing they do. The downside for celiacs is even though you've been told the product you're asking about is gluten-free, there will be some legal gibberish attached to the answer. Stuff like "there *could* be gluten or other allergens in this product . . . it is impossible to say positively that gluten or any other offending substances may not have entered the manufacturing process . . . someone who touched your food may have once eaten a slice of bread." One company, in an inspired burst of obfuscation, actually sent as its response a list of products that were definitely *not* gluten-free. They fudge, they obscure, they cover their you-know-whats. Don't take these responses literally. These are not dire warnings. This is simply a sign of our lawsuit-happy society. Bottom line: use common sense. If the label lists no wheat or gluten, there probably isn't any. If you have a reaction, stop using the product.

Basic Rule No. 3

Read labels carefully. **NEVER** *eat a meal or a packaged food if you don't know what's in it. If there's no label, ask for it. It it's not available, don't risk it.*

This can be a problem on airlines, at salad bars and catered affairs, and in chain restaurants, fast-food establishments, school cafeterias, and weight-loss programs such as Jenny Craig, L.A. Weight Loss, Nutri-System, and others that sell their frozen meals and diet products directly to clients. Such programs are not required by law to disclose any nutritional information, including calorie and fat content and ingredients, which is why I believe so many people fail on these plans and regain the weight. They have no idea what they've eaten and the minute they resume eating normal food, they overeat.

The point is, whenever you are a captive audience—where you have not specifically requested a gluten-free meal, the chef is unavailable for consultation, or the ingredient label is missing—you are in real danger of consuming hidden gluten. Don't risk it. Eat before you go or fly with a banana and a bag of nuts. It's going to be better than what they give you anyway.

Basic Rule No. 4

Look for gluten in unexpected places.

Yes. Someone out there right now is working on a pill, patch, or a patent for some kind of gene-altering device that will make all of this academic. At least I like to think so. But let's be honest with ourselves, there are other cures a bit more urgently needed. For now, CD can pose a problem not only at mealtimes, but on Sunday mornings as well. My doctor told me about another patient who continued to be sick even though she followed the gluten-free diet scrupulously. Just as more tests were ordered to rule out refractory sprue (a rare condition in which the villi simply do not heal), the devout Catholic woman volunteered that she attended Mass and took Communion every day. Bingo. More about that later.

Some other little-known facts. Don't try to lick your gluten problem in the stationery department. The glue used on some envelopes and mailing labels (most of them imported) may contain wheat. Since glue is not a food to those of us over the age of four, this source is easily overlooked. It's smart to use a damp sponge, self-sticking envelopes, and to buy self-stick U.S. postage stamps, or forget the whole thing and let somebody else in the family pay the bills.

Many celiacs are sensitive to chemicals as well as to gluten. Those with dermatitis herpetiformis (a skin reaction to gluten described in chapter 16, "The Seven-Year Itch & Other Associated Disorders") should be careful using furniture refinishers, craft kits, paste and spray waxes, and cleaners. Try to avoid using these substances and, if you must, only do so wearing a mask and in a well-ventilated area. It's important for highly sensitive celiacs and those with skin reactions to avoid wheat germ oil in cosmetics and in many personal products like skin creams, lotions, potions that could end up being swallowed. Even toothpaste and false teeth fixatives must be scrutinized.

Watch out for imitation seafood commonly found in many take-out food stores, salad bars, and restaurants. These products often start out gluten-free, but unsafe binders are added to help mold the product into shrimp, crab, lobster, or scallop shapes. Look for gluten-free imitation seafood and always ask if the shrimp or lobster salad is mixed with imitation seafood in a restaurant or deli. And don't forget to ask the dental hygienist what's in the prophy paste used to clean your teeth.

On the plus side, a trip to a winery will be a special joy for the gluten-impaired, because pure wine in all its glorious variety is gluten-free. This includes sherries, ports, cognacs, brandies, and sake, Japanese rice wine. Do watch for fortified and flavored wines. Just as food companies use wheat in the manufacturing process, wineries use additives, too.

Beer is a no-no. But you have the good fortune to be a celiac in the age of the gluten-free brew.

Basic Rule No. 5

If you don't understand it, don't eat it until you do. If you can't remember, carry a cheat sheet to the market until you do.

This is one time ignorance is not bliss, not to mention fiscally irresponsible. Don't spend your hard-earned money on foods that could make you sick. Let's review some basic food additives.

Caramel Coloring. In the United States and Canada caramel coloring is the dark brown liquid that results from heating dextrose, invert sugar (a mixture of dextrose and levulose found in fruits or that is produced artificially by the process of inversion), lactose, molasses, or sucrose from beet or sugarcane. This ingredient should always be questioned as it may be made from malt syrup or wheat. When in doubt, consider the country of origin and contact the company for specifics.

Dextrin. Not as common as maltodextrin made from corn, dextrin is an incompletely hydrolyzed starch that can be made from corn, potato, arrowroot, rice, tapioca, and/or wheat. It's used as a thickener, prevents caking of sugar in candy, and encapsulates flavoring in mixes. It is wise to question an imported product containing dextrin or that which is not labeled corn dextrin, tapioca dextrin, etc.

Glutinous Rice. The word *glutinous* just means sticky or gummy and should not be taken to mean containing gluten, as in *glutenous*.

Hydrolyzed Vegetable Protein (HVP), Hydrolyzed Plant Protein (HPP), or textured vegetable protein. These additives can be made from soy, corn, rice, peanuts, casein, or wheat. Always check with the manufacturer of a product containing HVP or HPP for the source of the protein. These are commonly found in canned foods like soups, sausages, hot dogs, and "mock" meats popular with vegetarians.

Malt or Malt Flavoring. These are made from barley malt or syrup and are often found in cereals, cookies, and candies. They are not gluten-free. If made from corn, of course, these flavorings are G/F.

Maltodextrin. Not to be confused with malt or malt flavoring (yes, it is easy to be led to conclusions by the word *malt*), the FDA describes this stuff as "non-sweet white powder or concentrated solution made from corn, potato, or rice." American products containing maltodextrin are gluten-free by regulation. However, it is always good to check the source when considering imported products.

Maltol. While its name may be misleading, it is a synthetic flavoring that contains no malt or gluten.

Mannitol. Used as an anti-caking, flavoring stabilizer and thickener in foods and Rx medications, this sweet substance is made most commonly from seaweed.

Modified Food Starch. This can be made from corn, tapioca, potato, wheat, or other starches, but in North America, corn is almost always used. Check with the manufacturer to be sure.

MSG or Monosodium Glutamate. Unless you are allergic to MSG (Chinese Restaurant Syndrome), you need not worry about this additive made from sugar beet or molasses.

Sorbitol. This sweet-tasting, poorly absorbed sugar alcohol is used in many sugar-free or "dietetic" food products. It is gluten-free, but even the tiniest amount can cause bloating, diarrhea, and abdominal pain in sensitive individuals, especially in those celiacs whose guts haven't yet healed.

Starch. When you see "starch" listed on an American food manufacturer's label, it means it is made from cornstarch only, in keeping with FDA requirements. If another starch is used, it must be disclosed, e.g., wheat starch or tapioca starch. No such rule for imported products.

Triticale. This grain is a cross between wheat and rye and, as such, is doubly bad for celiacs.

Wheat Starch. This substance is a part of wheat that is considered by some less toxic than flour. It is believed unsafe for celiacs in the United States and Canada, but in Great Britain and Europe, in accordance with the Codex Alimentarius, it is considered acceptable for those on the gluten-free diet.

Vegetable Gums. Even if you are in the oats-are-okay-for-celiacs camp, avoid any product that contains oat gum. If a vegetable gum is made from carob bean, guar gum, gum arabic, gum acacia, locust bean, cellulose gum, gum tragacanth, or just plain gum, while it may sound unappetizing, it isn't unsafe.

Basic Rule No. 6

It's better to look silly than to get sick. Remember, there are worse things to be called than "fussy."

Only a crumb would ask you to share a toaster. This may sound like Felix's fuddy-duddy behavior in *The Odd Couple*, but Newton's law of physics applies here. A toaster oven is a better choice than a conventional toaster because it allows your bread to toast flat, clear of the crumbs that normally drop off breads, muffins, and bagels and collect on the bottom, mixing with your gluten-free variety. Do not assume a french fry is just potato. Never succumb to the pressure of eating a meal that is unsafe, even if a friend has cooked it and you don't know what to say. Try saying, "I love you for making this and I'm sorry for not explaining my diet properly." And speaking of fuddy-duddy, if your sweetheart has just had two pieces of apple pie, no kissing until he or she has brushed and flossed.

Basic Rule No. 7

Make sure you know who or what is touching your food at all times.

People can spread gluten just like viruses, and, in fact, you can make yourself sick by not washing your hands after handling wheat flour. Watch inanimate sources of contamination, too, such as deep-fat fryers and grills and ice-cream scoops. Always ask the clerk at Baskin-Robbins to rinse the scoop before serving your cup (or the cone you've supplied) to avoid getting some cookie dough or other unsafe flavor mixed with yours. Find out if your french fries have been "beer-battered," coated in some other way, or cooked in the same oil as the breaded onion rings. Find out if the hamburger patty is all beef or if it has been mixed with bread crumbs (many establishments do this to stretch profits). By all means, bring your favorite pasta to your neighborhood Italian restaurant (only after you've asked if you can), but don't forget to ask that it be cooked in a pot of fresh water. When you barbecue at home or with friends, always make sure your food is first up on the grill; this way you won't end up with bits of grilled buns and other glutenous food on yours.

Basic Rule No. 8

Live by the Boy Scout motto—Be Prepared!

Right about now you're asking, "Will I ever eat again?" The answer is yes, and you will eat pretzels, pasta, pizza, lasagna, cookies, biscotti, and more varieties of bread than you ever dreamed because there is a whole world of mail-order gluten-free food companies and specialty stores out there. For now, though, and especially if you prefer to eat at home for the time being, you'll want to stock the basic pantry with the staples listed below. If space allows, set aside a place apart from the rest of the family's provisions. This way you'll always know what you've got, and limit the possibility of mixing things up.

Arrowroot. This thickening agent blends well with most gluten-free flours and makes for silky gravies.

Brown and white rice flours. Keep these on hand and use them for dusting, dredging, flouring hands, and mixing with other gluten-free flours for cooking and baking.

Baking mixes. There are many commercial gluten-free baking mixes you can buy to substitute cup for cup for wheat flour in your favorite recipes, or you can blend your own. *In More from the Gluten-Free Gourmet* (Henry

Holt), Bette Hagman suggests two parts rice flour, two-thirds part potato starch flour, and one-third part tapioca flour. Mix up a batch and keep on hand for baking.

Cereals. Breakfast is no longer "grab a Danish and dash," so always keep a box of gluten-free cold cereal, hominy grits, and hot rice cereal on the shelf. It's a good idea to keep individual bags of GF cold cereal at the office or in your work bag as well. Add your own nuts and raisins, mix with gluten-free pretzel pieces, and you've got a quick snack as well.

Corn Flour. This smoother version of cornmeal is the right texture for corn muffins and other baked goods or recipes requiring a lighter result than cornmeal alone can achieve.

Cornmeal. You'll need to keep this staple on hand for cereals, crusts, accompaniments to roasts, soft or grilled polenta, and gluten-free batters. Corn bread makes an excellent addition to stuffing, meat loaf, and other ground meat dishes and can often replace bread crumbs in standard recipes. There is nothing like cornmeal-crusted fish or soft-shell crabs sautéed in a little butter and olive oil.

Cornstarch. Like arrowroot, this is a great thickening agent for sauces and gravies and is less prone to lumps than wheat flour.

Crackers and biscuits. Always keep a quantity of brown rice, corn, or flaxseed crackers on hand for cheese, dips, crusts, munching, and taking to friends' houses, parties, etc.

Guar gum. According to *Webster's New Collegiate Dictionary*, guar gum is "a gum that consists of the ground endosperm of guar seeds and is used especially as a thickening agent and sizing material." Basically, this is the edible stuff used on your sheets and shirts to make them feel crisp and in foods as a filler. Eat as much as you like, guar gum is gluten-free.

Gluten-free breads. In mixes or premade, these are available in health food stores, whole foods markets, specialty stores, and by mail. Experiment with small orders until you find your favorites. Many of these breads are sold in shelf-stable packages and freeze well, so keep yourself stocked.

Gluten-free pastas. Gone are the days of limp, gooey ersatz pasta. Now there's spaghetti, lasagna, penne, fettuccini, ziti, and manicotti. These are a must for any celiac's pantry.

Oriental rice sticks, rice wrappers, and noodles. These are available in Asian markets and many specialty markets and require very little preparation, usually no more than soaking, for use in gluten-free cooking.

Potato flour. Don't confuse this with potato starch flour. Potato flour is made from the whole potato. A small amount goes a long way to refine the texture of coarser rice flours. For example, 1 teaspoon potato flour is enough to redefine the texture of ½ cup rice flour, or as little as one tablespoon can re-texturize 1 or 2 cups rice flour.

Potato starch flour. This thickener is interchangeable with cornstarch and can be found in most supermarkets, health food stores, or whole foods markets.

Rices. Stock up on as much white rice, brown rice, wild rice, sweet basmati rice, arborio, and all the gorgeous varieties of this delicious grain as you can afford. Play. Experiment. But avoid commercial rice mixes, many of which are unsafe.

Rice bran. This is the bran that comes from polishing brown rice. It's loaded with minerals, vitamins B and E, and fiber. Add it to cereals, muffins, cookies, smoothies, etc. The oil content makes it fragile, so store it in the freezer.

Rice polish. This is a soft flour made from the hulls of brown rice. Like rice bran, it's fragile, so buy a little at a time.

Soy or soya flour. As this can have a heavy flavor when used alone, it should be used in conjunction with other, milder flours. Since it is high in fat and protein, it can add nutrients and needed moisture to an otherwise dry recipe. For example, if a recipe calls for 2 cups wheat flour, use 1 cup rice flour, ¾ cup potato starch flour, and ¼ cup soy flour.

Specialty flours. You may want to keep on hand small amounts of flours made from lentils, peas, chickpeas, artichokes, acorns, bean, mung beans, manioc or cassava, almonds, hazelnuts, and pistachios, but unless you are going to use them consistently, they are best bought fresh. It is best to buy nuts for nut flours—used in many "flourless" cake and torte recipes. Grind them yourself, as the high oil content means they'll turn rancid when stored for long periods.

Sweet rice flour. This is usually found in Asian food markets and health food stores. Because it has more starch than regular rice flour, it makes an excellent thickening agent.

Tapioca flour. Use this flour in recipes where a light texture is required, as in pancakes and waffles. It is on a par with and, in some cases, superior to wheat flour.

Xanthan gum. This is used as a binder, thickener, or stabilizer. It is used commercially as a suspension agent in salad dressings and in pie fillings, canned gravies, and sauces to give these products a smoother texture. It is made by using the bacteria *Xanthomonas compestris* to ferment corn sugar. If you are planning to make your own gluten-free breads and baked goods, you'll need to stock up on it.

Note: All flours and meals should be tightly sealed and kept in the refrigerator to avoid rancidity and mealy bugs. Most freeze well and can be kept for months this way. Date everything you freeze. If you're like me, you'll forget when you put it in faster than ice can form.

A word of advice: Get thee to a dietitian. Better, a registered dietitian who can assess the nutritional damage of all those years of not absorbing your food and design a healthy diet that encourages healing. Your goal is to reach a normal weight and stay that way. Many GI departments offer nutritional counseling to their patients after diagnosis. Ask your doctor for a referral or contact the American Dietetic Associated listed in chapter 21, "The Resourceful Celiac."

Basic Rule No. 9

Never, Never assume the words Wheat-Free *on a label mean* Gluten-Free.

Wheat-free products may contain rye, oats, barley, or other unsafe ingredients. And some products are just Greek to you. The more you know about unusual or exotic foods, the better you'll eat. Here's a little homework before you head out to the store.

Amaranth. *Webster's* defines this ancient Aztec grain now enjoying a comeback as "from the Greek amaranton meaning unfading; any of a large genus of coarse herbs including pigweed which is also known as tumbleweed in certain parts of the country, and various forms cultivated for their showy flowers." In its commercial form as a breakfast cereal, amaranth is full of fiber and gluten-free, as long as it isn't mixed with any other unsafe grains.

Buckwheat. Some things bear repeating. Despite its unfortunate name, this gluten-free plant bears no relationship to wheat. It's a fruit, really, and it comes closer to the density of animal protein than any other plant. Consume it **ONLY** if you are sure it has been milled in a dedicated facility and is not contaminated with other glutenous grains.

Kamut. Prounounced *KA-moot*, this ancient Peruvian member of the wheat family is low in gluten and is touted as something tolerated by those who are allergic to wheat. Don't try this on a gluten-free diet.

Quinoa. Pronounced *keen-wah*, this is Inca for "the mother grain." According to legend, it was so crucial to the Inca diet that the king planted the first row of quinoa each season with a solid gold spade. Royal affluence aside, this tiny grain that is no bigger than a mustard seed dates back over five thousand years. Is it gluten-free? Absolutely.

Mochi. This sticky Japanese sweet rice cake is gluten-free as long as it does not contain any other unsafe grains or flavorings. Scored, cut into squares and baked, mochi puffs up as individual rolls or can be cut into strips and made into waffles.

Spelt. This is another way of saying a split piece of wood and the British past tense of the word *spell*. Webster's tells us it is also a form of wheat called *Triticum Spelta*. Wheat by any other name is just as dangerous.

Teff. Not the stuff in your nonstick pan, this is the smallest grain in the world and has, for thousands of years, been the grain of choice for the baking of *injera,* a traditional Ethiopian flat bread (see the recipe on page 227). As long as it isn't mixed or milled with forbidden grains, it's gluten-free.

Tempeh. This is not a place in Arizona. It is a low-fat, vegetarian source of protein made from soybeans that can be sautéed, steamed, baked, barbecued, used as a bread substitute in meatballs, or diced and simmered in soups and stews. It is gluten-free as long as it is sold in its natural state and is not mixed with other grains or wheat-containing soy sauce.

A final note: Remember that there is safety and support in numbers. Join a national organization and get on the gluten-free grapevine with newsletters, recipe sharing, and announcements of celiac-friendly restaurants, medical information, and the latest on ingredient labeling. You can Walk for the Cure, learn how to become a lobbyist, sample new products, attend gluten-free gatherings; it depends on how involved you want to be. These associations have local chapters all over the country and chances are there is a support group near you. It is especially important just after diagnosis to have a safe place to network with other celiacs, share information, and learn the ropes from the veterans.

In California there is the Celiac Disease Foundation with affiliates all over the country. The Gluten Intolerance Group of North America (GIG) is headquartered in Seattle with satellites in many cities and towns and CSA/USA (Celiac Sprue Association United States of America) is based in Omaha with chapters in each state. North of the border is the Canadian Celiac Association. These organizations and all their local affiliates are listed in chapter 21, "The Resourceful Celiac."

One more bit of basic advice. Never join the first club you call. Make sure the organization you choose shares your goals and can help you achieve them. Learn more about these groups in chapter 19, "How Many Celiacs Does It Take to Change a Label?"

attitude. attitude. attitude.

Some people walk in the rain . . .
Others just get wet.

—ROGER MILLER

Any streetwise inner-city kid will tell you, survival is 10 percent smarts and 90 percent attitude. With three squares, two snacks, and a midnight nibble at stake every day for the rest of your life, you're going to have to do a lot more than survive.

While it's true you may have enough wheat and gluten-free food stashed in your kitchen to last through the next millennium, you can't stay home and munch rice crackers forever. Sooner or later you must sit down to a meal with other humans. How well you do is going to depend heavily on your attitude.

Is your stomach half full or half empty? Are you half sick or half well? Do you see two perfectly poached eggs slathered in silky hollandaise beckoning to you from matching slabs of honey-baked ham? Or do you see only the English muffin?

Your answers to these and other important questions will determine how hard it's going to be for you to make your way in a world that is much more comfortable saying *no* than *yes,* that would have you suffer in silence rather than give you special treatment, and that would have you believe being different is tantamount to being sick or odd or needy.

The attitudinal trick is to see yourself as perfectly healthy or, to be more precise, no longer sick, in spite of the fact that your plumbing is peculiar at best, your immune system so weird it sees an innocent chunk of bread as a deadly poison. No matter that your genetic structure probably should be displayed in *Ripley's Believe It or Not.*

The problem is, other people often confuse healthy, which you are now, or soon will be, with normal, which you are decidedly not. Anyone who can't eat pizza, chocolate chip cookies, apple pie, hot dogs, hush puppies, hamburgers, and biscotti is not only considered abnormal in certain small towns and villages in America, but he or she may even be considered a threat to society. To decline the foods so symbolic of our national preoccupation with Mom, the flag, instant gratification, and empty calories is to be met with narrow-eyed suspicion at best.

My advice is to stop trying to pass yourself off as normal. To be accurate as well as politically correct, you are "nutritionally challenged." The sooner you digest this important distinction, the sooner you can stop seeing your diet as an obstacle to pleasure and start approaching it in a way that allows for maximum possibility. The goal is not simply eating, it's eating well; not merely getting a meal on the table, but getting a great one on the table. If this is to be achieved with any regularity, the solution must be as unusual as the problem. It's really as simple as that. The harder you try to fit in, the hungrier you get. Look at it another way: Your body has been eccentric for years, why shouldn't you be, too?

The night I slipped a demitasse spoon out of my evening bag and headed for the caviar was the first time I realized this. If I had insisted on seeing myself as normal, I would have behaved in a way that was appropriate to the situation. I might have spooned some caviar onto a cracker and tried to discreetly scrape off a bit of roe with my teeth, risking a potentially nasty spill, which is not a great idea in a new evening dress. Worse, I might not have tried at all and begun the New Year with a great big helping of self-pity.

By seeing myself not as unwell but as special and, by virtue of my peculiar and special genetic makeup, one who is allowed to break the rules, I was able to enjoy my fill of one of my favorite foods. In the process, I began the necessary shift in attitude that brings with it self-respect, self-reliance, a sense of adventure, a sense of being in control, and more than its share of good things to eat. By giving myself permission to be creative about my problem, I was able to apply the principle of old-fashioned positive thinking and come up with an elegant solution that fit the festive tone of the occasion.

It tickles me today to know that the other guests did not see my odd eating style for what it really was—a clever way around a tough problem. I smile when I see that others, thinking I am a connoisseur, have on successive evenings copied my caviar-eating style, waving their spoons and proclaiming their passion for the stuff. I once overheard a gentleman who witnessed my now annual descent-into-caviar-with-spoon dismissing the cracker, as well as the chopped egg and onion, as "irrelevant."

I admit this behavior may seem a bit crazy by some standards, especially to those poor souls who sleepwalk through life with a rule book bolted to their heads, but think of the alternative—a howling empty place in your stomach and in your heart that gets bigger and bigger with every treat denied. In light of that, does it really matter what others think?

If carrying your own spoon to cocktail parties isn't comfortable for you at first, start small. Carry two slices of gluten-free bread or your favorite roll to a restaurant, ask the waiter to toast it, then order a hamburger the way you like it (as long as you can be sure the other ingredients are gluten-free). Ditto for dipping, mopping, sopping, grilled cheese, tuna melts, Reubens, and ordering eggs Benedict, once you have thoroughly investigated the hollandaise, of course.

Forget plastic baggies. These will turn your bread into instant bread crumbs. Measure your favorite loaf and find yourself an attractive plastic container that holds two slices securely. Prowl the flea markets, pick up a campy child's lunch box from the fifties, and use that to keep your gluten-free baked goods fresh. Trust me, people will love your style, especially if you're lucky enough to find a vintage Hopalong Cassidy, Betty Boop, or Yosemite Sam. Why not have one made in metal or bright red plastic or wood? You're going to use it often, so why not splurge on something that looks great? (You had nice lighters when you smoked, didn't you?) Just make sure the waiter returns it. Some years ago, I found a lovely old miniature silver hinged box of the type Victorian women dangled from their belts and their bosoms. They filled them with mysterious things—lace hankies, a lock of a lover's hair, some snuff, a teensy vial of laudanum that I imagine gave them the dreamy looks they always seemed to wear. I slip mine on a velvet ribbon and wear it to parties. People are amazed to find such a lovely object home to my personal cache of gluten-free crackers.

For those occasions that warrant gooey cheeses, finger foods, and lots of dips, carry your favorite crackers and make sure you wear something with deep pockets or carry them in your purse (it's a good idea to line purse or pocket with plastic wrap to avoid stains). Slip them out one at a time (or ask for your own small serving bowl) and nosh to your heart's content. To avoid other dippers' crumbs, get there first and serve yourself a portion of the dip on a clean plate. And don't try to hide what you're doing. This is a great conversation starter as long as your don't belabor it and, God forbid, get trapped in a discussion of the medical reasons for your unusual social behavior.

For longer eating experiences, such as weekends at the beach or family visits, fill a bag with your own food. This may sound awfully self-centered, but it is really quite thoughtful, both for you and your host, who is responsible not only for your comfort and pleasure but for every guest's needs for the duration.

If I have to travel for business for an extended period of time, I ship a carton of my goodies to myself, care of the hotel, then alert the chef and the room service manager to my special requirements. It's amazing what a slice of toast with jam or a gluten-free muffin served on a tray can do for your spirits and your stress level when you are working away from home.

The idea is to do whatever it takes to help you feel as special as you are in every way possible and to put the power back where it belongs—with you, not with your diet. With apologies to the late John Fitzgerald Kennedy, "Yours is not to ask why, but to ask why not." Naturally, your new and more confident self will not emerge overnight. But if you follow these steps, you too will be packing small spoons, asking for sliced cucumbers (delicious with hummus), waving your bread at waiters, and demanding (always politely) that your special foods be presented to you with as much of a flourish as everybody else's. Carried off properly, the right attitude celebrates your uniqueness. It can, along with the right tone of voice and a well-timed chuckle, even offer a touch of sympathy for those unlucky enough to be ordinary.

Before you move ahead, however, you must go back—all the way back to the beginning—and adjust. How tough an adjustment this is really depends on who you are and how much self-esteem and confidence you possess. How much self-examination have you been exposed to, and where are you, high to low, on the risk-aversion scale? How seriously do you take yourself and your dietary circumstances, and how willing are you to appear assertive, even foolish, to strangers?

The important thing to know is that it is absolutely within your power to change in a more positive way, to become resourceful about your diet and forthright in presenting it to others. No major personal overhaul is required, nor is the prerequisite twenty or thirty years of painful therapy. At this important fork in your road, a few minor revisions in the way you look at life in general and your diet problems specifically can make all the difference. You may find you're a whole lot healthier than you ever imagined.

Attitude Adjustment No. 1

First you mourn.

It is so easy to feel guilty about grieving for something the rest of the world perceives as unimportant. After all, people are dying and all you have is a little problem with grain. Right?

Wrong.

If you haven't moaned and complained, kicked and screamed, whimpered, whined "Why me?" and refused to be in the same room with spaghetti, you must do so now. Without the sadness and the anger and the acknowledgment of how serious a loss this is for you, that it will be with you for the rest of your life, there *is* no new attitude. There is only the downward spiral of self-pity and denial, guilt and self-destructive behavior that leads to the never-ending cycle of more of the same. To use food terms, if you don't allow yourself to grieve openly, your resentment will simmer and boil over, eventually scalding everyone in its path. We all know people who'd have a great smile if it were not for the blood on their teeth. Wallow away.

Attitude Adjustment No. 2

Accept that you are powerless over your diet.

Beyond pain is acceptance and beyond that is recovery. I'm not talking about recovery in the look-Ma-I-can-eat-grain-again sense. I'm talking about recovering your balance, your good humor, your ability to see yourself not as ill but as a creative person who uses his or her natural resourcefulness to enjoy life and to maintain health, someone who can say "It's no big deal" and mean it. To borrow a bit of wisdom from Alcoholics Anonymous's twelve-step program, you can't develop a healthy attitude toward your food intolerance until you admit that you are powerless over it.

Like everyone who has ever had to face a disability—and yes, this is a disability only in the sense that it's not going away—the sooner you accept the unalterable fact of it, the sooner you can move beyond it to the strategy for coping with it creatively and positively.

Put another way, the energy it takes to deny the problem, ignore it, trivialize it, pretend it's not there, wish it weren't, and suppress your true feelings about it can now be used to a better purpose.

Attitude Adjustment No. 3

Don't complain. Explain.

We don't ask a person who is trying to quit smoking to empty the ashtrays, nor do we send a drinking problem to the liquor store for a nice California merlot. So why do we ask people on restrictive diets to prepare our meals?

I've seen this happen to people, usually women, who are trying to lose weight, eating almost nothing while continuing to prepare enormous, high-calorie meals for their families. The dieter weighs in with radishes and cottage cheese while the rest of the clan eat like longshoremen after a hard day on the docks. The same is true for those of us who must follow a grain-restricted diet. This is even more unfair because our problems won't melt away with portion control and exercise.

At my house, no one would dream of asking me to toast an English muffin, not because my family guessed that I can't bear that singular aroma and the way the butter disappears into all the little nooks and crannies, but because I told them exactly how sad it makes me feel. Waiting for people to magically understand your needs is always unrealistic, expecting a spouse or children or good friends to know at any given moment which food cues upset you is asking for trouble. And it's not fair to them.

I am reminded of the man who is working up the courage to ask his neighbor if he can borrow a ladder. He thinks about the chances of his neighbor lending it to him with generosity and thinks, "Well, after all, I loaned him my electric drill." A little while later he remembers the time the neighbor took a month to return a barbecue fork. And even later in the day, still worrying about whether his request will be met with a negative response, it occurs to him that his auto-buffing attachment has never been returned. Finally, several hours later, the man marches across his neighbor's lawn, rings the doorbell, and when the unsuspecting fellow answers, he shouts, "You know something, I don't want your damn ladder anyway!" and stomps off.

It's tempting to find fault with the people who ask us to cook for them. After all, that's selfish, isn't it? Not really. The blame lies not with those who expect us to continue making dinner, but with the one who doesn't complain or explain why it's selfish to ask. Adjusting to the gluten-free diet is tough enough, suffering in silence is stupid.

Attitude Adjustment No. 4

Communicate. Negotiate.

Dolly Parton once said, "Get down off that cross, honey, we need the wood." Sighing, eye rolling, and looks of martyred despair went out with Melanie and Ashley in *Gone with the Wind* and *My Little Margie*. Tell all the people who love you how hard it is for you to watch them butter a hunk of good French bread.

Old patterns must change and family traditions need to be adjusted if you are to succeed and your diet is to be acknowledged, not as an afterthought, but in a meaningful way. While everyone must understand how serious this is and how important the elimination of wheat and gluten from your diet is to your well-being and long-term health, it is your responsibility to tell them, not theirs to guess.

As with everything in life, no one is going to respond to your needs unless you communicate to them what those needs are. If you don't, believe me, you will find ways to make them pay for their lack of clairvoyance. The important thing is not to pile one resentment on top of the other in a kind of pousse-café of grievances until no one remembers, least of all you, how many layers of anger make up this lethal and destructive cocktail. Get those feelings out in the open, theirs as well as yours, as they occur.

Here are some ways to get off to a good start:

1. If you are the primary chef in the family, you may want to let go of this responsibility for a while and explain that preparing "normal" food is hard for you. In fact, you may find one meal more difficult to prepare for others than another. Breakfast and brunch are the most brutal for me because I still miss bagels and croissants and all those crunchy granola cereals that are the backbones of these grain-based meals. (Yes, I know there are gluten-free versions of all these foods, but we're talking about you handling the real thing.) Tell your family exactly how you feel when you watch them nibble a brioche. For a long time I unconsciously chewed along with people, like a passenger who brakes from the backseat.

2. Hold a family meeting to discuss food preparation options and develop a rotating schedule, so no one is ever stuck with fixing the same meal for longer than a week. Include everyone in the family, even the youngest members, so everyone plays a part. Review the schedule weekly or monthly as your own coping skills improve.

3. Discuss your sadness or feelings of deprivation when faced with specific food situations, such as family picnics, pizza night, mall food grazing, preparing sandwiches for school lunches, and special occasions. Talk about upcoming parties and holidays and ask everybody to think of ways they can be easier on you. This way you're less likely to be blindsided by the birthday cake you can't eat, or suffer a thankless Thanksgiving at your sister's if the whole tribe is on the same page.

4. If there is one food in particular, such as pizza, chocolate chip cookies, or marble pound cake that you can't stand to see being enjoyed, say so. Ask that friends, family, and receptive coworkers not eat these things in front of you.

5. Tell family members ahead of time that you will not be preparing multiple versions of meals. Be very clear in letting them know that the pasta that is good for you will have to be good for them and ask their understanding about this. Find out what their favorite brands are and be as inventive with their meals as you are with yours.

The more people enjoy your food, the less isolated you'll feel, so make a game of it. My husband has developed a real preference for rice now that I have learned to do so much with it, and his reaction when I prepare risotto or jambalaya can hardly be characterized as disappointment. Glee is more like it when I offer friends manioc bread sticks still warm from the oven. Grilled polenta with a savory sun-dried tomato and mushroom sauce and freshly grated Parmesan is always a crowd-pleaser. Who says selfishness is a bad thing?

6. Communication works both ways. Listen carefully to how other people feel about this change in their lives and try to be just as understanding and accommodating when loved ones express sadness or anger at losses resulting from your diet. While this may be easy to understand on an intellectual level, it's much harder to put into practice.

When your family tells you they're all going out for pizza and have not invited you so they can enjoy it without having to bear the guilt of gobbling it up in your presence, it's easy to feel sorry for yourself. Try to thank them for their consideration, even if you don't feel particularly grateful yet. A healthy attitude doesn't mean life is a one-way street in your direction. It means being sensitive to the needs of others as well as your own, even if it hurts, and it does.

7. Be open. Be willing to compromise, such as by saying, "I'll make lunch, if you take care of your own breakfast." Remember, children have very strong feelings about being cared for and nurtured, and they really can't understand a parent's problem unless they are directly told. Consider this talk with your

child as a lesson in becoming an adult who isn't afraid to ask for special attention. If you honor your children with their own importance in your happiness, they will honor you. They will also grow up honoring themselves. Never underestimate them.

When you are comfortable that your family understands this important change in your life, broaden the communication to friends, relatives, and coworkers. These are people with whom you are not necessarily intimate, but who may be in a position to cook or order food for you, such as the office lunch pool, cafeteria manager, secretary, or meeting planner. Here it is important to state the problem and what you require of people without baring as much of yourself as you have to your immediate circle. (Hint: Your office rival is not the one with whom to share your deep sense of loss over cheese Danish.)

A word of warning here—controlling someone's food is as close to controlling the person as it gets. Be prepared for some disappointments, even some nasty surprises. There will be people who will always find a reason to forget your special diet and never seem to have extra goodies on hand for you. Asking people to extend themselves may unearth some negative feelings toward you, ones that may have lain dormant until now.

If there are unresolved issues or negative feelings between you and the people you are asking for help, it may not be possible for them to extend themselves until those issues are brought out in the open. Be direct. Ask why this person never remembers your problem. You may be surprised at the answer. Be willing to hear it.

For some, the extra effort just may be impossible because what you're really asking them to do is change their behavior and many people simply can't or won't do that. Others can't accept it when someone in their circle changes, voluntarily or not. I've seen this happen in very serious instances where a friend is faced with a sudden change in economic status, a severe physical impairment, and even the tragedy of diminished mental capacity. In each instance the person has asked for support in accordance with the circumstances, and it may as well have never been said. Everyone listens, but not everybody hears. You too will expect the best and, sadly, discover the inflexibility of some people. In some cases the awakening will be rude. But for every disappointment, someone else you never expected to will come through and you will be blessed by a friend you never knew you had. If you'll pardon the expression, the wheat will separate from the chaff.

Attitude Adjustment No. 5

Never trivialize your problem or allow others to do so.

The word *just* no longer exists for you. Never use this sloppy little adverb to present your problem to the world. I'm referring to the popular usage, "Oh, it's just a little gluten problem" or "It's just an allergy." When you speak this way, you are belittling the importance of your needs, and it is a cue for others do the same. Besides, it is not "just an allergy."

People who minimize the importance of their diets remind me of the old joke that asks, How many martyrs does it take to change a lightbulb?

None. They'd rather sit in the dark.

Words such as *just, only,* and *merely* fly in the face of all that you are. Whenever you use them, you are begging the listener to turn off and not to take your request seriously. Habits like this are tough to break because something in your background is telling you you don't deserve the full attention of others, that your problems are not as important as theirs. Short of years of professional help, the following affirmation can help you see yourself differently. (An affirmation is something you say or write over and over until you begin to believe it.)

I, _____, am a unique and special person worthy of all the special attention, love, and understanding I ask from those around me.

Fill in your name and write this affirmation in a small notebook or on an index card that you can carry with you at all times. When you feel that you are about to trivialize your needs or reject special attention from people ("Oh, it's nothing, don't bother . . ."), take it out and remind yourself that you deserve only the best from yourself and from others.

Developing a new attitude means responding differently to old cues. People will tell you how lucky you are that it's "just" (there's that word again) a diet and nothing worse. There are many ways to deal with this, none of which includes agreement, because agreeing with someone else's judgment about how you should feel is tantamount to being rendered invisible and invalid. These depend on your relationship with and emotional investment in each person.

Over time you will develop your own responses to people who have treated you carelessly or behaved in a way you find unacceptable, disappointing, or intolerable. For now, here are some stock answers that will let others know you are not a person to be dismissed and will leave you feeling a whole lot better for having stood up for yourself. If someone is rude and/or dumb enough to say, "You know, you really should feel lucky it's just an allergy and not something worse," match the punishment with the crime:

1. "Maybe I will at some point, but right now this is really tough for me."
2. "I'll let you know when I do."
3. "Why don't you try my diet for a week, then tell me how lucky you feel."
4. "Do me a favor, don't visit someone who's just had a mastectomy, okay?"

As sure as the sun comes up, you will find yourself in food situations where someone in your family or circle of friends has forgotten you completely. Most people will apologize profusely and you should accept it as graciously as a growling stomach can. Some, however, will try to cover their embarrassment by saying something stupid and insensitive. Naturally, you must gauge your response to the intention and measure it according to how often this person has offended you.

My own experience is that most people usually forget once. After a gentle reminder, they will more than make it up to you the next time. Some will do this twice before they get it. But one or two may forget so often, you have no recourse but to question their motive, decline their invitation, and examine the shaky ground upon which your relationship is built. The subtlety or vehemence of your response naturally will depend on whether food is central to the occasion—you're not going to tell the recently bereaved at the funeral luncheon that she forgot to order you a gluten-free meal, nor are you going to tell the host of a surprise birthday party for someone else that it was tacky to serve cake. Let common sense prevail and let the punishment fit the criminal as well as the crime.

Sooner or later, someone is bound to say, "Oh, I forgot. You can't eat that." This is your cue to say:

1. "It's my fault. I really should have phoned ahead to remind you."
2. "If making special food is a problem for you, let me know and I'll bring my own food next time."
3. "Tell you what, next time you invite me, I'll forget to come."

Another common stupid comment is the one usually made by your brother-in-law Boomer or your Aunt Ethel after realizing you've been served a slice of flourless chocolate cheesecake (safe) with a cookie crust (not safe). Instead of apologizing profusely and getting you a dish of ice cream or some fruit, the guilty party compounds the problem by acknowledging the error in a way that gets him or her off the hook and you squarely on it. This little face-saving, guest-embarrassing tactic is a question you will hear much too often: "Why don't you just eat the middle?"

It's tough to remain unruffled, hang on to your dignity, and be firm in your resolve never to reduce yourself to doing any such thing. Why? Because no matter how carefully you remove the crust, the middle will most likely be contaminated.

Some good answers to this deflective and dumb comment:

1. "No, thanks. I'd really rather not risk eating something that might make me sick."
2. "No, thanks. I don't really enjoy picking my food apart."
3. "Great idea. Let's all scrape off our crusts!"

Of course, if you're really disgusted, have been asked this question once too often, or have given serious thought to the wisdom of accepting any further invitations from this particular person, you do have other options:

1. "Why don't you eat the middle, too, and let me know how *you* like it?"
2. "Clearly you enjoy watching me suffer."
3. "Why don't you just put my dish on the floor with the dog's (cat's)?"

Attitude Adjustment No. 6

Pity is not positive.

Reject negative attention politely and firmly. All that poor-you stuff does not contribute to a good attitude, nor does it inspire creativity.

Slowly and insidiously, the pity of others can erode self-esteem and may even contribute to a victim mentality. You may find yourself always presenting that needy side of yourself to the person who encourages it, and it also may result in being viewed as a victim and less than equal in other areas of the relationship.

It's easy to fall into this trap, especially right after diagnosis when you are feeling sorry for yourself. Beware the person who does not encourage you or offer ways to help you get back to your old/new self, who whispers to others about how hard it is for you to live on this diet, who is always there to pat your hand and remind you how badly you feel about pasta, and who, whether consciously or not, keeps you in that swamp so long, you start to see yourself only as the one who can't eat gluten. That's a pretty narrow view of yourself. Pretty soon, you, too, are forgetting all the wonderful things you are besides being a celiac.

Naturally, you must learn to distinguish between an unhealthy focus on your problems and genuine concern. The fastest way to do this is to see what action follows the talk. People who use pity to keep the people in their lives feeling as badly as they no doubt do often don't follow through with positive action. True compassion and healthy caring usually results in wonderful surprises, special foods, generous ideas, pantries permanently stocked with goodies for you, and very little talk about your diet beyond learning more about how to make it easier and more pleasant for you.

We pay dearly for being coddled. You simply have to be willing to give it up. You don't need it or the people who indulge your need for it. But you know that.

Attitude Adjustment No. 7

The harder you work, the better you eat.

From here on in, you have to participate in the process. Every meal at home. Every breakfast, lunch, and dinner out. Every bite on the road, at work, at the mall, in a plane, at the park. Every time. And it's work.

When we visit friends, we can't just hand them a list of foods we must avoid. We have to teach them how to make the foods we can eat, where to buy them, and how to keep them from touching the foods we can't eat. We have to make sure they're using the right thickeners, ice creams, spreads, and dips, that their corn bread is all corn, that their barbecue sauce is a safe brand, their soy sauce is gluten-free. If necessary, we must supply these things.

Suddenly, we can't just dash to the market for a few things. We have to take the time and extra expense to bake or mail-order gluten-free foods. We have to learn how to add extra chocolate and nuts, a layer of raspberry jam or a decadent icing to make a gluten-free cake or brownie as memorable as the ones we miss. We have to become expert at doctoring recipes, adding fresh fruit to muffin recipes, reinventing breakfast cereals with extra raisins, bits of dried fruit, and shredded coconut. If we want cheesecake, we have to show the cook how to adapt their recipes for us, using gluten-free ginger or cocoa cookies in place of their traditional cookie crust or learn how to bake something from scratch ourselves (see page 125 for the perfect piecrust). Often we are forced to prepare an entire dessert just because we crave one serving. If we don't trust ourselves to deposit the remainder in the freezer or if the recipe doesn't keep, we find ourselves hosting more than our share of dinners.

We have to know the ingredients in foods sold by vendors of every description well before we are struck with the urge to buy ourselves an ice cream, french fries, or a banana smoothie. We have to be willing to prepare the meal, host the party, do dessert, bring a casserole, roast the turkey, and make the stuffing in order to be sure we've got something to eat. If not, you will be disappointed. Guaranteed.

The adjustment to this new "interactive" eating can be daunting, but you have to realize the world cooks and eats a certain way. Fad diets and passing culinary fancies aside, it's not going to change for you.

The bottom line: You can no longer just show up, sit back, and be served. The desire to give up and eat something out of a can or a box will be very strong at times.

Attitude Adjustment No. 8

Assume nothing and never take yes for an answer.

Periodically, phone, fax, write, or e-mail any company that makes a gluten-free product you really like. Just because it was gluten-free when you read the label doesn't mean it will always remain so. Many food marketers buy their ingredients from different suppliers, and changes may not be reflected on labels that are printed well in advance of any such reformulation. You don't have to be paranoid, but you do need to be careful, especially if the product is a big part of your diet.

The operative attitude here is "I'm the customer and you are in business to please me and I need to make sure I don't get sick from something you have not told me about." While this may sound adversarial, it really isn't. The people who make your food have an obligation to tell you what's in it. As more and more food marketers are voluntarily labeling their products gluten-free, companies not willing to answer your questions need another kind of attitude adjustment. And, of course, you will always start a conversation by saying how much you love this product before you get down to business, won't you?

Attitude Adjustment No. 9

No one knows more about your problem than you do.

Understand that when it comes to your diet, no one is as clever, as resourceful, or as smart as you are. And no one has a better reason to be.

All too often, we sell ourselves short because we take the word of someone we presume to have authority. When the waiter tells us the chef uses flour to coat a cutlet or a plate of scallops, it's important to push past this negative information to the more palatable answer. Ask if that same dish can be prepared with cornstarch or cornmeal or simply grilled, baked, sautéed, or roasted unadorned. With few exceptions, you will see the lightbulb going on in the waiter's face, usually followed by an offer to consult the chef. Remember, the chef is an expert on the preparation of food, not the preparation of *your* food.

And don't always assume your doctor knows more about living with your condition than you do. With notable exceptions, most don't spend five minutes understanding the conditions they diagnose so expertly, especially if those conditions require no medical intervention. If you need proof of this, ask your doctor for his or her position on kamut or spelt. Better still, ask why, when you have had a short gastroenterological procedure like a colonoscopy or a follow-up small bowel biopsy, you are handed a package of peanut crackers along with everyone else. From now on, it's up to you to connect the dots.

Call me nuts, but I believe every one of us already knows all we need to know to create our own happiness and well-being. It can be of enormous help if you try to believe this, too. If the picture seems bleak right now, paint your own and use brighter colors. Ask questions, make requests, switch dishes, offer to cook with a friend, start every sentence with "What if . . . ," assume nothing, and trust that the other person can always say no. In my experience, when asked politely and from a place of truth, very few ever do.

Attitude Adjustment No. 10

Never ask what is offered when you can tell what you need.

If I sound like a hopeless idealist, I have learned that this is not a bad way to be. Yes, I know there are people who will mug you, steal your identity, steal your SUV, and, if you're not careful, deposit your life savings in a Swiss bank.

I'm not suggesting that you become foolish or naive, but I am suggesting that you give people the benefit of the doubt before you assume they are not interested in making your meals more pleasant.

If you're not sure, go to a public place such as a hospital or an office building and ask the receptionist if you can use the copy machine or phone simply by saying, "May I use your copy machine/phone for a minute?" You may get lucky, but most likely you will be politely told to go to a Kinko's or to the nearest phone booth.

Now go to another institution and ask the same question, this time starting with, "I hope you can help me. I really am in a tight spot and I wonder if you would be kind enough to allow me to make a copy of this/make a quick telephone call." Chances are the person will offer to make copies for you or hand you the phone and maybe even laugh about forgetting her cell phone just when she needed it.

The lesson is simple. The better your ability to ask a question in a way that encourages the other person to do the right thing, the better your chances of hearing the answer you want. The trick is asking it in a way that brings out the other person's natural instincts to help you. "You have no idea what a treat it would be for me to have your wonderful Bolognese sauce on my gluten-free pasta."

Learning to do this is not so simple. Practice on your family: "Darling, it would mean so much to me if you took out the trash/changed the cat's litter/passed that math test/lowered the stereo . . ."

thinking like a celiac

Don't lose
Your head
To gain a minute,
You need your head,
Your brains are in it.

—*Burma-Shave roadside ad, 1925*

Special diets create special challenges. They force us to be creative, inventive, ingenious, canny, and clever, to think outside the box, to go "against the grain." In short, you've got to use your noodle—your rice noodle, that is.

Living gluten-free is a state of mind. Once you get the hang of it, it becomes second nature. You ask yourself, What can I do to make this diet easier, to pamper and honor myself, save some time and money and eat well in the process? The idea is to know how to do it so well that you hardly have to think about it. Herewith are some shortcuts, ideas, strategies, and just plain smart thinking to help you save money and time, and maybe even yourself and your family in a real emergency.

Not all celiacs are carnivores. Some of us are strict vegetarians. And others are laissez-faire, eating eggs, poultry, or fish but drawing the line at red meat and dairy. No matter, we all have one thing in common. Our digestive systems have not operated properly for quite awhile, some of us for most of our lives. To compound the problem, often a diagnosis of CD leaves us temporarily lactose intolerant. In my own case, this problem disappeared after about six months, but wreaked its own form of havoc in that time. In our impatience for the return of good health, we forget we are temporarily wounded, some of us worse than others. Not only do we have do be vigilant in the hunt for hidden gluten, we need to be patient. Bodies don't bounce back as quickly as we'd like. Some of us heal more slowly than others.

One of the best ways to foster healing is to temporarily avoid gluten-free versions of our old favorite dishes and eat soothing, easy-to-digest foods during the transition. It helps to pretend you are a child who has just been weaned and learning to eat solid foods for the first time. Try one food, then another, adding slowly until you are confident each food agrees with you. Save the cookies and the sugary treats, and any experiments with questionable foods like oats, for when you feel better.

With its polish intact, brown rice is a healthful alternative to white rice, full of fiber and good nutrients. Prepared in a pressure cooker the way the macro chefs do it, it is also one of the easiest foods to digest. Mixed with some calcium-rich kale that's been sautéed in a bit of toasted sesame oil, it can make for a soothing supper. Add some beans (cook them well to aid digestion and don't forget the Beano) and you've got a complete protein. Use the leftover rice to make breakfast porridge with some soy milk, a little maple syrup, and a few raisins. Or add fruit, a bit of honey, and some toasted almonds.

Miso soup is also one of the all-time comfort foods and couldn't be easier to fix. With its mineral rich wakame (sea vegetable in the kelp family), protein-rich tofu, and warming broth or dashi, few dishes are as strengthening or as soothing. Miso soup is a traditional breakfast in Japan, but you can enjoy it anytime. Never allow the broth to boil after the miso is added or you will destroy its beneficial digestive enzymes. This recipe is from Christina Pirello's *Cooking the Whole Foods Way* (HP Books).

Minute Miso Soup

4 Servings

   3 cups spring or filtered water
   1 3-inch piece of wakame, soaked and diced
   1 small onion cut lengthwise into thin slices
1½ teaspoons brown rice miso
      Small handful of fresh parsley, minced

1. Bring water to a boil in a medium saucepan over medium heat.
2. Add wakame and simmer 1 minute.
3. Add onion and simmer 1 to 2 minutes more.
4. Remove a small amount of broth, add miso and stir until dissolved.

5. Stir mixture into soup and simmer 3 to 4 minutes more.
6. Serve garnished with fresh parsley.

Okay, so it takes 6 minutes. It's still easy. Experiment with other whole, low-fat foods like azuki beans, a staple in Japan where they are eaten for their healing properties and high vitamin B_{12}, potassium, and iron content, a smart idea after years of poorly absorbing these important nutrients and especially if you've been anemic. Learn to cook with fresh or dried daikon, a peppery Japanese radish said to aid in the digestion of fats and protein. Sea vegetables are full of protein, calcium, potassium, and iron and are great way a to replace lost or depleted minerals. Look for delicate wakame, crisp and salty dulse, sushi nori and hiziki, traditionally used in pressed salads.

To learn more about other healing whole foods, health seminars, and cooking classes and where to buy the highest-quality, hand-harvested, sun-dried sea vegetables, contact the Kushi Institute, (800) 975-8744 or go to www.kushiinstitute.org.

The Gluten-Free Kitchen

Like that pesky sock drawer we never seem to get around to, we're always promising ourselves we'll clean out the refrigerator and defrost the freezer (what *is* that petrified lump underneath the frozen spinach?). Someday, we

Use Your Noodle

Many celiacs are quick to blame gluten for every reaction, unnecessarily eliminating foods from an already limited diet. Taking it easy, going slowly, and adding foods one at a time not only allows your gut to heal, it helps you to understand what foods are difficult or easy for you to digest. It allows you to know which ones create a sense a well-being, give short or long-lasting energy, put weight on, take it off, and which foods give you a problem. Testing the trouble foods (lactose and fats are the big ones) at monthly intervals will tell you if these are going to be permanent problems or if you are simply not ready for them yet. Heal. Experiment. Use your noodle.

Use Your Rice Noodle

. . . .

Miss fried chicken? Brush chicken pieces (skin removed) in gluten-free ranch dressing, then roll in potato flakes and bake in a preheated 450-degree oven. Turn the oven down to 350 degrees and bake for about 25 minutes or until juices run clear. No flour, no fuss, less fat.

say, we'll organize the cupboards, rearrange the drawers (do I really need that twist-tie collection?), replace the crummy old shelf liners, and throw out the canned beans that expired before the turn of millennium. Well, someday is here. No better time than now to organize a smooth functioning, safe cooking, separate but equal, gluten-free kitchen.

If you are going to cook gluten-free for everyone, as I do, there's not much need for separate equipment. My husband loves rice and has grown quite fond of my brown rice pasta, so any meal that I prepare for two or for guests is going to be gluten-free. All sauces are thickened with cornstarch, recipes that call for flour get either rice flour or gluten-free baking mix. For dessert, there is usually fresh fruit, ice cream or sorbet, and our favorite almond paste cookies. On special occasions, including birthdays, there is gluten-free lemon pound cake with strawberries and whipped cream or a chocolate torte with raspberries and powdered sugar. For dinner parties I like to fill small matching vases with breadsticks—regular on one end of the table, gluten-free on the other. Unless I get a special request for Carr's water crackers (once a year my husband gets a yen for these) appetizers are spread onto Glutino flax crackers with sun-dried tomatoes and onions or lightly salted Hol-Grain brown rice crackers. Our friends prefer these to the usual kind.

But even I will make the occasional sandwich, serve the odd croissant, leave a basket of brioches and muffins on the kitchen counter for weekend guests to nibble on when they get up. I put the jam in a little glass dish, so as to prevent a sticky spoon from leaving crumbs in the jar. Ditto for the butter. A small serving dish keeps the rest of the stick pristine.

How do I make sure no gluten served to guests makes its way to my lips? It starts with a few simple rules to help polish your organizational skills.

Rule #1: Everybody learns the rules.

This way nobody has to shoulder the entire burden. If everyone knows what foods and utensils should touch what, there's a better chance to avoid a gluten accident. It's also a wonderful family lesson about looking out for each other.

Easy for me to say with our boys grown and out of the nest and only two adults, as the saying goes, to keep the cookie from crumbling. I realize that in big families where some members are gluten-free and some aren't and meals are fixed on the fly, it isn't that simple.

Rule #2: Establish "Gluten-Free Only" Equipment.

Some equipment you might want to have two of in a mixed-use kitchen:

Cutting board
Toaster (to avoid the extra expense and use of space, many gluten-free cooks use toaster ovens because household crumbs drop to the bottom, away from gluten-free bread)
Flour sifter
Colander
Spatula
Pans with nonstick coatings like Teflon
Cast-iron frying pan
Sugar bowl
Wooden spoon (time to dispose of old spoons that may have a lifetime of gluten in the cracks)

A good idea is to buy a pretty crock or pitcher and keep your gluten-free spoons, forks, spatulas, egg turners, tongs, etc., away from the drawer that contains gluten-mixing utensils.

To save having to buy separate cookie sheets or baking pans, keep an extra roll of tin foil for heating and baking gluten-free foods where pizza or cookies may have been baked.

Use your head. If something that contains gluten regularly touches your food, buy a new one and use it only for gluten-free cooking. If it's glass or metal and washed properly in lots of hot water after each use, it's fine to use for both.

Rule #3: When it doubt, wipe it down.

This means counters, cutting boards, sinks, anything that might have come in contact with gluten. The rule is simple and unbreakable. Never spread butter, cut a sandwich, slice cheese, fry an egg, flip a burger, cut up a chicken, or scoop ice cream with the same utensil that has touched gluten. In my kitchen, putting a knife or a spoon or any object that has come into contact with bread or flour, etc., goes directly into the dishwasher or is promptly washed by hand. It is something we don't have to remember anymore. It's reflex.

Rule #4: Divide and conquer.

How separate should gluten-free food be from the rest of the family groceries? Think church and state. A separate cupboard or shelf is a good idea. Keep a supply of cereals, crackers, mixes, soups, special flours, cookies, pretzels, and other treats and snacks on hand. If space allows, dedicate a shelf of the freezer for individual gluten-free pizzas, frozen macaroni and cheese, and other entrees, bread, rolls, muffins, etc. This will help other family members understand that these foods are off-limits to them (unless invited to share) and you always know what you have and when it's time to restock. In a big family and if space and budget allows, it's wise to buy duplicates of things like jam, peanut butter, and dips too easily contaminated by the spoons and knives and chips of non-celiacs. This also makes keeping an inventory of your favorite products much easier. Tack price lists to the inside of the door and jot down typical delivery times, so you aren't caught short between orders.

Use Your Noodle

If the price tag on packaged gluten-free baking mixes seems a bit rich for your blood, baker Rebecca Bunting (see pages 125 and 418) suggests mixing up 6 cups of brown or white rice flour (she prefers brown for flavor and nutrients) with 2 cups of potato starch and 1 cup of tapioca flour. Store in a coffee can or plastic container in the refrigerator if you don't bake often, on the pantry shelf, if you do. Substitute cup for cup in recipes calling for wheat flour, i.e., thickening sauces, muffins, cookies, etc.

Of course, you will be generous with your goodies (after all, don't you want more family members eating your way?), but only to a point. At these prices, special foods are just that—*special*—too rich for the munching and grazing habits of ravenous teenagers, hungry toddlers, or the midnight prowling of snacking adults.

And speaking of expenses . . .

The Cost of Living Gluten-Free

No way around it, gluten-free food is expensive. For some, paying extra for special food is merely annoying. For others, it means scrimping on something else, and for still more, it is a downright hardship. Some companies have begun to coupon their products, much the way mainstream food processors do, rewarding their customers with price-off incentives. Frequent buyer cards and quantity discounts are beginning to make competitive sense to gluten-free companies. Many of you are forming food co-ops and pooling expensive orders, especially those that cross the border from Canada and other places with hefty shipping charges. This is best done through a support group with a central drop-off point and a system for distributing the individual orders. Another way to avoid high freight costs is to convince a local market that there is enough demand to warrant ordering these products through a commercial distributor.

Profit will be built in, of course, but these foods will be a bit cheaper without your having to bear the shipping costs all by yourself. If, despite your best efforts, the gluten-free diet is still too much of a burden, or if you feel shouldering the extra expense adds insult to injury, you can always deduct the extra costs of these items from your income tax return.

U.S. Tax Regulations

Is the gluten-free diet tax deductible? More to the point, is it a medical expense? Yes. According to IRS publication #502 and as of 2003, medical expenses are "the costs of diagnosis, cure, mitigation, treatment, or prevention of disease, and the costs of affecting any part or function of the body. Medical care expenses must be primarily to alleviate or prevent a physical or mental defect or illness. Medical expenses include dental expenses. Medical expenses do not include expenses that are merely beneficial to general health, such as vitamins or a vacation."

Most tax professionals agree that celiac disease, requiring special food in order to avoid disastrous consequences, definitely does qualify as a medical expense

> *if* you don't take the standard medical deduction, but rather itemize your medical deductions. . . . And only *if* your medical and dental expenses exceed more than 7.5% of your adjusted gross income, which means some years you'll deduct gluten-free expenses and some years you won't.

If you qualify, you are allowed to deduct the difference between so-called normal food and the higher-priced items and *only if* the food is used for your sole consumption. If you share meals with non-celiacs, you must determine the fraction you consume then figure the price difference—an accounting nightmare, if you ask me.

It's critical to save all receipts (and some register tapes showing the cost of non-gluten-free items against which to compare) and have a certified letter and a prescription from your doctor stating the medical necessity of your gluten-free diet and the consumption of special (and more expensive) foods. I would add that it's a good idea to have that letter and prescription updated from time to time and rewritten if you change doctors, which is likely to happen in the course of a lifetime. Keep all this handy in case of an IRS challenge. Most tax preparers will tell you deducting a medical expense as esoteric and unfamiliar to the IRS as gluten-free food may flag your return for a closer look, which is why you may come to the conclusion, as I have, that deducting gluten-free food is more trouble than it's worth.

To order a copy of IRS Publication #502, contact the Internal Revenue Service, (800) 829-1040, www.irs.gov.

Canadian Tax Regulations

According to the Canadian Celiac Association, individuals who suffer from celiac disease are entitled to claim the incremental costs of purchasing gluten-free products as a medical expense for the year 2003 and subsequent tax years. These individuals, as the Canada Revenue Agency points out, are not entitled to claim the disability tax credit for the "inordinate" amount of time it takes to shop for or prepare GF products.

The incremental cost is the difference between purchasing GF products and the cost of similar non-GF products. This is calculated by subtracting the cost of a non-GF item from the cost of a GF one.

Generally, the food items are limited to those produced and marketed as specifically gluten-free, like GF bread, bagels, muffins, and cereals. Intermediate items, like rice flour and other gluten-free ingredients, will also be allowed where the celiac uses the foods to make GF items for their exclusive use.

The operative word here is *exclusive*. If several people consume the products, only the cost related to the parts of the product consumed by the individual with celiac disease are to be used in medical expense tax credit. Try to keep track of that!

All of this assumes you have a certificate from a medical practitioner that states you require a GF diet because of celiac disease. Without it, deductions are ineligible. A receipt for every item purchased during the year is required to make your claim. For example, 52 loaves of bread, which should cost $1.49 each, but cost $3.45 each, would result in an incremental cost of $1.96, resulting in a total of $101.92 for bread for the year.

And so on . . . and so on.

For more information and questions, contact the Canada Revenue Agency, (800) 959-8281, www.ccra-adrc.gc.ca.

Use Your Noodle

Don't wait until April 14 to organize receipts for gluten-free foods. Print up a schedule of favorite and frequently purchased items. In one column, print the regular price, in another the cost of its gluten-free counterpart, and don't forget special flours and mixes for baking breads, cookies, cakes, muffins, etc. As you are putting away groceries (unpacking a mail-order shipment) scan all register tapes and receipts for gluten-free items and highlight in yellow. Use your price sheet to note the difference in cost. Toss in a shoe box or basket kept in the kitchen. At the end of the year, all you need is a calculator.

Celiac Preparedness Plan

Hurricanes, tornadoes, earthquakes, floods, ice storms, blizzards, heat waves, power failures, and sadly, after September 11, 2001, all manner of man-made catastrophes. We live in a world where the weather is getting wilder and anything can happen out of a clear blue sky.

We can't do anything about what we don't know is coming, but we can be reasonably prepared for most emergencies. The last thing you want to do is get to a shelter and find there's nothing to eat but donuts, peanut butter crackers, and bologna sandwiches. You don't want to be trapped at home with no way to shop for food. With a little advance planning, the well-prepared celiac can leave the future to a higher power, knowing you've done all you can do to weather the storm. When you remember your umbrella, it never rains.

With gluten-free adaptations from yours truly, the American Red Cross suggests the following:

- One gallon of water per person per day (two quarts for drinking, two quarts for food preparation).
- At least a three-day supply of water for each person in the household (don't forget to include pets).
- Store at least a three-day supply of nonperishable gluten-free food. Select foods that require no refrigeration, preparation or cooking and little or no water, i.e., gluten-free canned beans, tins of tuna fish or salmon, canned fruits, vegetables, shelf stable soy milk, canned juices, and gluten-free soups. If you must heat food, pack a can of Sterno. Don't forget staples like sugar, salt, and pepper and high-energy foods like peanut butter, jelly, gluten-free crackers, gluten-free energy bars, cereal, and trail mix.
- Don't forget to pack a supply of vitamins, formula for infants, and special foods for any elderly people in your household.
- Comfort/stress foods like gluten-free cookies, pretzels, candy, lollipops, instant coffee, and tea bags.
- Assemble a first-aid kit for your home and one for your car with the following items: sterile adhesive bandages in assorted sizes, adhesive tape, scissors, tweezers, needle, moistened towelettes, antiseptic, thermometer, petroleum jelly, safety pins, soap, 2 pairs of latex gloves, sunscreen, aspirin or non-aspirin pain reliever, anti-diarrhea medication, antacid, syrup of ipecac (used to induce vomiting if advised by the Poison Control Center), laxative, activated charcoal (if advised by the Poison Control Center). Don't forget prescription medications, especially heart and blood pressure medications and insulin, contact lenses and supplies, extra eyeglasses, denture supplies.
- Assemble a quantity of necessities like toilet tissue, liquid detergent, personal hygiene items, garbage bags and ties, plastic bucket with a tight lid, disinfectant, and chlorine bleach.

- Also good to have on hand—paper cups, plates, and plastic utensils, battery-operated radio and extra batteries, flashlight and extra batteries, cash or traveler's checks and change, non-electric can opener, utility knife, small cannister-type fire extinguisher, pliers, tape, compass, matches in waterproof container, aluminum foil, plastic storage containers, signal flare, paper and pencil, medicine dropper, shut-off wrench to turn off household gas and water, whistle, plastic sheeting, and a map of the area.
- Include at least one change of clothing and footwear for each person.
- Niceties include games and books.
- Keep all important family documents like wills, insurance policies, deeds, stocks, bonds, passports, Social Security cards, bank credit card account numbers, and immunization records in a waterproof portable container.

The American Red Cross further recommends that you keep all these things in an easy-to-carry container in a place known to all family members with a smaller version of your supply kit in the trunk of your car. A good container is a large, covered trash can, a camping backpack, or a duffel bag. Always keep items in airtight plastic bags. Change your stored water supply every six months, and always rotate stored food at the same time. Establish a family plan, i.e., decide how people will stay in contact, meeting places, emergency phone numbers, teach children how and when to call 911 or other local emergency services, etc. Practice the plan from time to time and if you don't know them already, get to know your neighbors.

Politely thank the Red Cross people for their snacks and give them to your non-celiac neighbor to enjoy. And while you're at it, don't forget about your gluten-free kids at school, who may not be able to get home during an emergency. Give them an emergency supply of crackers, peanut butter, trail mix, juice boxes, GF protein bars, a couple of cans of beans, beef stew, tuna fish, etc. (don't forget the can opener) to stash in their school lockers. Up to you what story you will tell the little ones (a snowstorm is always good, unless you live in Florida, in which case it could be a hurricane). You don't want to scare them with something that may never happen.

The Gluten-Free Dinner Party

Don't rush in to gluten-free cooking as if it were a crash course in survival. And don't, as the saying goes, "throw the baby out with the bathwater." There are many dishes you already know how to make that can be converted.

Dredge meat and poultry for stews and ragouts with gluten-free flour and thicken with cornstarch.

Substitute gluten-free pasta—ravioli, lasagna (see recipe on page 143) spaghetti, linguini, shells, penne, etc, for your old kind. Check all labels on canned and jarred sauces and learn how to make a great, gluten-free tomato sauce of your own.

Substitute cup for cup gluten-free flour mix for the wheat flour in your favorite recipes.

Broil, bake, sauté, and barbecue, and avoid thick sauces.

Find a good marinade recipe or two—one for fish and one for meats—and make your own to avoid overly processed or outrageously expensive store-bought varieties. Buy gluten-free rolls and breads until such time that you are moved to learn how to make your own. Or compromise and buy prepared mixes. Make sure all your drinks and mixers are gluten-free and keep a supply in the bar. Buy only fresh, ripened cheeses or aged cheeses that have not been doctored or processed in any way. Find the freshest vegetables and fish you can, which should go without saying.

Some of us are better at certain courses than others. Don't think you have to bake a dessert or concoct a complicated starter you're not comfortable with. It's perfectly acceptable to add fresh fruit, whipped cream, or ice cream to a store-bought gluten-free cake or a box of GF cookies.

Lose the idea that a dinner party involves several formal courses. It's perfectly fine to serve a family-style meal to one's guests and, in fact, it can result in a better time had by all.

Whatever you do, don't think you have to master something before you serve it to your friends or family. What's the worst that can happen? Order up sandwiches or pizza (at this point you toast your own bread, put your individual pizza in the oven) and have a story everyone can laugh about for years to come. I'll never forget the leaden peach crisp I tried to carry off the summer I was diagnosed. People stared at the soggy mess and politely tried to eat it. Somebody laughed, then somebody else, then another, and before you know it, there was a rollicking dumping ceremony. Ice cream was served and the whole episode slipped into "remember the time you baked a peach cobbler that weighed more than the Liberty Bell?"

Your friends are not spies for Michelin, they are willing subjects for your gluten-free experiments. Not only will they love you for being so adventurous and support your efforts to feed yourself and them with style and grace, they can be a valuable source of non-celiac feedback on the success of each dish. (Nothing is worse than asking another celiac who hasn't had a baguette in a dog's age if you've succeeded making a gluten-free version.) As long as you set

---

Use Your Noodle

. . . .

Why buy expensive crackers when you can toast your own corn tortilla chips? These are wonderful in chili, soups salads, salsa, guacamole, and other party dips.

For about 40 strips, cut 8 corn tortillas into 1-inch-wide strips.

1. Preheat oven to 375 degrees.
2. Spread tortilla strips in a single layer on a baking sheet.
3. Bake until crisp and just beginning to turn golden, about 5 to 10 minutes.
4. Let cool. Keep in an airtight container at room temperature for up to 2 days.

---

ground rules—do not be polite and tell the truth—you've got your own gluten-free lab. Encouraged and empowered by their thumbs up as well as their nixes, you can build a repertoire of dishes for tougher and less candid audiences, i.e., dinner for the boss, the new in-laws, brunch for the new minister.

Need a good reason to go to all this trouble? With every successful gluten-free dinner you serve, you virtually guarantee gluten-free reciprocation. Master one complicated recipe at a time and do them often enough that they become second nature. (The Chicken Crepes on page 134 or the Goat Cheese Cake with Nut Crust and Lemon Curd on page 141 are all showstoppers).

If you could do one food to perfection, let it be rice. Once you've mastered this richly satisfying grain, perfected a creamy risotto, or achieved the fluffiest basmati possible, there is no end to the dishes you can produce.

If you are preparing a time-intensive and rich entrée, serve something light with drinks, like olives, salsa or celery stuffed with guacamole, or a bit of proscuitto wrapped around small slices of melon, and go easy on dessert. Not only will it save you time, your guests will appreciate not being stuffed into their coats at the end of the evening.

When I invite friends who are watching their fat and cholesterol intake (who isn't?), I combine a scant ounce of a good, full-flavored chèvre with an entire package of silken tofu. Tofu, as you may know, is the chameleon of foods, absorbing the flavor of whatever it is mixed with. Allowed to marinate

Use Your Noodle

An interesting change from the usual gluten-free breads are these savory Parmesan crisps from chef Bryan Sikora of Django Gypsy Cafe. The secret is using a good Parmesan Reggiano that's been aged over a year. Don't use Asiago, processed, or pre-grated cheese, the rennet in them will make them rubbery. This is the sort of thing people rave about with virtually no effort on your part. They substitute wonderfully for biscuits in stews and chilis; place them on top of the casserole to add texture to the dish.

1. Preheat oven to 350 degrees.
2. Line a baking sheet with parchment paper.
3. Place a cookie cutter or ring form or any other shape you like (stars and hearts are my favorites) on the baking sheet and sprinkle grated Parmesan in one layer within the outlines of the form. Fill form evenly until you can't see the parchment paper through the cheese. Repeat.
4. Bake for 8 to 10 minutes or until golden brown.
5. Remove baking sheet from oven and let sit in a warm place for ten minutes. They will crisp up as they sit.

overnight, the spread takes on the wonderful flavor of the cheese. I never use the T-word. I just put it in a pretty dish with some healthy flax crackers, and people cannot believe they're not eating something naughty.

One of my favorite gluten-free company desserts, written on an index card that is as old as I am, is fresh figs and a creamy cheese like St. Andre or Brie. Cut an X into 12 figs, taking caring not to smash the fruit, and stuff a teaspoon of cheese into each fig and sprinkle with a pinch of thyme. Roast the figs, cut side up, on a baking sheet in a 400-degree oven for about 5 minutes (less for really ripe figs). Season with a grind of pepper and serve. Depending on your stuffing technique, the whole deal takes about 10 minutes. Heaven.

Another easy dessert is vanilla ice cream topped with brandied cherries and a drizzle of syrup from the jar. Add a sprinkling of slivered almonds and crushed almond cookies and serve in oversized martini glasses (who says martini glasses have to hold alcohol?) for a spectacular effect.

F.Y.I.: Brandied cherries are expensive, but a little goes a long way and they keep forever. Well, maybe not forever. Buy them just after the holidays when gift foods go on sale and keep them in the pantry for special occasions.

And speaking of food . . .

Gluten-Free Doesn't Mean Home-Free

Just because you've sought out and destroyed every molecule of gluten in your life, doesn't mean your diet is ideal. In fact, banishing toxic grains won't do you much good if you replace them with equally empty calories and fat. Refined flour, bad fats, and sugar, whether gluten-free or not, can be just as health-zapping as the other stuff.

When you consider you're coming from behind and haven't been absorbing the vitamins and minerals in your for a good long time, depending on how old you are at the time of diagnosis, eating well becomes even more important. Not only that, absorbing food properly can be a recipe for weight gain.

Sugar

While you're examining labels for gluten, ferret out excessive sugar, which can be listed as anything but. Corn syrup, fructose, dextrose, glucose, high-fructose corn syrup, fruit juice concentrate, high-maltose, molasses, invert sugar, sucrose, and just plain syrup are all synonyms for the sweet stuff. And just because the product is labeled "all fruit" or "no added sugar" doesn't mean it's good for you, says *Consumer Reports*. Artificial sweeteners are a billion-dollar industry. Do you really think anybody's going to tell you they're bad for you?

Use Your Noodle
. . . .

Have a baseline bone density scan (DEXA) and repeat once a year. If you are developing osteopenia or osteoporosis, you can get started on bone-building medications (provided they're right for you) as soon as possible. And don't think you need a fancy set of weights to work your bones. Use a resistance band and a doorknob. Or pump canned food. Start with peas and work up to big cans of tomato juice. Do a few jumping jacks every day. What matters is doing it, not how it's done.

Calcium

Bone up on your calcium. Years of undiagnosed CD can deplete this important mineral. Eat yogurt, low-fat cheese, spinach, and other greens like kale and collards and try to do some weight-bearing exercises every day. Talk to your doctor about supplementing calcium, magnesium, and zinc.

Other Nutrients

We live in a society that's always looking for the quick fix. The diet du jour is always the one that makes all others obsolete. For years, we drank black coffee and ate cottage cheese. Then there was grapefuit and hard-boiled eggs, an alternating exercise in heartburn and constipation. Then the damn burst with fruit, enough of it to found a banana republic. Some of us keeled over (literally) from high-protein drinks. We tried being macrobiotic, but who had time to soak beans? And for almost a decade, we rid our lives of every ounce of fat. It's amazing our systems worked at all. Not only that, we reduced our collective HDL to skiddingly low levels and ate so much pasta we ended up with insulin resistance and worse. We got even fatter.

Now we're demonizing carbohydrates—so much so that every food producer in America is offering a low-carb alternative to their own products. Pasta makers are filing for Chapter 11 and beer companies are filing suit against those who use the term "beer belly." Our current obsession with carbohydrates will go, as all fad diets eventually do, the way of the buffalo. One day we'll all wake up to learn that low-carb bars cause crankiness in rats. But, by then we will have moved on to the Next Big Thing. Maybe it will be uncooked foods or maybe it will be okay to consume anything (except gluten) as long as it fits in one small bowl or is eaten standing on one leg.

In the meantime, dear friend, remember this. You've dodged a bullet. And good health is not about chemicals, even if those chemicals contain not a scintilla of gluten.

In "10 Foods That Pack a Wallop," *Time* magazine lists superfoods that possess important disease-fighting properties. They are, in order of importance:

Tomatoes. Rich in lycopene, these are the most powerful of the antioxidant carotenoid-containing fruits and vegetables.

Next comes spinach with its iron and folate, which can prevent neural-tube defects in newborns and can lower levels of homocysteine, an amino acid linked to heart disease. This is especially important for celiacs who have been and may still be deficient in this important B vitamin. Spinach also contains phytochemicals that may ward off macular degeneration.

Use Your Rice Noodle

· ·

If portion control is a problem for you, get smaller plates.

A few glasses of red wine per week can help raise good cholesterol (HDL) and may also help reduce the degenerative condition we call hardening of the arteries.

Nuts are full of fat (the good kind), but they're also full of protein and can lower your LDL or bad cholesterol, while raising the good HDL. Nuts trigger a process called apoptosis, in which cancer cells kill themselves. But don't go nuts—a handful a day is enough.

Broccoli, brussels sprouts, and bok choy. These are the big three cruciferous vegetables and they're loaded with cancer fighters like beta-carotine, fiber, and vitamin C.

Oats. Despite the problem of cross-contamination, oats may lower your blood pressure and contain a soluble fiber that makes short work of cholesterol. If your doctor feels these are safe for you, use only whole oats grown in dedicated fields. The last thing you want to do is feel them.

Salmon is full of omega-3 fatty acids that help keep arteries from developing plaque and may even protect brain cells from the diseases of aging. Ditto for bluefish, herring, and mackerel.

Garlic is one of the great health wonders of the world. Not only will it keep vampires and colds away, it can make blood less sticky and less likely to form clots. Smash it, mince it, or mash it to release its power, but don't overcook it. My favorite way to eat it is roasted with a little olive oil, then spread on a slice of toast (gluten-free, of course). If you take aspirin or other blood-thinning drugs, be careful. You can have too much of a good thing.

Green tea or even black tea may help to prevent cancer, and some say it even inhibits cavity-causing bacteria. This is good news for those of us prone to dry mouth and other conditions related to CD.

Blueberries are good for the eyes, heart, immune system brain, sweet tooth, and soul.

Eat some of these foods every day and limit the gluten-free treats. Why? Because as much as we wish to meet our quota for health problems, life is just not fair. A steady diet of pizza and mac and cheese, even if it's gluten-free pizza and mac and cheese, isn't exactly a recipe for health.

Use Your Noodle

· ·

Balance your gluten-free snacking with nutrient-packed superfoods. Eat blueberries with your gluten-free cereal. Stir broccoli into the mac and cheese. Declare Sunday as Salmon Day. Make a spinach frittata with hormone-free eggs. Reach for a handful of nuts, instead of a cookie. And pour yourself a nice glass of merlot every now and then. You may be nutritionally challenged, but you're not dumb.

"Dear Friends and Family . . ."

Some support groups advise writing an open letter to one's friends and family after a diagnosis of CD telling them essentially what you can and can't eat, and that you would like to be invited to their houses despite your diet restrictions. In it, you're supposed to tell people how important it is to you that you be allowed to visit (the key word here is *allowed*) and that you don't mind bringing your own food and how lucky you feel not to have anything life-threatening or contagious. I've read these letters and, well, they sound as if they've been written by someone who's trying to sound cheerful, but would happily strangle the family dog if he ate a biscuit in front of her. I came across one such letter published in one of the newsletters that actually suggested saying, "*Please let me come to your house. It is more important to me that you let me visit with you than you feed me.*"

I don't know about you, but I'm not comfortable begging for emotional crumbs, even if those crumbs are gluten-free.

Of course you'll be trouble. Everyone is a little bit of trouble. Friends decide friends are worth it. And pals don't let pals go hungry. Besides, if you have to write a letter asking to be invited to a friend's house, there's something worse than gluten gumming up the friendship. If you have fallen off the A-list because of food, I would venture to say the friendship was in trouble well before your need for rice crackers and a clean cutting board got in the way.

You can't blanket the neighborhood with form letters and expect to feel good about going to a barbecue. Besides, it's kind of presumptuous to infer that if you're not invited it's because of your diet. If the situation were reversed, think how smarmy you'd feel if you got a letter asking that you not exclude a certain celiac from your table. Any time you had a gathering and didn't invite this person, even if it was dinner for the cousin from Brooklyn nobody likes, or your husband's boss, or your daughter's new boyfriend, you'd feel like a criminal, not to mention deeply shallow and biased against the grain-challenged.

Writing a letter to someone you already know as a general announcement strikes me as more than odd and all that "please invite me" stuff smacks of martyred complaint. Nothing substitutes for eye contact when you tell someone who claims to love you what you require. Second best is the telephone. Third best is e-mail: "You'll never guess what just happened to me!"

By all means, follow up with a list of no-no's and yes-yes's, especially if there's a dinner party imminent. By all means, send instructions if you're going to visit your sister in Minneapolis for a week, and include a supply of gluten-free foods so she doesn't go completely nuts trying to plan meals. And while you're at it, don't forget an extra-special house gift for all that extra attention. That's the way you get invited back, not by asking to be invited back.

Use Your Noodle

In our time-consumed world, the holiday letter is now considered an acceptable substitute for individual correspondence regarding family news. This is a great way to announce your gluten-free status in the context of the year's news. Do have fun. People are supposed to be cheered by these things. (Really sad news should never be sent out as a blanket mailing.) Do mention the foods you can't have and do mention the other friends and family members who have risen to the challenge of your diet. That should be enough to give people the idea without your actually having to ask to be fed properly.

Obviously, the following letter is made up. I've had some fun with it and so should you. (If you can't be upbeat about being gluten-free, who can?) The idea is to let your friends know you're okay, but that they have to feed you differently and do it in a way that's memorable. There's nothing like humor (and a little manipulation) to get people on your side. They wouldn't dare forget your special food after being lumped in with the good guys.

Dear Friends and Family:

Oh, what a year this has been!

After two years as a shampoo girl for Mr. Phyllis, Becky Ann finally got her own chair at the beauty parlor, a miracle considering that incident with the henna we wrote about last year. She celebrated by giving the whole family a permanent wave and you should see her proud father in his new curly 'do. The twins dyed their hair pink in her honor (they have decided to dress alike at college this fall and we support that decision) and I baked a cake in the shape of a pair of scissors.

A good time was had by all until yours truly spent the rest of the day in the bathroom. At first I thought my reaction was limited to novelty cakes, but after quite a few of these episodes (I'll spare you the details) and many visits with the doctor, it turns out I can't tolerate anything with gluten in it. Turns out I'm a celiac. At first, I was as confused by this as the next person, but now I know this means I can't tolerate anything with wheat, rye, barley, possibly oats (don't even ask about that!), and any derivatives thereof. Who knew all those Ring-Dings I ate in college were killing me!

The family has been wonderful. After they got the jokes about celiacs out of their systems—silly yak, celiac rhymes with maniac, etc., etc.— they made a big sign declaring the kitchen a **Gluten-Free Zone**. Billy (or was it Brad?) looked up gluten in the dictionary to see if it has anything to do with glue. It doesn't. Just flour and pasta, bread and cookies and most gravies, and beer and packaged cereals, soy sauces, commercial gravy and beer, all the things most of us like. Well, it sounds impossible, but it isn't. There are so many companies that make bread, spaghetti, cookies, and muffins without gluten; you could get fat just reading the list. The kids make a game of going to the market and finding new ones for me.

We made a little funeral for the veggie burgers (hydrolyzed vegetable protein) and the Spaghetti-O's (the twins wrote a wonderful eulogy), and I must say, this brought us all closer as a family. For our anniversary, Bob took me on a gluten-free cruise. Who knew they had such things?

Best of all, Sissy and Dan down the street gave a barbecue this summer and none of the other guests even knew it was gluten-free. This Thanksgiving Mom surprised me with a great gluten-free sage stuffing everyone loved. We are blessed to have such a wonderful family and friends like these, friends like you.

We send our love and prayers for health, prosperity, world peace, and gluten-free labeling.

The Bickersons—Brenda, Bob, Billy,
Brad, Becky Sue, and Barker, the Dog

Now that's using your noodle.

Myths, Misconceptions, and Grains of Truth

Somebody, I don't know who, but it could have been Joan Rivers, once said, "If it tastes good, spit it out." That's the way this gluten-free life of ours can feel sometimes, confusing and dangerous, with gluten lurking in the oddest and most unsuspected places.

You have questions. And well you should. Celiac disease is confusing at best, and there is quite a bit of folklore out there, including some misconceptions coming from professionals who should know better. While there is solid research telling us how common CD really is (and getting commoner, it seems, every day), the condition is still grossly misunderstood. The presence of gluten in any given food or substance has taken on the proportions not of science but of myth. No wonder celiacs fret about the safety of tea bags, dental floss, dog food, airborne contaminants, cheese, sticky rice, and whether or not it is safe to breathe while passing a bakery. We ask if there's any truth to the rumors of a cure. Is a pill, patch, or vaccine in the pipeline? Is celiac disease a bona fide disability or is it just plain annoying? Some even confess to gluten dreams that are nightmarish and menacing, full of killer bagels and gnocchi the size of the Brooklyn Bridge chasing them down an endless food court. Fond memories full of longing for our forbidden foods rise up out of the soup of our collective subconscious. If pressed, more than one celiac will admit to harboring unkind thoughts about those who can eat pasta with impunity. Others wonder why if it's possible for medication to get into the body via a skin patch, why not gluten?

For starters, let's agree that we are among friends and there's no such thing as a dumb question. These, taken straight from letters from readers, Internet postings, and other places where celiacs gather to chat and share information, are some of the most commonly asked questions from newbies and veterans alike. Herewith, a few myths debunked, misconceptions corrected, and some grains of truth.

Food and Drink

Q: Since my diagnosis, I have been drinking at least three cups of coffee a day. Now I'm getting coffee nerves about whether or not my jolt of java is gluten-free.

A: It depends.

Coffee and tea are naturally gluten-free as long as you are a purist and drink plain, unflavored brews. However, many instant coffees and decaffeinated coffees contain cereal fillers, which make them unsafe for celiacs. Be careful, too, of the flood of fancy flavored coffee coolers and drinks and teas on the market, especially those sold in retail outlets like Starbucks. Many of them contain wheat-based flavorings and syrups. Ask before you imbibe, especially if you have a favorite company for your daily brew. Or, take your joe straight.

By the way, Melitta tells me there is no gluten in any of their coffee filters and no tea company I talked to admits to glue in tea bags. If they're not folded and stapled, they're pressure sealed. Of course, you could forget the whole thing and brew leaf tea the old-fashioned way.

Q: I've got a hankering for a nice, big hunk of Maytag blue cheese. It's natural, unprocessed cheese, so why can't I have it on the gluten-free diet?
A: Blue mold.

It isn't the cheese, I'm told, it's the way it's made. Rich, veiny cheeses like Maytag and Gorgonzola are made from mold, which, in the grand and highly secretive cheese-making tradition, is started from bread. Until the food researchers get around to investigating the gluten content of such a starter, not high up on their lists I'd imagine, we can comfort ourselves with a nice, runny triple crème Brie, a tangy chèvre, or a sharp English cheddar.

Q: Is it possible to inhale gluten and have a bad reaction?
A: Yes and no.

This is like the president's marijuana question. I tried it, but I didn't inhale. If you walk into a cloud of anything, most likely you're going to sneeze, wheeze, or cough. You don't have to be a celiac for that.

Let's say you're walking down the baking aisle and a bag of flour explodes (not likely) or you rear-end a flour truck and are buried in an avalanche of the stuff (even less likely). You may have a reaction, not because you're breathing, but because you've swallowed some. A big enough face full of any substance, e.g. pollen, dust, etc., is going to cling to the back of your throat and you're going to swallow. If you are cleaning up the mess yourself, a small amount may get under your nails and find its way, via a circuitous and completely unconscious route, into your stomach.

This is something you shouldn't worry about, unless of course you work in a bakery, in which case I respectfully suggest a change of career, maybe a job in a gluten-free enterprise requiring the same skills.

Q: I thought tuna fish salad was safe to order out, but heard that some diners use white bread. Is this true?
A: I'm afraid so.

I asked at a local diner and had to promise I wouldn't use their name before they 'fessed up. You've heard of Hamburger Helper? Well, this is tuna surprise. Or chicken surprise. Or even shrimp and crab or seafood surprise. Bottom line: Expensive ingredients go further when stretched with bread filler. Always, always, always ask how a dish is prepared before ordering any food that can be doctored, enhanced, or plumped in any way, even those that sound innocent enough.

My source tells me the biggest offenders are diners, delis, food courts, and truck stops. Profit margins are very slim in these places. Other areas of potential problems are omelets in chains like International House of Pancake (IHOP), which may contain batter. Do they do it to make the eggs go further or to enhance the taste? Your guess is as good as mine. Batter on french fries is another potential pothole and it's becoming commonplace.

A good rule to follow is if you can't get a straight answer about how a dish is made, don't order it. If you've ordered it and you suspect there is bread or batter or other gluten in it, send it back and eat something else. And for heaven's sake, don't pay for it.

Q: If food doesn't cause a reaction, does that mean it's gluten-free?
A: Absolutely not.

This should be obvious, but to a newly diagnosed celiac, it is not. Hidden gluten may be present in a food in such small amounts that it doesn't cause a reaction. Or, it could be you are one of the unlucky celiacs who don't react in an overt way to gluten. (I say unlucky because it is much easier to conform to the gluten-free diet when it's an antidote to suffering.) No matter, experts agree. The effect of gluten on the intestine and on the general health is cumulative. Over time, eating gluten can cause problems. Always check and eat only those products or foods you know for sure are gluten-free.

This is one time when a little bit *can* hurt.

Medical Matters

Q: My doctor says celiac disease is a rare childhood disease. Is this true?
A: Not on your life.

Alas, many doctors have not caught up with the latest research and remember only what they learned about celiac disease in medical school. To compound the problem, CD was considered rare at one time, or rather the full-blown condition many American physicians were trained to recognize was rare. At the 2004 National Institutes of Health Consensus Development Conference, experts agreed that only a small percentage of celiacs fit the classic picture. They tell us that so-called asymptomatic adults can suffer from osteoporosis, anemia, infertility, and related autoimmune disease. Complaints can be vague and seemingly unrelated to the gastrointestinal tract and can range from bloating, abdominal pain, skin rash, and neurological problems. Many doctors simply have not been trained to look beyond the symptoms they studied for the many signs related to celiac disease. A proper diagnosis can take as long as twelve years.

Case in point: A good friend who had been experiencing unexplained weight loss and a strange, floppy foot worried that he may have celiac disease. After a CT scan and a colonoscopy ruled out other problems, he asked his gastroenterologist to test him for CD. "Impossible," said the doctor, "you don't have diarrhea and you're fifty years old." Fortunately, my friend pressed his case. Concerned that his physician might not know what blood tests to order, he ordered a kit from a specialty lab to return with his drawn blood for analysis.

My friend did what everyone who suspects he or she might have celiac disease (all those with a celiac in the family) should do. He insisted on the proper blood tests and he helped create physician awareness by making his doctor an instant expert. Never fault a doctor for being wrong. Help him or her to get it right.

Q: If a dermal patch can deliver medicine through the skin, why can't gluten be absorbed the same way?
A: Sounds logical, but it doesn't work that way.

It's easy to make that assumption, but gluten and skin patches are apples and oranges in the highly engineered world of dermal drugs. Kays Kaidbey, M.D., retired University of Pennsylvania Adjunct Professor of Dermatology, explains:

> Several drugs can be delivered to the systemic circulation through the skin and these are usually relatively small molecules that are incorporated

in specially formulated and highly complex vehicle systems designed to maximize drug release to the stratum corneum [skin's outermost layer] via patches. The ability of chemicals or molecules to penetrate the skin is determined by several factors, including the size of the molecule, its solubility in lipids or fats, and by its physico-chemical properties. Most proteins, as well as glutens, are simply too large to penetrate the skin.

Translation: Gluten has to get into your gut to cause trouble.

Q: I've heard there are patents pending for pills, patches, and a vaccine for CD, true?

A: They're working on it, but don't give up your frequent gluten-free buyer card any time soon.

A story in the June 21, 2003, edition of *Science News* features Stanford University biochemist Chaitan Khosla, who has every reason to work on a cure—his wife and six-year old son are both celiacs. Khosla's work focuses on understanding the disease's biological mechanisms and he has isolated three potential molecular targets for potential drugs, aiming for a prescription pill for celiac disease by the time his son goes to college twelve years from now.

In the June 2002 issue of *Gastroenterology*, Willemijn Vader and Frits Koning identified several amino acid sequences on peptides that survive digestion and appear to trigger celiac disease in some children. It is these that Dr. Khola's experiments are attempting to block.

John H. Griffin, chief scientific officer of Pharmix Corp., a small biotech firm in Redwood Shores, California, suggests that some of the therapies already approved for other immune disorders of the gut like ulcerative colitis and the inflammatory condition called Crohn's disease, might prove capable of serving double duty against celiac disease.

Researchers reported in the journal *Nature*, November 7, 2002, that statins, typically used to combat heart disease provided a benefit to patients with multiple sclerosis. "If statins can achieve this effect by clogging the receptors of misbehaving immune molecules," says Dr. Khosla, "they may also confer benefits in celiac disease." I do not pretend to understand the science behind all this vigorous work, but I do know this. Those who work for love, not merely the profit motive, succeed faster. We will have a pill or a vaccine one day because somebody loved somebody else enough to figure it out. Isn't that how most good things happen?

Bodily Functions

Q: This is a tacky question, but is it normal to have a bowel movement every day?

A: Not necessarily.

There's a lot of "toilet talk" in the celiac community, mainly because that's where many of us notice our first symptoms and it's where we know if we've gotten some inadvertent gluten. When Beano first hit the market, celiacs definitely started the buzz. This is how the fuzzy logic goes: If we manage to force our habits into what we think is an acceptable normal, maybe we'll be normal in other ways. Sorry, but there's no such thing.

According to the National Digestive Diseases Clearing House Web site, "The frequency of bowel movements among normal healthy people varies from three days a week to one a day, and some people fall outside both ends of this range."

And guess who might typically fall outside both ends of the range? You, that's who. Strike the word *normal* and *should* from your vocabulary. If you suffered from diarrhea, you may be more prone to frequent bowel movements than those who may have experienced constipation and bloating.

On the other hand, don't give yourself a hemorrhoid trying to force the issue. Self-medicating with laxatives or habitual use of enemas can, over time, impair the natural muscle action of the intestines, leaving them unable to function properly. Better to skip a day or to go after each meal than to obsess. If there's really a problem—and you will know it if there is—seek medical attention. Otherwise, accept that we are individuals who cannot be quantified, categorized, and normalized.

Societal Issues

Q: Is it possible to be a celiac and still serve my country?

A: Yes, but your country may not serve you.

According to the Department of Defense, any person with a special dietary need that can be confirmed as a medical problem is disqualified from joining the U.S. Army, Navy, Marine Corps, Air Force, Coast Guard, National Guard, or any other military service requiring a special haircut and a uniform.

A very good article in *Lifeline*, by U.S. Air Force Captain John Himberger, puts the military in perspective for celiacs. As a member of the armed forces, you are expected to go anywhere at any time to enforce policy or engage in conflict as necessary. This means that, as part of a rapid deployment force, you're going to have to take along a supply of prepackaged food, all of which is full of gluten, according to Captain Himberger. Put another way, it's not going to be convenient to call the company that produced the meal in your pack up in the mountains of Afghanistan. You're not going to get food you can eat in a tank.

There is no draft—for now, anyway. Besides, if you are determined to enlist, you'll lie about CD and end up serving no one, least of all yourself. Getting sick under battle conditions could have dire consequences, not only for you but for your comrades, whose lives depend on clear thinking from everyone. Risking your life in battle only to die slowly from the food is not using your rice noodle.

The more difficult question is the one rarely asked: What happens if I'm diagnosed while in the military?

According to the good captain, the answer here is not so clear-cut. The armed forces varies in its policies toward those with medical conditions, depending on the mission and the branch of the service. The definition of "fit to deploy" is a relative term, especially as it pertains to celiac disease. Some cases are not well defined and mild, while others are disabling. Once the diagnosis of CD is made, officials decide whether the individual will be retained in the military or released to the civilian community.

The most influential factor in the decision to retain is the amount of time the individual has invested in the military and vice versa. Just like a corporation, the military will weigh its investment. If you are fresh out of basic training, says Captain Himberger, you can pretty much expect to be jettisoned. If you are a seasoned veteran and have been a productive member of the military for many years, your chances of being kept on are higher. If there is a shortage of personnel in your area and you are considered indispensable, all the better.

One prerequisite for retention is the soldier's resolve to be in compliance with the diet—drinking beer and going to sick bay for four days is not considered compliant. As far as military families are concerned, medical facilities with an understanding of celiac disease are "adequate." Read into that what you will.

Q: A celiac friend was sentenced to a year in a federal prison for a white-collar crime. The prison is more like a camp than a penitentiary. Will he be able to get a gluten-free diet?

A: No, you won't. I mean, no your friend won't.

Not even Martha Stewart has enough pull to order gluten-free French toast in a federal prison. Cushy or barbed wired, locked down or wide open, the rules are the same. Alan Schwartz, Regional Food Director for the Federal Bureau of Prisons, tells me the only diets available to prisoners are those eaten for religious purposes, e.g., kosher for Jewish prisoners and followers of Islam and vegetarianism, or as the prison system so quaintly calls it, "no flesh."

Whether it's wheat, gluten, lactose, peanut, tree nut or casein, diabetes, low-cholesterol, or low-salt, I am told it is incumbent upon each inmate to manage his or her special diet by asking to see the ingredient labels, which will be made available and to self-select the proper food. Prison is punishment. They don't go out of their way to make it easy. A way around this, according to Mr. Schwartz, is to contact the prison doctor and he or she will assign a medically necessary diet, which is then put into the computer and reviewed periodically. Care must be taken not to downplay the repercussions of getting gluten; otherwise a celiac may find he or she is doing time in a prison hospital. Officials would not comment when I asked what would happen to a gluten-sensitive inmate who was caught carving a rice cake into the shape of a key.

If you are so far gone as to be in a position of having to choose a last meal, gluten is the least of your worries.

Q: What happens to celiacs in nursing homes, homeless shelters, psychiatric wards, and other places where there is "captive feeding"?

A: The news is not good, I'm afraid, for people who cannot insist on a gluten-free diet.

Many of the consumers of such services are not well enough, sane enough, or strong enough to make their wishes known. The mentally ill are especially vulnerable, and we all have a story of an elderly resident of a nursing home who has been the recipient of a serious error in care. Phone calls to various facilities assured me all special diets are honored, and I believe many reputable managers of such places do their best in light of the fact that many of their residents cannot ask for a gluten-free meal. Exacerbating the situation is the sad fact that many residents are difficult, lacking in family visits, and subject to careless employees.

There is no way of knowing how many of the homeless in this country are celiacs because medical services are usually the first to go on a downward spiral into poverty. Malnutrition combined with malabsorption is a terrible cross to bear.

For many, church and community groups and food charities are often the only source of food for the needy, homeless, homebound, and chronically ill. Observing my neighborhood church's efforts on this score, food packages are carbohydrate-intensive.

I wish I had the answer to this terrible problem for "invisible celiacs." I don't. Here and there celiac volunteers make GF food packets, but at this point, it is not a national effort. I would love to see the day that gluten-free companies, joined by national celiac organizations, fund a food program for the thousands of elderly, needy, and homeless celiacs around the country. I spoke with a representative from an international organization called Nourish the Children which distributes a gluten-free rice and lentil meal in a pouch called VitaMeal to the poor all over the world. I have no financial interest in this company, but it did occur to me that with so many professional gluten-free kitchens in business, such a product could be developed and made available to celiacs who can no longer cook or look after themselves. Why not market to caregivers, institutions, and food charities right here at home? A kind of meals-on-wheels for the gluten-free.

While most of us will never have to face homelessness, we are all going to get old. Why not start planning the gluten-free future now?

Friends and Family

Q: My dog is not a celiac as far as I know, but his food is loaded with gluten. Poor thing doesn't understand why I wear rubber gloves to feed him. What do I do?

A. Could be gluten-free kibble is in Fido's future.

Man and woman's best friend not only eats, he slobbers, drools, licks the hand and the face that feeds him, and fetches your slippers on occasion. What's the point of having a pet if you don goggles and rubber gloves and treat him like a furry Three Mile Island?

One way to solve the problem is to go for a zero-tolerance household and feed the family pet one of the gluten-free pet foods like Sensible Choice or Nutro. Some owners report their dogs are healthier and their coats are glossier on this diet, while others complain the soy-based foods give some breeds more than a bit of a gas problem. If you don't go with gluten-free dog chow, keep food bowls separate from the family utensils and always wash your hands after feeding or cleaning out the dishes. If yours is not a single household, give the non-celiac the dog-feeding duties. If the celiac is a child and loves to feed the family pet, as many toddlers do, it's especially important to teach hand-washing the minute the chore is accomplished. The fastest way for gluten to get into a tummy is via fingers that go into mouths after touching Fido's dinner.

Like humans, dogs and cats need cuddling and love. If you can't deliver on your end of the bargain because of gluten fears, don't have a pet in the first place.

PART II

Now You're Cooking!

a walk down the aisle

Caveat emptor.

—PROVERB

Food shopping . . . what was once a boring and repetitive weekly chore is now an exciting adventure. Once upon a time you could do it in your sleep, multi-tasking on your cell phone as you filled your cart with the bread, milk, butter, cereal, frozen pizzas, and the usual snacks. Now you are on a mission. You are a gluten sleuth, alert and hypervigilant. Labels are required reading, as you learn to sniff out unsafe ingredients. Yes, it's work and it can be time-consuming, at least until you get the hang of it, but finding something you can eat is a real thrill. I'm still spinning from my latest find—Southern Homestyle Tortilla Crumbs, gluten-free Mexican "bread" crumbs. And if you're willing to venture beyond the traditional supermarket, it gets even more exciting.

Okay. Grab your shopping list and your cheat sheet of ingredients covered in previous chapters, and don't forget, along with your coupons and specials, to check cupboards and clear the fridge of all those little plastic containers of things best not opened. Clean your glasses, it's time to for a short course in Marketing 101.

The Supermarket

Double coupons, cash back, two-for-one-deals, and frequent buyer cards aside, the average American supermarket is still not the friendliest place for a celiac to shop. There are notable exceptions—slick new stores with organic produce departments alongside those foods grown according to conventional methods. There are wonderful new prepared food departments with freshly cut *bento* boxes of sushi, barbecued chicken, salads, soups, and entrees ready to take home. There are new counters purveying fresh fish, meats, and smoothies for the road.

Despite these welcome advancements, the supermarket is where major food processors (the key word here is *processed*, not prepared) sell products that are not only riddled with additives, stabilizers, fillers, emulsifiers, and preservatives, many of which are sources of hidden gluten, they serve up more fat, sodium, sugar, calories, artificial colors, chemicals, and palm kernel oil than your average toxic spill. Much of what you will find in boxes, bags, cans, pouches, and single-serving freezer trays have little nutritional value and barely resemble the foods they purport to be. Not to be an alarmist, but employees of a certain popcorn company got sick breathing in the "butter." It gives one pause. Obesity and ill health is a growing problem in America, and for good reason. Many of us are not eating real food, food that is alive with vitamins and minerals and natural energy. We think we are, but we're not. To make matters worse, livestock and poultry are fed hormones and antibiotics that cannot be good for the people who consume them. Regulation is lax and legislation favors the big producers and agri-giants, not the consumer. It's enough to make a cow mad.

What's more, within the food industry are powerful distribution chains that vie for the lucrative and all-important shelf position. This is why you won't find the same brands of cereals or cookies that are available in independent health food stores and chains like Wild Oats, Whole Foods, and others. Small companies like Pamela's, Erewhon, and The Gluten-Free Pantry are just not going to have the same kind of distribution clout as R.J.R. Nabisco, Kellogg's, and Betty Crocker. A handful of gluten-free food companies are making inroads, but there is still a long way to go.

I know this is not what you want to hear. You want to know how to substitute your favorite foods for similar gluten-free products. It is possible in the supermarket, but not as easy, as in other venues. You are a brand-new person, one with a chance to heal all the problems caused by undiagnosed celiac disease. Like a new baby, you will eat what you tolerate, little by little, until you build back to health. Why not use this opportunity to start fresh? Once your gut begins to heal and health returns, the idea is to maintain a normal weight (be neither too thin nor too stout), eat a well-balanced diet of foods that are not only gluten-free, but contribute to overall health. Use the gluten-free goodies you find on these pages as sparingly as you would any other treats.

The point is this: Just because something is gluten-free doesn't mean it's free of fat and chemicals. Just because it's gluten-free doesn't mean it's good for you.

Caveats aside, let's explore the geography of the modern-day supermarket. Obviously, chains carry similar brands, but vary slightly by region and local tastes. As far as organization and large national brands, there aren't too many differences. To navigate safely, it helps to think of yourself as a kind of grain Geiger counter. I'm not talking about good whole grains that contain no gluten, like rice and corn, quinoa and pure buckwheat. I'm talking about dead, white flour. You hear a quiet tick-tick at the perimeter of the store where fresh meats, produce, dairy, and deli are found. It gets louder as you move toward the aisles on either side, going full tilt as you find yourself in Soups, Cake Mixes, Cereals, and Dips, losing its little mind in Pastas, Cereals, and Snacks, virtually exploding in frozen foods.

A good rule to follow is that the more processed the product, the more risk it contains for you. Conversely, the fresher the food and the closer to its natural state, the better your chances are of being able to eat it. Many supermarkets are attempting to compete with the large natural foods stores and can be a good source of competitively priced hormone-free, free-range eggs, poultry and meats, and organic produce. You finally got healthy. Why not try to stay that way? If yours is a savvy supermarket skewed toward special diets, you may find Amy's gluten-free line of frozen lasagna, macaroni and cheese, pizza, or Van's Gluten-Free Waffles, or my fiber-filled favorite, Mesa Sunrise waffles by Nature's Path. Don't hang out near the freezer cases any longer than you have to. The Stouffer's frozen dinners and all Sara Lee cakes are not going to make you feel better. Before your fingers get blue, especially those of you with Raynaud's, grab your favorite gluten-free flavor of Ben & Jerry's and the bag of Green Giant frozen peas (but not Green Giant peas and rice) and get out of there.

As you consider your old friend the supermarket in the new light of your diet, try to remember these simple rules:

1. It is always better to buy the ingredients and assemble a meal yourself than to buy one that has already been boxed, bagged, canned, hermetically sealed, or rendered shelf-stable. The truth is, it's just as easy to bake or broil a juicy chicken breast with a little garlic and olive oil as it is to warm one that's already cooked, sauced, and full of gluten, unnecessary calories, and chemicals. It's also healthier for the budget.
2. Buy a coupon organizer. Add a list of all the gluten-free products as you discover them, along with its price-off coupon. You're already paying through your stomach, why pay through the nose?

3. Just as the words *fat-free* scrawled across a package do not mean sugar and calorie-free, neither do *wheat-free* and *all natural* necessarily mean gluten-free.

4. Always do homework at home. Lighting and other conditions conducive to reading are not exactly ideal in a supermarket aisle and, at peak shopping times, may even be dangerous. The more you know ahead of time, the faster it will go.

5. Understand that products and conditions will vary according to regional tastes, test markets, and from store to store. Formulations can change without warning, even on a product that has been declared gluten-free. Understand that a food company may change its formula without necessarily reprinting the label. Check periodically with the manufacturer.

6. Don't forget to use the toll-free numbers or Web addresses in "The Resourceful Celiac" (chapter 21) to verify periodically that your favorite product is still gluten-free. A good example of this is the Boca Burger. One day it was, the next day it wasn't.

7. Just because it is written down doesn't mean it won't change at some point. All products stated here as being gluten-free have been declared so by their makers and, in some cases, listed as such by the stores that carry them. This means *at this writing*. Check, check, and check again. This is the cross every celiac must bear.

Okay. Get rid of the cart with the wheel that needs oiling, and let's go shopping.

Alcoholic Beverages

If you live in a state that allows supermarkets to sell beer and alcoholic beverages, beware of beer and any malt-containing drink, as well as flavored and otherwise trumped-up wine. Read labels carefully in this department, and remember that anything that weakens your resolve, especially when you're just starting out, may not be a good idea.

Baby Food

Gluten-free varieties of Beech-Nut Stage 1 baby foods include Beef and Broth, Butternut Squash, Chicken and Broth, Chiquita Bananas, Golden Delicious Applesauce, Instant Rice Cereal, Tender Sweet Carrots, and Yellow Cling Peaches, among others. Stage 2 Apples & Bananas, Apples & Pears, Apples &

Blueberries, Beef Dinner Supreme, Jar Rice Cereal & Apples, Turkey Rice Dinner, Vegetables & Beef are all gluten-free. Ditto for Stage 3 Applesauce, Apple Cobbler, Broccoli & Potatoes with Cheese, Vegetable Chicken Dinner, and Vegetable Turkey dinner.

Gerber's, too, offers a wide variety of foods for the gluten-free baby. EnfaCare formula, Enfamil, Lactofree, Next Step Toddler Formula in Regular or Soy, Nutramigen, and Pregestimil are all gluten-free.

Baking Needs

Gluten-free baking products include Arm & Hammer baking soda; Kraft Calumet baking powder; Baker's, Ghirardelli, Hershey's, Nestlé baking chips; Baker's German baking squares; Ghirardelli milk, mint, and dark chocolate baking squares; Premium unsweetened cocoa; and Nestlé cocoa and chocolate syrup. Betty Crocker almond paste, marzipan, and chocolate and rainbow sprinkles are gluten-free, as well as Duncan Hines Homestyle frostings.

Canned Goods

Most canned vegetables and juices are gluten-free unless there is evidence to the contrary on the label. All varieties of B&M beans are gluten-free, as are Bush's, except for Bush's Best Chili Beans and Bush's Chili Magic. Don't forget to pick up some Beano; your friends will be relieved to know it is gluten-free.

Bumble Bee tuna is gluten-free, as is StarKist and Crown Prince salmon, sardines, oysters, anchovies, kipper snacks, and crab meat. Tins of Hormel breast of chicken, ham, turkey, and chicken are safe, as is Libby's Chicken Vienna Sausage, Roast Beef Hash, Corned Beef Hash, and Potted Meat Vienna Sausage. Ditto for Swanson Premium Chunk White Chicken.

Marketing Strategy #1

What you can't read on a label *can* hurt. Carry a magnifying glass for print finer than your prescription can handle. Or better still, put a small magnifier on a ribbon and wear it around your neck for closer scrutiny.

Cheese and Deli Items

The safest way to approach cheese is to buy it as close to its natural state as possible. A block of aged, pure cheddar is a good choice. Kraft, which has voluntarily begun to label its gluten-free products, declares their Natural Cheddar Swiss, mozzarella, Colby, ricotta, and Monterey Jack gluten-free. Ditto for Kraft Singles. Many celiacs avoid Roquefort and blue cheeses because the mold culture that makes veined cheeses is begun on bread crumbs. Nobody's ever done a study as to how much gluten is really in the cheese after the cheese matures. Until such time, it's best to be safe than to be sorry. Breakstone regular cottage cheese and Kraft Philadelphia regular cream cheese are gluten-free as well. Some of you (and you know who you are) just can't imagine life without Velveeta. This cheesy stuff is many things, but glutenous is not one of them. At the deli counter always remember to ask the counter person to wipe down the slicer before filling your order (and make sure there are no crumbs on the scale—yes, I know this is picky, but. . . . And make sure the cheese, ham, or turkey you are buying is from a gluten-free source. Boar's Head bologna, ham, and turkey ham are safe choices, as are Oscar Meyer ham and cheese loaf, baked cooked ham, and Genoa salami.

Coffee and Teas

Pure coffee is gluten-free, but do watch out for the fancy flavored ones, as well as instant coffee made from cereal. Stick with leaf tea or plain tea in tea bags. There has been quite a lot of buzz about the glue in tea bags. As far as I can tell, there is *no* glue in tea bags.

Condiments, Cocktail Sauces, and Dressings

Olives, pickles, pure honey, Heinz ketchup, Lea & Perrins Original Worcestershire Sauce, HP Steak Sauce, and Original Barbecue Sauce are all gluten-free. Dijon mustard, Hellmann's mayonnaise, all Smucker's jams and jellies, preserves, marmalades, low-sugar and Simply 100% Fruit Spread are gluten-free, as is Polaner All-Fruit jelly, jam, and preserves, and Watkin's preserves. Arrowhead peanut, almond, and cashew butters are safe. There are many salad dressings to choose from, but beware of low-fat dressings. When something is taken out, something else is usually put in to make the dressing palatable. Read labels carefully. Annie's Natural dressings are a good choice, for taste as well as safety. So are Newman's Own, with an extensive gluten-free list for consumers.

Ice Cream and Frozen Desserts

Life is short, so eat dessert first. Remember one simple rule: never eat ice cream that contains mix-ins like brownies or cookie dough or not-so-obvious ingredients such as nuts and chips that may have been dusted with wheat flour. See Baskin-Robbins gluten-free flavors in chapter 5 and stock up. Edy's, or Dryer's in some regions, offers a long list of gluten-free flavors, as does Kemps, Dove Bars, Rice Dream dairy-free ice cream in chocolate, vanilla, or plain carob, Soy Dream, in all flavors except chocolate fudge brownie, and Weight Watcher's Chocolate Mousse Bars, Orange Vanilla Treat, and Chocolate Treat. Kemps and Blue Bell make gluten-free frozen yogurts as well. As flavors change with the fashions, my best advice is this: make a list of your favorite flavors, check with the company to make sure yours is indeed safe, then pass out the spoons.

Meat/Meat Substitutes

The rule here is simple. If it comes from a fairly recognizable part of a cow, sheep, pig, or chicken and nothing has been added, it's okay to eat. If the meat is preserved in any way or is an unspecified blend of animal and other ingredients, check with the butcher and look at the label before you buy it. If you can't vet the product, don't put it in your cart.

Pastas and Breads

Some celiacs are so afraid of consuming gluten accidentally that they won't even breathe near the pasta and bread aisles. A good exercise is to march proudly up and down past the stacks of empty and refined carbohydrates and say (repeat after me), "You can't hurt me anymore." If someone overhears you, tell him or her it's an aversion therapy exercise. You won't be bothered after that. Besides, there are so many wonderful pastas, breads, and muffins outside the realm of the average supermarket, you won't care what people say.

Beware of Veggie Burgers!

They almost always contain wheat gluten (seitan), which gives them the taste and texture of meat.

Soups

Where can gluten hide in a clear broth? As a new celiac, this was my question, too. I have since learned that gluten is a master of disguise. My favorite chicken broth was one such example. Better to buy Progresso, Healthy Valley, Pacific Foods, or just buy a chicken and make it yourself. Herb-Ox and Edward & Sons are good choices for bouillon cubes.

Snacks

Plain, unadulterated nuts with a little salt should be self-explanatory and you don't want my opinion on puffs, popcorn, etc. That aside, Lay's Classic potato chips, Ruffles potato chips, Utz unflavored potato chips, and Homestyle potato chips are all gluten-free. *Si Si* for Baked Tostitos tortilla chips, Doritos Baja Picante and Toasted Corn, and Utz Black Bean and Salsa Tortilla Chips, as well as Low-Fat Baked Tortilla Chips and White Corn Tortilla Strips. Barbara's Bakery makes a gluten-free blue corn chip, and all unflavored varieties of Frito's corn chips are safe as well. How hard is it to mash up an avocado with some lime, chopped tomatoes, and cilantro? If you must buy a commercially prepared dip, choose Ortega Thick & Chunky Salsa in three temperatures, or Garden Valley salsas. Athenos hummus is quite good and gluten-free.

The Health Food Store: Gluten-Free Heaven

With rare exceptions, gone are the open bins of tofu, Birkenstock sandals, and hippies with stringy hair, carotene-stained palms, and superior airs. Many of us know the difference between kudzu and kombu (the former is a gluten-free thickener, the latter a kind of seaweed used in soups and stews to make them more digestible, also gluten-free). Health food stores are the happening places in many neighborhoods. Here you can buy holistic and herbal medicines, cruelty-free cosmetics, all manner of wheat-, dairy-, chemical-, casein-, pesticide-, and hormone-free, organically pure, environmentally safe, and really great-tasting, as well as good-for-you products. Many of these new markets offer grind-it-yourself peanut butter, back rubs, food tastings, neighborhood events, book signings, coffee from self-sustaining farms (not agri-businesses) around the world, fruits and vegetables, cards, flowers, handmade soaps, exotic oils, aluminum-free cookware, colorful handmade brooms from Guatemala, and, yes, a huge inventory of gluten-free products.

Essene Natural Foods Market & Cafe. One of the finest independently owned whole food emporiums in the country is a mere two blocks from my home in Philadelphia. I know how lucky I am. People drive hundreds of miles to get to it and not merely for gluten-free food; it is one of the important centers of the macrobiotic cooking movement in the United States. I take a break from my shopping to sit in their café and enjoy a bowl of miso soup (made with brown rice miso) or a cup of Ku Kicha (roasted twig) tea, feeling both virtuous and guilty, knowing I have several snack-sized bags of Energy Foods' gluten-free pretzels in my bag, along with a box of Tinkyada gluten-free spaghetti and a bag of masa harina for my homemade tortillas. There are Gluten-Free Pantry baking mixes, Bob's Red Mill gluten-free chickpea, teff, and tapioca flours, and Mesa Sunrise cereal. The shelves are stocked with Health Valley soups, gluten-free black bean and vegetable, lentil and carrots, Edward & Sons brown rice snaps in cheddar, onion garlic, tamari seaweed, tamari sesame, toasted onion, and plain. I always keep a supply on hand for guests and an extra bottle of San-J wheat-free soy sauce to keep in the pantry and to take to the Japanese restaurant.

It's good to know I don't have to load up. I can come here anytime. I chat with the tourists and every now and again, spot a newly diagnosed celiac, introduce myself and give her a gluten-free tour of the place. 719 South 4th Street, Philadelphia, PA 19147, (215) 922-1146, www.essenemarket.com.

When Away from Home

There are wonderful, independently owned markets all over the country. One of my favorites is Nature's Food Patch in Clearwater, Florida. When I visited my parents, we would stop there first to load up on gluten-free foods for my stay and have lunch in the Bunny Hop Café. My favorite away-from-home trick is to shop first, open a loaf of gluten-free bread, and give it to the café server for a fresh and terrific sandwich. The country is dotted with these wonderful, celiac-friendly places.

Viva's Healthy Dining Guide, published by Viva Center for Nutrition and written by Lisa Margolin and Connie Dee, is a great way to find similar markets in towns and cities all over America. Find the one nearest you and don't forget to pack your copy for car trips.

Sunset Foods. According to an article in *Living Without* magazine (a must, by the way for news, recipes, and perspective on the gluten-free life; see page 477 for details), at one time this Chicago grocery store was below average in terms of the availability of gluten-free foods. That was before Lisa Addis, mother of a newly diagnosed celiac, decided her local grocer should know how to get special food for her family. Thanks to her chutzpah, Sunset Foods is now home to Glutino bagels, Kinnikinnick breads, Foods By George Crumb Cake, donuts from Gluten-Free Delights, Midel cookies, Pamela's biscotti, millet bread, and apple cinnamon raisin buns. Not only do they offer a full-range of great gluten-free foods, they've even become a sponsor of the University of Chicago Celiac Disease Program. 1127 Church Street, Northbrook, IL 60062, (847) 272-7700.

Trader Joe's. This no-frills West Coast phenomenon has migrated east, and we couldn't be happier. Not only do they carry a great selection of gluten-free items, the freight is kinder and gentler than many of the pricier specialty natural foods stores. Their catalog is called the "Fearless Flyer" and falls somewhere between *Consumer Reports* and *Mad* magazine in tone. It's a cheeky, fun read and the prices are amazing. Where else can you find frozen asparagus spears at $1.99 for a 12-ounce bag or roasted whole almonds at $3.29 a pound, naturally gluten-free, or smoked salmon for half the supermarket price? The trail mixes alone are cause for shopping cart gridlock, and there is, of course, the most wonderful chocolate in the world—a 3.5-ounce bar of Valrhona extra dark chocolate bars (an unheard of 71 percent cacao) for $2.59. Trader Joe's offers a list of gluten-free items, but as you should wherever you shop, look carefully. You are sure to find items not on the list that are perfectly safe.

A word about this. It is common for employees who compile these lists to overlook products that are not made specifically for the wheat and gluten-free market, missing items that are just plain safe for us to eat, but not marketed as such. Companies are catching up, but for now, keep reading those labels.

Marketing Strategy #2

. . . .

Always point out your favorite gluten-free products to your non-celiac friends. Good friends love to know how to please you when you come for dinner.

When you find something, ask that it be put on the gluten-free store list to make it easier for those who follow you.

As with all company gluten-free lists, double check. There is always the possibility of human error. If it doesn't sound right, ask.

Among the many gluten-free items are Trader Joe's brand canned garbanzo beans and organic refried pinto beans, After Eight chocolate mints, Trader Joe's chocolate espresso beans, Puff 'n' Honey cereal, Mesa Sunrise cereal, Boursin cheese, Patisserie de France tiramasu, and Muffaletta olive spread. Where in Arizona, California, Illinois, Ohio, Pennsylvania, New Mexico, Michigan, Massachusetts, New York, New Jersey, and Washington, D.C., is the nearest Trader Joe's? Go to www.traderjoes.com and find out.

Wegman's Food Market. Started in Rochester, New York, in 1915 with a pushcart and some fruit, Wegman's has become an empire. There are rolls, pie shells, and the new premade pizzas by Gillian's, as well as a huge list of gluten-free items in this temple of natural and artisanal foods. There are stores in New York, Pennsylvania, New Jersey, and Virginia and there is an online shopping service. For information, www.wegmans.com.

Whole Foods. Four blocks west of me is a gigantic new market. This wonderful corporation with stores all over the country is where gluten-free is codified, pamphleteered, and elevated to a shopping art form. Ditto for wheat-free and dairy-free as well. This is where neighbor meets neighbor at the prepared foods counter, café, or 15-minute massage chair, where shopping seems to take longer as friends turn up, ingredients labels are perused, and cheeses sampled.

The new Manhattan store in the Time Warner Center at Columbus Circle recently opened to movie premiere press and is the largest of its kind in the country, maybe even the world. (A bit too big to absorb, in my humble opinion, but certainly worth a stop on any celiac's New York itinerary.)

In the works is the Whole Foods Market Gluten-Free Bakery created by the Chapel Hill store's celiac chef Lee Tobin (see page 424 for his gluten-free holiday fruit cake). Soon it will possible to buy fresh baked goods in stores up and down the East Coast. No, you are not dreaming.

The Whole Foods Market gluten-free product list is vast and ever changing in response to customer requests. Case in point: I asked if my local store would carry Amy's frozen gluten-free pizza and it was stocked within the month.

In the baking aisle, gluten-free products include Arrowhead Mills blue or yellow cornmeal, gluten-free flours, pancake and baking mix, Ener-G egg replacer and tapioca flour, Fearn rice baking mix, and Gluten-Free Pantry muffin mixes, and quick breads, gourmet baking mix, piecrust mix, and

---

Marketing Strategy #3

. . . .

For gluten-free shopping that's kinder on the budget, divide your list between commodities found in the supermarket, i.e., organic produce,
meats, and fish, and what is really worth the extra money you'll spend in
a specialty store or by mail.

---

brownie mix. Lotus Foods rice flour comes in several types—Bhutanese Red,
Forbidden, and Roasted Kaipen. Also available are Pamela's gluten-free gourmet pancakes and baking mix and Ultra Chocolate Brownie Mix.

Beverages include Ceres fruit juices (don't look for sugary sodas here),
Naturade Total Soy Calcium 1000, Total Soy Ready to Drink in chocolate and
Vanilla, and Organic Soy in chocolate, banana, and coffee bean.

The cereal selection is huge with 365 Brand Honey Frosted Flakes, Arrow-
head Mills Puffed Corn and Puffed Rice, Barbara's Bakery Frosted Corn Flakes,
Breadshop's Crispy Rice 'n Corn Flakes, Erewhon Corn Flakes and Rice Twice,
Health Valley Organic Blue Corn Flakes, Lundberg Hot 'n Creamy Rice Cereal,
Nature's Path Mesa Sunrise Cereal, Envirokidz Amazon Frosted Flakes and Go-
rilla Munch, Pacific Grain Nutty Rice Cereal, and Pocono Cream of Buckwheat.

There is Health Valley Chili and Bearito's Low-Fat Premium Black Bean
Chili, Barbara's Bakery Cheese Puffs, and Good Health Olive Oil Potato Chips
in plain, rosemary, lemon, garlic, trio, blue, black pepper, and sweet potato.
This is where I buy my Glutino pretzels in big, fat, family-sized bags.

Condiments include Bragg Liquid Aminos, Eden Organic Tamari Soy
Sauce, Lotus Foods Kaipen Pressed Fresh Water Green Algae, Miso Master
Organic Miso in Mellow White, Traditional Red, Nasoya Nayonaise, and Fat-
Free Nayonaise, San-J Wheat-Free Soy Sauce, Westbrae Miso (Brown Rice,
Genmai, Hatcho, Mellow Red, Mellow White), and Whole Foods Soy Sauce.

The cookie aisle yields Pamela's Gluten-Free cookies and biscotti, Midel
ginger snaps, Hol-Grain brown rice crackers, and there are Kozy Shack puddings in chocolate, rice, and tapioca, Lundberg Rice Pudding Mix in cinnamon
raisin, coconut, and honey almond, Morinu Mates Chocolate Low-Fat Pudding
Mix, and Azumaya Tofu Spoonables in almond, chocolate, and vanilla.

The frozen case yields a real bonanza in gluten-free items. Cedarlane
makes a Three-Layer Enchilada Pie, Natural Feast Blueberry, Cherry, and

Marketing Strategy #4

. . . .

Don't get more than you paid for. The Environmental Working Group says U.S.-grown red raspberries, strawberries, apples, and peaches, and Mexican cantaloupe are often contaminated with pesticides. POP (persistent organic pollutants), forbidden in organic agriculture, are found in butter, cucumbers/pickles, meat loaf, peanuts, popcorn, radishes, spinach, summer and winter squash. Go organic for these foods.

Pumpkin Pie, Nature's Hilights Soy Cheese and Vegetarian Beans Tostada Rice Crust Pizza, and Amy's Cheese Pizza, as well as Mexican Tamale Pie, Shepherd's Pie, Lasagna, and Rice Mac and Cheese, Nature's Path Buckwheat or Mesa Sunrise waffles, Van's gluten-free waffles, and Taj Gourmet Indian entrees—Bean Masala, Channa Bhaji, Chicken Korma, Chicken Tikka Masala, Dal Bahaar, Eggplant Bhartha, Palak Paneer, and Vegetable Korma.

In the International Section, all of Asmar's Mediterranean Foods are gluten-free, as are Tamarind Tree and Thai Kitchen brands.

For vegetarians, Whole Foods Market lists Lightlife Foney Baloney, Tofu Pups, and Soy Tempeh, Garden Vege Tempeh, and Wild Rice Tempeh as gluten-free. Ditto for Nasoya Tofu, New Menu Tofu Mate Eggless Salad, Northern Soy Not Dogs, and Vegetarian Breakfast Links, Vitasoy Tofu, and White Wave Tempeh in Original Soy, Sea Veggie, Soy Rice, and Wild Rice.

Gluten-free side dishes include Road's End Organics Dairy-Free Brown Rice Penne and Cheese, and Tasty Bite Agra Peas and Greens, Bombay Potatoes, Jaipur Vegetables, Jodhpur Lentils, Madras Lentils, Simla Potatoes, and Tasty Kashmir Spinach. In addition, all varieties of Ginny's Vegan Foods are gluten-free.

The pasta aisle is a carb-lover's dream, with Ancient Harvest Quinoa Pasta, China Bowl Cellophane Noodles, DeBole's Brown Rice Pasta, Eden Foods 100% Soba Japanese Buckwheat Pasta, Pastariso Brown Rice Pasta, Tinkyada Rice Pasta Elbows, Fusilli, Penne, Spaghetti, Spinach Spaghetti, Spirals, Vegetables Spirals, and Lasagna Noodles, and Westbrae Natural Brown Rice Noodles and Spaghetti-Style Corn Pasta.

Most of Annie's Naturals salad dressings are gluten-free, as are Nasoya Veggie Dressings in Creamy Dill, Creamy Italian, Garden Herb, Sesame Garlic, and Thousand Island.

As if this were not enough, a careful inventory of the bakery department yields low-fat chocolate chews, pure almond paste cookies, miniature and full-size flourless chocolate cakes, and, depending on the season, Passover cookies and cakes without a scintilla of gluten.

To find a Whole Foods Market near you, go to www.wholefoodsmarket .com.

Wild Oats Natural Marketplace is another great source for gluten-free products, organic produce, herbal remedies, health information, and giant pecan and chocolate cookies and mini pecan pies made by Foods By George, Frookie's Cookies, Midel, and Healthy Times Brown Rice Cereal for Baby. There is a huge selections of pastas, as well as Barbara's Instant Mashed Potatoes, Muir Glen Ketchup, Taste Bite Indian Dinners, Annie Chun's Rice Noodles, and Thai Kitchen Rice Noodles. My favorite Hol-Grain Brown Rice Crackers are found here, as are Gillian's new premade gluten-free pizzas and Lifestream Wildberry Buckwheat Waffles. There are baking mixes by Ener-G Foods, Lundberg Farms, Gluten-Free Pantry, Arrowhead Mills, Sylvan Border Farms, and Bob's Red Mill. In the Natural Living department, there is gluten-free Ultimate Meal Powder, Wild Oats brand supplements with gluten-free varieties clearly marked, as well as Solgar, Rainbow Light, and Source Naturals Supplements, all gluten-free varieties clearly marked. While you're checking these out, grab a Newman's Own Organic Chocolate Bar; Wild Oats lists it as gluten-free.

This is a company that cares about the environment and gives back to the community, which is wonderful as long as you have to spend money anyway. Every three months, a different local nonprofit gets 5 percent of the day's pretax sales total. The Wooden Nickel Program gives you a nickel for every sack you reuse and the e-Scrip Giving Program makes sure 5 percent of your monthly total goes to your favorite charity. With outposts in Arizona, Arkansas, British Columbia, California, Colorado, Connecticut, Florida, Illinois, Indiana, Kansas, Kentucky, Maine, Massachusetts, Missouri, Nebraska, Nevada, New Jersey, New Mexico, Ohio, Oklahoma, Oregon, Tennessee, Texas, Utah, and Washington, it shouldn't be hard to sow your Wild Oats.

For locations and a downloadable gluten-free list, go to www.wildoats.com.

Gluten-Free Markets, Specialty Stores, and Bakeries

Illinois

The Gluten-Free Market
Buffalo Grove Town Center
Route 83 and Lake Cook Road
Buffalo Grove, IL 60089
(847) 419-9610
www.glutenfreemarket.com

With more than 360 brands of gluten-free products like Enjoy Life Foods (delicious sesame, onion, and plain bagels, snack bars and Big cookies), Bette Hagman's Four Flour Blend, her Featherlight Flour, and other baking staples by Authentic Foods, Amy's Kitchen heat and serve soups, Kinnikinnick, Cybros breads and dinner rolls, Dietary Specialties frozen entrees, and a huge selection of cookies, crackers, sauces, cereals, desserts, snacks, this store is a celiac's dream come true. While you're waiting for your order to be filled, browse the books and have a chat with the certified nutritionist on staff. Too far to drive? Log on to their Web site and put in your order.

Goodday Gluten-Free
514A North Western Avenue
Lake Forest, IL 60045
(847) 615-1208

Fred Lehman is the proprietor of this division of Goodday health food stores. Many of the best gluten-free brands are to be found here, and if it isn't convenient to drop by, Fred puts out a mail-order catalog. Three or four times a year, Mr. Lehman contacts the folks at the University of Chicago Celiac Disease Program, gives them an empty carton, and tells them to go on a shopping spree for their gluten-free care package program. Kudos to this company for helping to make sure it is a good and gluten-free day for celiacs everywhere.

Michigan

Celiac Specialties
48411 Jefferson
Chesterfield Township, MI 48047
(586) 598-8180
www.celiacspecialities.com

    This newly opened Detroit area gluten-free bakery is just like the one you remember. Cakes, pies, cookies, English muffins, and corn bread are among the sweet and savory baked goodies offered by Michelle Fuller, the owner and baker behind the take-and-bake pizza from "On the Grapevine" at *Living Without* magazine. Too far to drive? They will ship anywhere.

Minnesota

Bittersweet
2105 Cliff Road
Eagan, MN 55122
(651) 686-0112
www.bittersweetgf.com

    Andrea Hawkinson is the inspiration behind this new gluten-free and dairy and preservative-free bakery in the Land of Lakes. There are lemon and pumpkin bars, almond Bundt, carrot and chocolate cakes, banana, cranberry and pumpkin raisin tea breads, oatmeal, chocolate chip, and spice cookies, and everything is made fresh daily.

New Jersey

Sorella Bakery
1595 Imperial Way, Unit 110
West Deptford, NJ 08066
(856) 848-8383
www.sorellabakery.com

    Brand-new at press time, this gluten-free bakery specializes in the biscottines our grandmothers brought with them from the Old Country. These Italian cookies are smaller and more moist than biscotti, and creator Phyllis Moffo has combined her restaurant and pastry-making experience for treats that have to be tasted to be believed. Hand-crafted Sorella biscottines are available through Miss Roben's and other specialty retailers.

New Mexico

The Great Harvest Bread Co.
11200 Montgomery N.E.
Albuquerque NM 87111
(505) 293-8277
www.greatharvest.com

If you're in the neighborhood, Sunday is the day to get freshly baked loaves and other gluten-free goodies from this franchised bread company. Their second gluten-free location in Albuquerque is 6301 Riverside Plaza Lane N.W., (505) 922-8817.

New York

Josef's Gluten-Free Bakery
1712 Avenue M
Brooklyn, NY
(718) 336-9494

This is the bakery of choice on The Celiac Chicks, a clever Web site designed by two hip young women who work in Manhattan and live in Brooklyn, devoting themselves to living a full and fabulous gluten-free life in New York. Walk in, have a piece of cake, or phone in your mail order. Review and details at www.celiacchicks.com.

Schick's Gourmet Kosher Bakery
4710 16th Avenue
Brooklyn, NY 11204
(718) 436-8020
www.schicksbakery.com

This mail-order bakery offers a huge selection of gluten-free items, which means a long list of gluten-free cookies, cakes, macaroons, jelly rolls, and specialty items not just for Passover. Call for prices and ordering information.

North Carolina

Whole Foods Market Gluten-Free Bakehouse
Morrisville, North Carolina
www.wholefoodsmarket.com

Oh, to walk right into a grocery store and pick up a loaf of freshly baked bread. Brainchild of Whole Foods Market chef, master baker, and resident celiac Lee Tobin, the new Bakehouse will let you do just that—with a selection of breads, cookies, brownies, scones, biscuits, cakes, pies, pizza crusts, corn bread, and much more. In southern and mid-Atlantic Whole Foods Market locations and in all northeast and Florida locations in winter 2005. For information and Bakehouse locations, go to the Whole Foods Market website.

Ohio

Kathy's Creations
460 E. Main Street
Alliance, OH 44601
(330) 821-8183 or (866) 821-8183

This is a gluten-free, made-to-order bakery, with cakes, cookies, muffins, and more—just like you'd bake if you had the time.

Pennsylvania

The Dietary Shoppe
4436 Ridge Avenue
Philadelphia, PA 19129
(215) 242-5302
www.dietaryshoppe.com

Oh, what a time to be gluten-free with knowledgeable and friendly people like Chelsea Smith (a registered dietician) stocking every gluten-free product imaginable. Of course, you can e-order, but if you can get there in person, it's worth a trip to stock up on gluten-free bagels, breads, muffins, cookies, individual frozen pizzas, ravioli, and stuffed shells. There are pizza crusts from Kinnikinnick, hot dog buns, hamburger buns, English muffins, donuts, biscotti, gluten-free licorice, vitamins, weight gain shakes, snack bars, gift certificates, gift baskets, books, and a complete inventory of casein, sugar, lactose-free and low-carb products.

The Grainless Baker
3276 Birney Avenue
Scranton, PA 18505
(570) 689-9694

The Minooka Pastry Shop has been a family business for as long as Jane and Dan Trygar can remember. Jane, a talented baker and newly diagnosed celiac, got around the cross-contamination issue by setting up her own bakery in the basement of her home. Some neighbors go straight to the house, but you need to call Minooka for gluten-free breads, cookies, sheet and layer cakes, hot dog and hamburger rolls and savory pesto rolls.

Mr. Ritt's
709 E. Passyunk Avenue
Philadelphia, PA 19147
215-627-30334
www.mrritts.com

Once upon a time, yours truly walked into this newly opened neighborhood bakery and asked if they carried anything that was gluten-free. There were puzzled looks and questions. After a few months of explaining what exactly gluten-free is, supplying reading material, and volunteering to taste the early experiments, the rest is history. I have no financial interest in this gluten-free bakery, but living literally around the corner, I do have a selfish one. This is a must stop on any trip to Philadelphia, and I love to pop in and say hello to fellow celiacs while I pick up my favorite brownies and lemon pound cake. It's amazing how many loaves of bread, cakes, pizza shells, ice-cream cones, waffles, cookies, scones, and biscotti you can get into a tiny shop.

Washington

Flying Apron Organic Bakery
4759 Brooklyn Avenue N.E.
Seattle, WA 98105
(206) 526-2903
www.flyingapron.com

Customers come back for the fudgey chocolate triangles. This vegan, wheat- and gluten-free organic bakery offers dairy and sugar-free delights as well. Among them, homemade goodies, tarts, cupcakes, freshly made gluten-free bread, and an honest-to-goodness layer cake.

Wheatless in Seattle
15700 Dayton Avenue
Shoreline, WA 98133
(206) 440-4147
www.wheatlessinseattle.com

    This totally gluten-free bakery and café will serve you entrees, desserts, breads right from the menu, prepare a meal for takeout, or will ship their homemade goodies directly to your door.

Wisconsin

Gluten-Free Trading Co.
604-A West Lincoln Avenue
Milwaukee, WI 53215
(888) 993-9933
info@gluten-free.net

    The premise is intriguing: "Imagine a store where nothing is off-limits, a store where someone has already read all the labels and made all the calls. Pasta from Italy. Soup from England, rice from Bhutan. Chocolate from the Ivory Coast. Cookies from that little bakery in New Jersey . . ." If you can make it to Milwaukee, don't come on a Monday or on weekdays from 1 P.M. to 2 P.M. when they are closed for lunch (gluten-free, we presume). Phone and e-mail orders taken gladly.

Canada

Panne Rizo
1939 Cornwall Avenue
Vancouver, BC V6J 1C8, Canada
(604) 736-0885
www.pannerizo.com

    This bakery/deli serves soup, sandwiches, pizza, pannini, and all manner of gluten-free goodies. Every delicious morsel here is baked from scratch in a gluten-free kitchen. A great place for lunch while vacationing in Vancouver. Short of a visit, you can order online. They ship 2-day FedEx to the United States every Wednesday from Bellingham, Washington.

Specialty Food Shop
555 University Avenue
Toronto, ON M5G 1X8, Canada
(800) 737-7976
www.specialtyfoodshop.com

In addition to carrying a huge selection of gluten-free products from all over the world, this shop specializes in low-protein, low-sodium, and other medical diets, as well as medical equipment, nutritional supplements, and books. Dieticians are on staff; phone and Internet orders accepted.

Cyber-Shopping

There's nothing quite like being a mouse click away from all your favorite gluten-free products. Do remember, though, to review a company's security before submitting your credit card number. Know how much you are expected to pay for shipping, and how long you may have to wait for your order. (With tight border regulations causing frequent delays, this may be an issue you want to discuss with the company before placing an order.) Familiarize yourself with the company's policy regarding spoilage or other reasons for dissatisfaction. If you do return a product, who pays? If all meets with your approval, send yourself goodies periodically and do as I do. When visiting a friend or family member in another state, I like to send a care package ahead of my arrival. The leftovers will remind your host to reorder for your next visit. Gift baskets are a great idea, too, especially for someone who's just been diagnosed, moved, or is in the hospital.

Cecilia's Gluten-Free Grocery. This Nevada-based online grocery boasts over 300 gluten-free products from over 40 manufacturers. Information on the gluten-free lifestyle and a recipe database, www.glutenfree grocery.com. Phone orders, too: (800) 491-2760.

Chef's Pantry. Organic, natural, wheat- and gluten-free foods, www.lees market.com.

Gifts of Nature, Inc. This Montana company offers their own brand of gluten-free baking mixes, as well as other gluten-free brands, www.gifts ofnature.net or (406) 961-1529.

Gluten-Free Bakery. This is the place that carries Pies by Maria. In addition to gluten-free breads, cookies, and other baked goods, there are egg- and casein-free products and a Snack of the Month Club. For a complete listing, www.glutenfreebakery.com, or (781) 440-0875.

Gluten-Free Cafe. This company specializes in instant prepared meals, side dishes, desserts, and the like that are freeze-dried and specially packaged for a long shelf-life for camping, hiking, traveling, emergencies, etc. No preservatives or MSG. www.alpineairefoods.com, or (800) 322-6325.

The Gluten-Free Cookie Jar. Bagels are a specialty in this Pennsylvania bakery, as are assorted buttery cookies like the kind we all remember. www.glutenfreecookiejar.com or (215) 355-7991 for phone orders.

Gluten-Free Delights. This company offers dinner rolls, English muffins, cookies, donut holes, mini pies, cranberry bread, and all kinds of gluten-free baked goods. www.gluten-freedelights.com, phone orders (888) 403-1806.

The Gluten-Free Pantry. Glastonbury, Connecticut, is headquarters to some of the finest gourmet baking mixes around—from flaky piecrust to cookies, cakes, bagels, brownies, and breads designed to be made with or without a bread machine. The staff is friendly and knowledgeable and will help with information on gluten-free baking. There is a quarterly newsletter with recipes and ideas, and its gluten-free founder, Beth Hillson, is a booster of all things celiac with profits from premade sandwich bread, cinnamon raisin bread, and hamburger/sandwich rolls going to support the American Celiac Task Force and Food Labeling Reform. www.glutenfree.com or (800) 291-8386.

The Gluten-Free Mall. They call themselves "your special diet superstore," and for good reason. There are dozens of products, not only for the gluten-free diet, but for wheat-, lactose-, and cassein-free diets as well. Surf their vast product list at www.glutenfreemall.com.

Gluten Free Supermarket. Authentic Foods baking and cake mixes, flours, flour blends, and recipes from Bette Hagman, Rebecca Reilly, and Karen Robertson. www.gluten-free-supermarket.com.

Gluten-Solutions. According to their Web site, this is the nation's first online grocery store dedicated to wheat- and gluten-free foods. They say they keep everything in stock for low shipping costs and fast delivery. The site is a bit difficult to navigate, but the frequent buyer rewards program should more than make up for it. www.glutensolutions.com.

Mimi & Me. This is "the little bakery from New Jersey" that the Gluten-Free Trading Company talks about in their ads. Wheat-free, gluten-free, lactose-free, casein-free, and kosher cupcakes, sandwich cookies, marble loaf, and other goodies with that bakery taste. Prepared by Mimi Davis, a celiac, and her partner Ardith Hodes in a wheat-free environment. www.miminme.com or (888) 758-9464.

Shop By Diet. This Internet company offers hundreds of gluten-free foods, as well as a product search by multiple dietary restrictions, www.shopbydiet.com.

Food Cooperatives and Buying Clubs

With prices what they are, buying in bulk is always a good idea, especially if your family is large and goes through food like "Grant took Richmond," as my mother used to say. Even if you just want to stock up for yourself, it's smart to share with other celiacs and save money. One of the biggest of these clubs in the Midwest is **United Natural Foods** (formerly called Blooming Prairie), which sells to gluten-free specialty companies as well as to individual consumers. The list of gluten-free foods and vitamins is long and the quantity discounts considerable. Buy only what you love. You're going to have a lot of it. For a club near you call (800) 323-2131 or www.unitedbuyingclubs.com.

Oregon's **Ashland Food Cooperative** is one the oldest in the nation. Here the focus is on organically grown produce and foods in bulk. 237 N. First Street, Ashland, OR 97520, (541) 482-2237 or www.acfs.org.

To find a food cooperative or buying club near you, go to the **Coop Directory Service,** 1254 Etna Street, St. Paul, MN 55106, (651) 774-9189 or www.coopdirectory.org.

Learn More

For information on gluten-free labeling legislation and other efforts on behalf of American celiacs, American Celiac Task Force, www.capwiz.com/celiac.

U.S. Department of Agricultur, www.ama.usda.gov/mop.

Information about all things organic, www.organic.org.

Learn more about whole foods at www.localharvest.org.

Environmental news from the Environmental Working Group, www.ewg.org.

Eco-friendly consumer topics, www.care2.com.

U.S. Food and Drug Administration (FDA), www.fda.gov.

Council of Better Business Bureaus, www.bbb.com.

Our teachers taught us never to write in our books, but they didn't know we would grow up to be busy, resourceful, and very hungry celiacs. Jot down your picks in the space below (this way all your gluten-free favorites will be in one place), and if you discover some new ones not listed here, let me know. I'll put them in a future edition.

My Discoveries

_____

_____

_____

_____

_____

_____

_____

_____

_____

_____

_____

_____

_____

_____

_____

_____

_____

_____

_____

_____

_____

and the winner is . . .

You like me, you really like me.

—SALLY FIELD,
accepting Best Actress Oscar for Norma Rae

In the dark days of stale rice cakes, corn spaghetti that turned into an indigestible ball, and bread that could double as wallpaper paste, finding a good gluten-free meal was as easy as finding an oat in a sack of buckwheat. What you got was lumpy, gummy, and heavy, with a kind of slippery-mouth feel and weird aftertaste one gets from too much rice flour. But you ate what you got and you were glad it wasn't bananas and rice. I remember, just after my own diagnosis, going to my first big celiac meeting in Chicago where conferees began to perspire as it got close to the hour or so given to gluten-free vendors and trays of free samples. No other way to describe it—otherwise well-mannered celiacs lunged and shoved and participated in what could only be called a feeding frenzy caused by a dearth of quality gluten-free foods. Hundreds of carbohydrate-starved celiacs were determined to get home with as much cake, muffins, cookies, and bread as they could carry (I held a pie in my lap all the way back to Philadelphia). I remember thinking that if we could only harness all this pent-up energy, we would really have something. Even better, if we could get some really talented chefs on the case like the pioneers at that early meeting, we would have something worth eating.

Sometimes you *do* get what you wish for. These days, there are thousands of products to choose from. And every day more and more gluten-free companies pop up on shelves, in catalogs, and on Internet lists. Both large businesses and small have seen the bottom-line possibilities of perfecting and investing in the growing gluten-free market. We may have put on a few pounds in the onslaught of all the goodies arriving every day, but it's always better to have too much, rather than too little. New problems arise, though. Given the high price we pay for our special foods, it can be daunting to know which products are worth the expense and which ones are not so hot. Herewith, ways to get on the grapevine, my personal picks, an insider's guide by category to the best gluten-free products available, and a gluten-free directory to find out where to buy them.

Word of Mouth

One way to get the latest dish is at your local support meeting. Vendors usually set up their booths before the program gets under way, and it's a great opportunity to sample products before you purchase and chat with other members about what foods they've tried, which ones they've passed on and which ones are favorites. Plan on arriving early. Today's celiacs may not be as desperate as we were years ago, but they are still hungry for what's missing. Booths fill up fast and lines can snake out the door. Ask a veteran long past the need for support why he or she comes to meetings and you may find that beyond interest in the latest in research, conference news, or the draw of an especially popular speaker, most people attend regular meetings just to find out what's new to eat. This is, after all, a disease completely managed by diet. It makes sense.

Another way to research before you buy is to post a question to the Celiac listserve (see the Resource Guide for Internet addresses) or on one of the Internet message boards. As a courtesy, posters are asked to summarize the responses they get, and many of these summaries exist in the archives of the message boards for your surfing pleasure. Of course, tastes vary, as well as opinions on how to interpret information and legal disclaimers. Look for large summaries in which many people responded to one item, the "best bread," for example. The more positive responses attached to one product, the more likely it is worth a try. Look for feedback on delivery and return policies as well. It doesn't matter how good the product is if it arrives moldy or otherwise inedible. Bear in mind that just because you read it on the Internet doesn't mean it's true. As the listserv owner-moderators are careful to point out, not everything you read is gospel truth. There are wide-ranging views on these bulletin boards where visitors express strong feelings, even the occasional declaration that is dead wrong. Despite warnings not to "flame" others, fights do break out about what is or what is not safe to eat.

Another way to do your shopping homework is to have a chat with one of the specialty store owners. Ask what products are the most popular and why. These proprietors know they are going to make a sale—you're a celiac, aren't you? What they want, as all good business people do, is for you to come back, for you to feel good about their recommendations, happy with your purchases and for you to tell your friends. And don't be shy about asking for a taste. How else will you know if you like it?

Look for product reviews in your local support group newsletter. These are great sources of feedback on gluten-free food companies, often with comments about how the non-celiac friends and family enjoyed the product. If the goal is a totally gluten-free household, you must aim to please everybody in it. And do contact a reviewer to ask questions not covered. This is your budget and your life.

Another good way to get some consensus is to order back issues of *Living Without* magazine or one of the other newsletters (see page 477 for contact information) and see what products, services, restaurants, food companies, books, etc., have been featured in articles and reviews.

And, if you're still not sure which cookie or muffin is going to do it for you, phone one of the many specialty foods companies listed in this chapter and ask for a sampler of their products before you buy in bulk. Some companies will sell you a sampler, generous (*and* smart) ones will send you a free package. If the diet is for life, so is the customer.

Only the Best in My Kitchen

Why don't I start with what's in the freezer and on the pantry shelves Chez Lowell. Obviously, this is subjective. There are no toddlers or teenagers at my house these days, so I get to indulge my preference for foods that are not overly sweetened or full of heart-clogging fats like palm kernel oil, corn syrup, and the like. We use olive oil instead of butter, eat a lot of fish and veggies, and never deep-fry. We're not saints, though. Like most people, I find bone-deep comfort in anything chocolate. Ditto for carbohydrates, and I indulge in the occasional gluten-free bagel, pasta dinner, pretzel, brownie, or slice of lemon pound cake. Knowing this weakness, I use the freezer as a fail-safe mechanism. I will splurge, for example, on one of **Mr. Ritt's** lemon pound cakes (fabulous with fresh strawberries or blueberries and a bit of whipped cream or vanilla ice cream), cut the whole cake into individual slices, wrap the slices, and freeze them. This way, I've got a spectacular dessert for unexpected guests and keeping it out-of-sight helps to minimize temptation.

My favorite dinner party trick is to serve the pound cake with all its extras, then serve myself a slice just as other people are ooh-ing and aah-ing over it. It never fails. Until I take some, nobody believes it's gluten-free.

I do the same thing with **Gluten-Free Pantry** chocolate truffle brownies and Favorite sandwich bread, two other favorite staples of ours. I'll bake up a pan, put a few out for the evening and freeze the rest. By the way, always slice a loaf of bread and wrap it in packages of two slices for easy defrosting and sandwich making. Have I mentioned that celiacs can and do gain weight like everybody else?

I do like to keep on hand a supply of **Glutino** bagels and **Foods By George**, especially his pizza and crumb cake. When we have weekend guests, I set up a tray of fruits, juice, butter, jams, poppy seed bagels, and crumb cake for people to nibble when they get up. Sunday breakfast with the papers doesn't get better than this, unless, of course, I decide to make a frittata or French toast. For impromptu graham cracker-like crusts I always have a box of Health Valley Rice Brand Crackers or **Kinnikinnick Foods** crackers in the pantry. **Mi-Del** gluten-free ginger snaps do nicely, too. In fact, with the addition of butter and sugar, any number of GF cookie crumbs, from lemon to vanilla to chocolate chip, make a perfectly decadent crust.

Dowd & Rogers makes a really good cake mix of Italian chestnut flour in Dutch Chocolate, Dark Vanilla, and Golden Lemon flavors. It's pricey, but worth it, I think, for the birthday emergency. Whip up a silky ganache and you've got something truly spectacular.

There are dozens of uses for **Chebe** bread mixes (an exotic blend of flour made from manioc or cassava)—pizza dough mix, garlic and onion bread mix, and cinnamon rolls to name a few, but my specialty is breadsticks. The secret: lots of fresh rosemary and tarragon and no cheese for a crispy outside/soft inside. Our friends polish off these savory little sticks (more like a fat little cigar than a stick) faster than you can ask, "Are these really gluten-free?"

Jax's List of Must-Haves

Glutino Pretzels. Nothing else does it when you've got a Jones for a pretzel, and these are the crunchy, salty real thing. If you're self-controlled, buy them in big family-size bags, otherwise get them in snack sizes. Mail order or in specialty or health food stores.

White Eagle Bakery authentic Italian almond paste cookies are the hands-down winners. Soft and chewy and made with nothing but almond paste, sugar, and egg whites. Studded with slivered almonds and not as sweet as the usual, these are the perfect foil for ice cream or fresh fruit. At Whole Foods Market.

Mesa Sunrise Waffles. This is my standard weekday breakfast, from Nature's Path. Toast one of these high-fiber waffles and spread with protein-rich peanut butter, add some sliced fresh fruit on the side. Tea, vitamins, and hello day.

Tinkyada Spaghetti. For making quick meals at home or bringing to my local neighborhood Italian restaurant, where the chef puts on a fresh pot of water to boil the minute I arrive, and bingo, a meal I wouldn't bother with myself. Friends and family prefer the nutty brown rice taste and the wonderful texture to the glutenous and more refined white stuff.

San-J Wheat-Free Tamari Sauce. I always have a bottle of this on hand for cooking, salad dressings, marinating, etc., and also take it (in a small plastic squeeze bottle) to our favorite Japanese restaurant.

Glutino Flax Crackers in tomato and onion and **Hol-Grain** lightly salted brown rice crackers. These are standard company fare at my house. The former contains no flour, just flax seeds and little bits of embedded onion and tomato (torn up in random pieces, they look gorgeous on an hors d'oeuvre tray). The latter are good for their spreadability, crunch, and texture for cheeses and spreads that require a cracker that won't overwhelm them.

A-Maizing Corn Snack. Whole corn kernels, salt and soy oil, no sugar or preservatives. I always have a bag on hand for unexpected company or when the mood strikes. Positively addictive. At health food stores.

Foods By George or Dietary Specialties include individual prepared pizzas. There's always two or three in the freezer for lazy days or a fast dinner with an added salad. Like most things, I spike the entree-size pizzas with hot pepper flakes, a little of my own sauce, and add toppings like anchovies, veggies, and thin slices of cooked sausage. I will occasionally take one of the pizza crusts listed below to the neighborhood pizza parlor for the real deal.

The Envelope, Please: The Best of the Gluten-Free Products

What do celiacs think are the best products out there? Which ones deserve the gluten-free Oscar? The following informal customer poll comes from readers, magazine editors, specialty store owners, support groups, and Internet posters. The best, by category . . .

All-Purpose Mixes

It's easy to mix up a batch of all-purpose gluten-free flour that works for you, and in fact you should experiment until you find the one that gives the taste and texture you prefer. With so many good packaged mixes available in health food stores and by mail order and with shelf space at a premium in so many family refrigerators (you do have to refrigerate these flours to avoid rancidity), there's plenty to choose from. Among the most popular, in alphabetical order:

> Bette Hagman's Gourmet Featherlight Rice Flour Blend
> Bob's Red Mill All-Purpose Baking Flour
> Ener-G Foods Gluten-Free Gourmet Blend
> Gluten-Free Pantry All-Purpose Sugar-Free Baking Mix
> Kinnikinnick All-Purpose Celiac Flour
> Mr. Ritt's All-Purpose Flour Mix
> Sylvan Border Farm

Bread Winners

Let's be honest. As long as you have your memories, there is no such thing as the perfect loaf of bread. So far, most would agree, no one has achieved the crunchy perfection and chewy interior of the baguette or its whole-grain Italian cousin. Yet as I speak someone somewhere is buttering a hot yeasty newcomer and shouting "Eureka!" Word has it the new Montina flour developed by the Amazing Grains Grower Cooperative is creating a sensation in terms of duplicating the flavor and density of wheat. It's only a matter of time, my friends. For now, many people recommend the Gluten-Free Pantry French Bread and Pizza Crust Mix, and others bake with Bette Hagman's French bread recipe, using only egg whites to get as many air holes in the loaf as possible.

Home baking aside, there are some very good packaged loaves out there. There are breads for toasting, breads for making sandwiches, and breads for getting some extra fiber. We love our bagels, English muffins, and dinner rolls as well. The following brands score well among discerning celiacs.

PACKAGED BREADS
Kinnikinnick Foods breads, English muffins, and bagels
Ener-G Foods Seattle Brown Bread

Enjoy Life Cinnamon Raisin English muffins
Foods By George English muffins
Gluten-Free Cookie Jar Bagels
Sterk's Bakery high fiber bread

BREAD MIXES

Cause You're Special Mock Rye Bread Mix
Gluten-Free Pantry Favorite Sandwich Bread and Bagel Mixes
Glutino breads, bagels, and English muffins
Manna from Anna bread mix

Breakfast Cereals

When they take away your morning bowl of farina or cream of wheat, your inner child howls in protest. You ask, as any questioning person would, "How will I ever grow up to be big and strong without my Wheaties?" No need to whine on a winter morning—there is enough gluten-free cereal to fill breakfast bowls from here to Timbuktu. When I'm not smearing my waffle with peanut butter, my cold-weather treat is whole-grain corn or brown rice porridge, slow-cooked overnight or made from dinner's leftovers and stirred with maple syrup and raisins. There are grits and quinoa, and for those of you who have decided to eat them in moderation, oats—as long as you remember that the source is as important as the substance, and avoid any cross-contamination with wheat. For stick-to-the-ribs power, these whole grains are unparalleled. In summer, there's nothing like crisp cold cereal swimming in a bowl of blueberries and milk. No reason to forgo a healthy start. The following cereals are considered excellent in the breakfast category.

HOT

Arrowhead Mills Puffed Brown Rice Cereal and Rice and Shine Hot Cereal
Kinnikinnick Bucky Hot Buckwheat Cereal
Lundberg Sweet Almond Hot Rice Cereal
Pocono Cream of Buckwheat Cereal

COLD

Enjoy Life cinnamon raisin cereal
Erewhon Rice Twice and Aztec Crunch Corn & Amaranth
EnviroKidz Organic Amazon Frosted Flakes and Peanut Butter Panda Puffs

Glutano Muesli
Health Valley Corn and Rice Crunchems
Nature's Path Mesa Sunrise Multigrain Flakes
Nutty Rice by Pacific Grain

Cake Mixes

Oh, those iced wonders. All silky sweet, candles blazing, ganache shining like a deep lake. Memories of birthday parties, strawberry shortcake, devil's food, black and white cakes, dense chocolate pound cake, butter cream trifles, raspberry jam cakes, seven-layer affairs, creamy towers, and ice-cream extravaganzas. The best of our gluten-free bakeries work their magic from that nebulous place called "scratch." Mr. Ritt's Bakery offers melt-in-your mouth bliss, Panne Rizo gladly ships the glories produced in its kitchens, Whole Foods Market's Lee Tobin pipes his wedding cakes with handmade roses, and there is always that dense, flourless miracle, the David Glass Ultimate Chocolate Truffle Cake. But it is still possible to bake a cake, and cupcakes, too, off the shelf as we used to do on rainy days in our mother's kitchens. Lick the bowl, make a wish and blow out the candles, the following companies take the cake:

Danielle's Chocolate Cake Mix/Gluten-Free Pantry
Dowd & Rogers Mixes
Kinnikinnick Cake Mixes
Miss Roben's Cake Mixes
The Ruby Range Mixes

In a category all its own: Baskin-Robbins ice-cream cakes.

Energy Bars

Are you envious of those souls who can grab a power bar and dash to the day-care center, then on to the next meeting with no energy drain? No need. *Living Without* magazine has featured the best of the hand-held meals in the gluten-free world. Stash some in the pantry to take on shopping trips during your lunch hour, put one in the gym bag, glove compartment, school lunch box, backpack, briefcase, and purse. Some are sweet, some are packed with seeds and fruit, and others are just plain decadent. These are the gluten-free best, bar none:

ANDI Bars. Gluten-casein-corn-soy-GMO-artificial flavoring and preservative-free; made by the Autism Network for Dietary Intervention

Bliss Bar. Macadamia Madness, Cosmic Combo, Heavenly Hazel, Brazil-Pine Divine, or Almond-Cashew

Bumblebar. Original, Chocolate Crisp, Lushus Lemon, or Chai

Ener-G Foods Granola Bar

Glutano Break Bar. Decadent chocolate and biscuit reminiscent of KitKat

Nutiva Organic Chocolate Flaxseed or Flax & Raisin

Organ Bars. Soft and chewy, a lot like a Fig Newton.

Soy Fields Bars. Marshmallow Soy, Peanut Butter, Cinnamon, gluten- and soy-free

Ice-Cream Cones

I scream, you scream, we all scream for ice cream . . . It's true there are many good, gluten-free flavors and brands of ice cream to choose from and, of course, there's always a dish or a cup or, if all else fails, a spoon and the carton. But sometimes you just want your scoop or two on a real ice-cream cone. Remember that wonderful combination of cold and creamy, crisp and crunchy? Keep them in the pantry or put one in your purse or backpack (carefully) and march right up to the counter of your local ice-cream parlor. And remember, for home dipping there's nothing like pulverized gluten-free cookies or brownies as topping. The ice-cream cone of your dreams can be found in gluten-free markets, ordered through companies like the Gluten-Free Pantry, or in many local health food stores.

Cerrone Waffle Cones
Barkat Round Cones

Pasta

Some say spaghetti, others say macaroni, not to mention penne, vermicelli, tagliatelle, angel hair, fusilli, fettuccine, rigatoni, spirals, corkscrews, twists, shells, lasagna, and just plain noodles. You can toss a quick spaghetti dinner with garlic and olive oil, or you can spend the day and have a gorgeous pan of lasagna for your trouble. The best in the category hold up to sauce, do not break down or get mushy, and, most important, please the whole family, not just the celiac. Gluten-free pastas tend to take longer to prepare, so always factor that into your timing. Whether swirled onto a spoon or twirled around a fork, these are some of the most popular pasta brands.

d and Rogers Le Veneziane

ls By George

Glutano

Lundberg Family Farms

Mrs. Leeper's

Pastariso

Tinkyada

Pizza, Pizza

We Americans love our pizza. I don't know about you, but I still miss the occasional gooey, cheesy, real thing with some red pepper flakes and a Diet Coke to wash the whole thing down. Not so good for the waistline, but never mind. Gone are the sticky rice-crust pizzas you had to scrape off the cookie sheet. Gluten-free chefs, bakers, and food companies large and small have focused a stunning amount of talent on this task. Some are premade and others require some assembly. Those who prefer to assemble their own favor homemade pesto, tapenade, sun-dried tomatoes, and goat cheese, among other inventive toppings. Again, in no order of preference, for being the chewy, yeasty, wonderful treat we remember, the pizza prize goes to . . .

CRUST ONLY

Golden Wave of Grains Pizza Crust

Mr. Ritt's Bakery Pizza Crusts (plain or rosemary-scented)

DO-IT-YOURSELF

Gillian's Foods Pizza Dough

MIXES

Gluten-Free Pantry French Bread & Pizza Crust Mix

Kinnikinnick Foods

Chebe Pizza Mix

Miss Roben's Biscuit Mix for pizza crust

Really Great Food Company Pizza Mix

FROZEN

Dietary Specialties individual frozen pizzas

Foods By George individual frozen pizzas

And yes, Virginia, you can have a nice cold glass of beer:

Ramapo Valley Gluten-Free Honey Lager. For ordering information, www.ramapovalleybrewery.com

Bard's Tale Beer Company, LLC. For ordering information, www.bardsbeer.com

The Gluten-Free Pages: A Company Directory

Consider the following list of specialty food companies your personal, gluten-free Yellow Pages, a directory of all the best companies that make the products listed in this chapter. Let your fingers do the walking or let your mouse do the clicking. Many of these specialty food companies will sell to you directly; others will give you a list of stores that carry their brand, many of which are listed in the previous chapter. Ask for catalogs, samples, delivery policies, and lobby your local grocery store to start stocking your favorites. Think about starting a buying club with friends or buy through a support group to save the freight.

Allen's Gourmet/Gluten-Free
Licorice
118 Houston Street
Nelson, BC V7A 4V4, Canada
(250) 352-3576

Amaizing Corn Snacks
35584 County Road 8
Mountain Lake, MN 56159
(800) 692-6762
www.gladcorn.com

Amazing Grains Grower
Cooperative/Montina Flour
405 Main Street, S.W.
Ronan, MT 59864
(877) 278-6585
www.montina.com

Amy's Kitchen Frozen Dinners
P.O. Box 7868
Santa Rosa, CA 95407
(707) 578-7270
www.amyskitchen.com

Ancient Harvest Quinoa
Corporation
P.O. Box 279
Gardena, CA 90248
(310) 217-8125
www.quinoa.bigstep.com

ANDI Bars
(609) 737-8985
www.autismndi.com

Annie Chun's Rice Noodles
54 Mark Drive, Suite 103
San Rafael, CA 94903
(415) 479-8272
www.anniechun.com

Annie's Naturals Salad Dressings and
Mustards
(800) 434-1234
www.anniesnaturals.com

Arrowhead Mills Mixes
110 South Lawton
Hereford, TX 79045
(806) 364-0730
www.arrowheadmills.com

Aunt Candice/4 the Kidz
Gluten- and casein-free
cookies/brownies
P.O. Box 1457
Wilsonville, OR 97070
(503) 682-8733
www.auntcandicefoods.com

Authentic Foods Baking Mixes
1850 West 169th Street, Suite B
Gardena, CA 90247
(800) 806-4737
www.authenticfoods.com

Barbara's Bakery
3900 Cypress Drive
Petaluma, CA 94954
(707) 765-2273
www.barbarasbakery.com

Banducci & Daughters—
meringue cookies
627 Webster Street
Palo Alto, CA 94301
(888) 207-1429
www.angelkisscookies.com

Bionature Gluten-Free Pasta
from Italy
Imported by Euro-USA Trading Co.
5 Tyler Drive
North Franklin, CT 06254
(609) 955-3218

The Birkett Mills—buckwheat
163 Main Street
Penn Yan, NY 14527
(315) 536-3311
www.thebirkettmills.com

Blue Diamond Growers Nut
Thins
1802 C Street
Sacramento, CA 95814
(800) 987-2329
www.bluediamondgrowers.com

Bob's Red Mill—specialty flours and
baking mixes
5209 SE International Way
Milwaukie, OR 97222
(800) 553-2258
www.bobsredmill.com

Bone Suckin' Sauce
1109 Agriculture Street
Raleigh, NC 27603
(800) 446-0947
www.BoneSuckin.com

Bouchard Family Farms—
buckwheat
RR 2, Box 2690
West Kent, Maine
(800) 239-3237
www.ployes.com

Breadshop's Natural Foods
16007 Camina de la Cantera
Irwindale, CA 91706
(800) 423-4846
www.hain-celestial.com

Bumblebar
(888) 453-3369
www.bumblebar.com

Butte Creek Mill Stone-Ground
Cornmeal
402 North Royal
Eagle Point, OR 97524
(541) 826-3531

Casabe Rainforest Crackers
and Cookies
(305) 661-8198

'Cause You're Special!
P.O. Box 316
Phillips, WI 54555
(866) NO-WHEAT
www.causeyourespecial.com

Cedarlane Natural Foods
1864 East 22nd Street
Los Angeles, CA 90058
(323) 758-1063

Chebe Manioc Bread Mixes
P.O. Box 991
Newport, VT 05855
(800) 217-9510
www.chebe.com

Cook in the Kitchen Soups
P.O. Box 3
Post Mills, VA 05058
www.cookinthekichen.com

Cornito Pasta
1133 Broadway, Suite 706
New York, NY 10010
(212) 613-1647
www.cornito.com

Cybros, Inc.
P.O. Box 851
Waukesha, WI 53187
(800) 876-2253
www.cyrosinc.com

David Goodbatters
P.O. Box 102, Dept. M
Bausman, PA 17504
(717) 293-7833
www.goodbatter.com

De Boles Pasta
P.O. Box 2059
Hereford, TX 79045
(800) 749-0730
www.hain-celestial.com

Desserts by David Glass
(860) 769-5570

Dietary Specialties, Inc.
10 Leslie Court
Whippany, NJ 07981
(888) 640-2800
www.dietspec.com

Don Pancho Mexican Foods—
gluten-free wraps
3060 Industrial Drive N.E.
Salem, OR 97303
(503) 370-9710
www.donpancho.com

Dowd & Rogers, Inc.
1641 49th Street
Sacramento, CA 95819
(916) 451-6480
www.dowdandrogers.com

Eden Foods, Inc.
701 Tecumseh Road
Clinton, MI 49236
(888) 769-6455
www.edenfoods.com

Edward & Son's Rice Crackers
P.O. Box 1326
Carpinteria, CA 93104
(805) 684-8500
www.edwardandsons.com

Ener-G Foods/Bette Hagman's
Gourmet Blend Mix
P.O. Box 84487
Seattle, WA 98124
(800) 331-5222
www.ener-g.com

The Enochs Mill and Family Farm—
cornmeal
84 Enoch Road
McEwen, TN 37101
(931) 582-3218

Envirokidz Organic Cereals
9100 Van Horne Way
Richmond, BC V6X 1W3, Canada
(604) 248-8777
www.envirokidz.com

Erewhon
200 Reservoir Street
Needham, MA 02494
(800) 422-1125
www.usmillsinc.com

Enjoy Life Foods
(888) 503-6569
www.enjoylife.com

Fantastic Foods, Inc.
580 Gateway Drive
Napa, CA 94559
(800) 288-1089
www.fantasticfoods.com

Fearn Natural Foods—baking
products
www.modernfearn.com

Foods by George
3 King Street
Mahwah, NJ 07430
(201) 612-9700
www.foodsbygeorge.com

Food for Life Baking Co.
2991 East Doherty Street
Corona, CA 92879
(800) 797-5090
www.foodforlife.com

Frookies
2070 Maple Street
Des Plaines, IL 60018
(800) 272-2537

Gardenspot's Finest Baking Mixes
438 White Oak Road
New Holland, PA 17557
(800) 829-5100
www.gardenspotsfinest.com

Genisoy Protein Bars
2351 North Watney Way, Suite C
Fairfield, CA 94533
(888) 436-4769
www.genisoy.com

Gibbs Wild Rice
10400 Billings Road
Live Oak, CA 95953
(800) 824-4932

Gillian's Rolls, Mixes, Pizza Dough,
and Shells
82 Sanderson Avenue
Lynn, MA 01902
(781) 586-0086
www.gilliansfoods.com

Glutano, Gluten-Free Foods Ltd.
Cereal, breads, Barkat ice-cream
cones
www.glutano.com

Gluten-Free Cookie Jar
(888) GLUTEN-O
www.glutenfreecookiejar.com

1-2-3 Gluten-Free Baking Mixes
7545 Fernwood Drive
Cincinnati, OH 45237
www.123glutenfree.com

The Gluten-Free Pantry—
gourmet baking mixes
P.O. Box 840
Glastonbury, CT 06033
(800) 291-8386
www.glutenfree.com

Glutino Foods
3750 Francis Hughes
Laval, QC H7L 5A9, Canada
(800) 363-3438
www.glutino.com

Golden Waves of Grains Bakery
10801 Blondo Street
Omaha, NE 68164
(402) 496-1835

Govinda's Fitness Foods/Bliss Bars
2651 Ariane Drive
San Diego, CA 92117
(800) 900-0108
www.govindabars.com

Grainaissance—mochi and amasake
1580 62nd Street
Emeryville, CA 94608
(800) 472-4697
www.grainaissance.com

Gray's Grist Mill
638 Adamsville Road
Westport, Massachusetts
(508) 636-6075

Hain Foods/Health Valley
16007 Camino de la Cantera
Irwindale, CA 91706
(800) 423-4846
www.hain-celestial.com

Hol-Grain Crackers
307 Ann Street
New Iberia, LA 70560
(800) 551-3245
www.conradmill.com

King Arthur Flours
P.O. Box 876
Norwich, VT 05055
(800) 827-6836
www.kingarthurflour.com

Imagine Foods
734 Franklin Avenue, #444
Garden City, NY 11530
(800) 434-4246
www.imaginefoods.com

Kingsmill Foods
1399 Kennedy Road, Unit 17
Toronto, ON M1P 2L6, Canada
(416) 755-1124
www.kingsmillfoods.com

Kinnikinnick Foods
10940 120th Street
Edmonton, AB T5H 3P7, Canada
(877) 503-4466
www.kinnikinnick.com

Lotus Foods—rice
921 Richmond Street
El Cerrito, CA 94530
(510) 525-3137
www.lotusfoods.com

Liberty Licorice Company
1360 Industrial Avenue
Petaluma, CA 94952
(800) 881-2347

Lundberg Family Farms
P.O. Box 369
Richvale, CA 95974
(530) 882-4551
www.lundbergfarms.com

Manna from Anna Bread Mix
(877) 354-3886
www.glutenevolution.com

Marlene's Mixes
P.O. Box 1821
Whitehouse, TX 75791
(903) 839-3892
www.marlenesmixes.com

Minn-Dak Growers—buckwheat
Highway 81 North
Grand Forks, ND 58208
(701) 746-7453
www.minndak.com

Miss Roben's Baking Mixes
P.O. Box 1149
Frederick, MD 21702
(800) 891-0083
www.missroben.com

Mrs. Leeper's Pasta
(940) 321-2599
www.mrsleeperspasta.com

Mr. Ritt's Bakery
709 East Passyunk Avenue
Philadelphia, PA 19147
(215) 627-3034

Mr. Spice
20 Silva Lane
Middletown, RI 02842
(800) 728-2348
www.mrspice.com

Nature's Hilights
1604 West 5th Street
Chico, CA 95927
(800) 313-6454
www.natures-hilights.com

Nature's Path/Lifestream Cereal and
Frozen Waffles
7453 Progress Way
Delta, BC V4G 1E8, Canada
(888) 808-9505
www.naturespath.com

New Hope Mills
5983 Glen Haven Road
Moravia, NY 13118
(315) 497-0783
www.newhopemilles.com.

Northland Native American
Products—wild rice
1113 Franklin Avenue, E.
Minneapolis, MN 55404
(612) 872-0390
www.northlandvisions.com

Notta Pasta
(800) 243-0897
www.nottapasta.com

Nutiva Snack Bars
(800) 993-4367
www.nutiva.com

Nu-World Amaranth
P.O. Box 2202
Naperville, IL 60567
(630) 369-6819
www.nuworldamaranth.com

Orgran/Roma Foods Products
47-51 Aster Avenue
Carrum Downs, Victoria 3201,
Australia
+613 9776 9044
www.orgran.com

Pacific Foods/Westsoy Beverages
19480 97th Avenue, S.W.
Tualatin, OR 97062
(503) 692-9666
www.pacificfoods.com

Pamela's Cookies and Biscotti
335 Allerton Avenue
South San Francisco, CA 94080
(650) 952-4546
www.pamelasproducts.com

Pastariso Rice Pasta
8175 Winston Churchill Boulevard
Norval, ON L0P 1K0, Canada
(905) 451–7423
www.maplegrovefoods.com

El Peto Products—breads and
mixes
41 Shoemaker Street
Kitchener, ON N2E 3G98, Canada
(800) 387-4064
www.elpeto.com

Quejos—Brazilian-style pre-baked
manioc cheese buns
P.O. Box 814
Santa Monica, CA 90406
www.quejos.com
(310) 829-6802

Ramapo Valley Brewery
122 Orange Avenue
Suffern, NY 10901
(845) 369-7827
www.ramapovalleybrewery.com

Red Mill Farms—Jennie's
Macaroons
290 S. 5th Street
Brooklyn, NY 11211
(718) 384-2150

The Really Great Food Company—
mixes
P.O. Box 2239
St. James, NY 11780
(800) 593-5377
www.reallygreatfood.com

Rice Expressions
www.riceandrecipes.com

The Ruby Range—gourmet
baking mixes
(877) 787-1552
www.therubyrange.com

San-J International—soy sauce
2880 Sprouse Drive
Richmond, VA 23231
(800) 446-5500
www.san-j.com

Schär—crackers, bread sticks,
spaghetti
www.schaer.com

Soy Fields Snack Bars and Cookies
(888) 566-5431
www.midwestbakery.com

St. Claire's Organic Desserts by
EcoNatural Solutions
Boulder, Colorado
(303) 527-1554
www.econaturalsolutions.com

St. Julien Macaroons
White Oak Farms, Inc.
343 Main Street
Sandown, NH 03873
(800) 473-8869
www.whiteoaksfarm.com

Sterk's Bakery
3866 23rd Street
Vineland, ON L0R 1S0, Canada
(905) 562-3086

Sylvan Border Farms Mixes/
Mendocino Gluten-Free
Products, Inc.
P.O. Box 277
Willits, CA 95490
(800) 297-5399
www.sylvanborderfarm.com

Tamarind Tree/A Taste of India
Entrees
395 Main Street
Wakefield, MA 01880
(800) 432-8733; (781) 224-1172
www.tamtree.com

T.C.'s Gluten-Free Flour
6604 East K-4 Highway
Gypsum, KS 67448
(785) 536-4482

Thai Kitchen
30315 Union City Boulevard
Union City, CA 94587
(800) 967-7424
www.thaikitchen.com

The Teff Company
P.O. Box A
Caldwell, ID 83606
(208) 455-0375
www.teffco.com

Terra Chips
58 South Service Road
Melville, NY 11747
(800) 434-4246
www.terrachips.com

Tinkyada Pastas
120 Melford Drive, Unit 8
Scarborough, ON M1B 2X5, Canada
(416) 609-0016
www.ricepasta.com

Tropical Source Chocolate Bars
(510) 686-0116
www.tropicialsourcecandy.com

Van's International Foods—
waffles
20318 Grammercy Place
Torrance, CA 90501
(310) 320-8611
www.vansintl.com

Westbrae
16007 Camino de la Cantera
Irwindale, CA 91706
(800) 434-4246
www.westbrae.com

White Eagle Bakery—almond
cookies
501 Prospect Street, Suite 109
Lakewood, NJ 08701
(732) 886-0739

White Wave, Inc./Silk Soy Milk
1990 North 57th Court
Boulder, CO 90301
(303) 443-3470
www.whitewave.com

Big Food Companies and Processors

Beech-Nut Baby Foods
Box 618
St. Louis, MO 63188
(800) 523-6633
www.beechnut.com

Butterball Turkeys
(800) 323-4848
www.butterball.com

Campbell Soup Company
1 Campbell Place
Camden, NJ 08103
(800) 257-8443
www.campbellsoup.com

Carvel Corporation
(800) 322-4848
www.carvel.com

ConAgra Frozen Foods
P.O. Box 3768
Omaha, NE 68103
(800) 722-1344
www.conagrafoods.com

Dannon
P.O. Box 90296
Allentown, PA 18109
(800) 321-2174
www.dannon.com

Dole
1 Dole Drive
Westlake Village, CA 91362
(818) 879-6600
www.dole.com

Eagle Family Foods
735 Taylor Road, Suite 200
Gahanna, OH 43230
(888) 656-3245
www.eaglebrand.com

Empire Kosher—gluten-free turkeys
(800) 233-7177
www.empirekosher.com

General Mills
P.O. Box 9452
Minneapolis, MN 55440
(800) 231-0308
www.generalmills.com

Gerber Foods
Freemont, MI 49413
(800) 4-GERBER
www.gerber.com

H.J. Heinz
1062 Progress Street
Pittsburgh, PA 15212
(800) 577-2823
www.heinz.com

Hershey Foods
100 Crystal A Drive
Hershey, PA 17033
(800) 468-1714
www.hersheys.com

Jennie-O Turkeys
(800) 328-1756

Jimmy Dean Foods
P.O. Box 2511
Cincinnati, OH 45225
(800) 925-3326
www.jimmydean.com

Kellogg's
Battle Creek, MI 49016
(800) 962-1413
www.kellogs.com

Kraft Foods
(800) 323-0768
www.kraftfoods.com

Shady Brook Farms
(800) 233-8757
www.shadybrook.com

separating the wheat from the chef

'Tis an ill cook who cannot lick his own fingers.

—SHAKESPEARE
Romeo and Juliet

Whenever I have friends to supper, I put on an apron given to me by Beth Hillson, founder and president of the Gluten-Free Pantry, which boldly displays her trademark line exhorting the cook to "separate the wheat from the chef." This is not something I do to keep food from splattering all over the front of me, even though I am not the neatest cook in the world. I do it to entertain, to get a laugh, and use the opportunity to explain to a new acquaintance what a celiac is, what it means to go through life "against the grain." I wear it to put the world on notice that this kitchen and this chef (I use the term loosely) can produce a meal everyone will enjoy without using so much as a whiff of wheat. My apron with its little pin, "Celiacs Do It Gluten-Free," a gift from Elaine Monarch, founder of the Celiac Disease Foundation in Los Angeles, is my way of folding some awareness in with the egg whites as I wield my noncontaminated spatula. My apron wears its scars proudly (the borscht stains that never came all the way out, the time I got it caught in the refrigerator door, or used it to sop up a whole pot of spilled dal). It gives me the confidence to try anything once.

That its creator was once a travel and food writer and restaurant critic is delicious proof that we can make lemonade with the lemons we are given, that we can find joy and inspiration by not seeing the end of something, but rather the beginning. It reminds me again and again of how generous professional chefs are and, in particular, celiac chefs who have made it a cause célèbre to nourish us with their ideas, their refusal to take no for an answer, and their deep-hearted love of good food.

Life is too short for perky-sounding recipes meant to placate the poor soul who can't have the real thing—crustless pizza, mock apple pie, rolls that taste like hockey pucks fool no one. Nor do I relish the idea of eating my food from a plastic bag while everybody eats his or hers from a plate. And I certainly can't imagine cooking something glutenous for my friends and something else for me. If you can't enjoy a meal at your own table, where can you?

Give me something fabulous, something everyone at the table will love, and oh, by the way, make it gluten-free. Ten years ago, most of the celebrity chefs who took my challenge had no idea what gluten-free meant. Even so, they gave us recipes that have become classics. Who can forget Molly O'Neil's glorious Corn and Lobster Pie in a Chili-Polenta Crust or Alex Cormier's Bananas Financier, an exquisite almond torte with caramelized fruit. Kevin Smith's Mexican lasagna is a perennial favorite. When time is ample and the spirit is willing, these are miracles that still materialize in my kitchen; they never fail to amaze friends and family alike.

This time around there is very little need for explanation. Special diets are a way of life in professional kitchens. They are a challenge to a chef's very nature. Awareness and a willingness to please even the grain challenged, has given us mouth-watering choices.

As home cooks and as diners we, too, have become more sophisticated, more familiar with exotic foods and cooking techniques. Thanks to TV's Food Network, an explosion of cookbooks and magazines, the appetite for new recipes has never been more voracious. There's no reason to miss out on all the fun just because you're gluten-free. As often as not nowadays we find chefs who specialize in creating gluten-free meals because he or she or a family member or a good friend needed something wonderful to eat. It may be an old saw, but necessity is still the mother of invention; nurture is the impulse of all good cooks.

When I asked chef Johnny Alamilla, owner of the *nuevo latino* San Francisco restaurant Alma, to share his soul-satisfying and gloriously gluten-free quinoa and potato gratin, he couldn't have been happier to lend his genius to the cause. Globe-hopping chef Shola Olunoyo tried many gluten-free flours before he found one that would allow the cheese soufflé he made for me, the first I have enjoyed in twenty years, to rise to the occasion. The results were so spectacular that he baked a stunning and sinfully rich chocolate version for dessert. And Lee Tobin, the mastermind behind Whole Foods Market's gluten-free Bakehouse, a celiac himself, did not hesitate to contribute his magnificent homemade lasagna (*and* a cupcake in chapter 14). All of which confirms my belief that people who cook for other people are the most generous people in the world.

Once again, I have asked a dozen talented chefs, bakers, foodies, cookbook authors, restaurateurs, rock stars, and downright fashion plates to take my gluten-free challenge. The times have changed, but the criteria haven't. The dish (a) must be fabulous and not something a person would make every day; (b) must be something all assembled will love; and, of course, (c) must be gluten-free.

Here you will find the savory, the sweet, the hearty, the hip, and the healthy. You will find entrees, desserts, light lunches, and party fare from celebrity chefs and ones who are about to be. Some are old friends, most are new and all are celiac-friendly. Among them, whole foods queen Christina Pirello, Bobby Flay of *Boy Meets Grill* fame, Johnny Alamilla, Shola Olunoyo, and Bill Wavrin, executive chef of the fabulous Miraval Spa in Tucson, Arizona. And there is pie, the flaky sweet thing you dream about, from Rebecca Bunting, the newest star on the gluten-free horizon. If you had any doubt, these good and gifted souls will prove once and for all that there has never been a better time to be gluten-free. Read, learn, shop, chop, simmer, cook, lick your fingers, and share the results with those you cherish. Be glad you are that special.

With apologies to the bard, "Ah, what foods these morsels be . . ."

Johnny Alamilla

Alma, San Francisco

Alma is Spanish for soul. And that is exactly what chef Johnny Alamilla serves in abundance in his sizzling, electric blue restaurant in the Mission District. Here Alamilla combines the foods of the Caribbean, Spain, and Portugal with classic French technique and fresh ingredients and somehow ends up with something uniquely American. Coming from French ancestry myself via Haiti and New Orleans, I am particularly drawn to the French and African influence on Latin food. Alamilla grew up with the flavors of Columbia and Peru, learning to cook in his Honduran grandmother's kitchen. Later, he distinguished himself at Postrio, Boulevard, and Farallon before opening his own shop. This is humble food. It is immigrant food, spiced with the flavors and culture and influences of all of Latin America. Alma is the kind of place where you can order *un poco de todo* (a little of each) and find yourself in the company of hip San Franciscans as well as Hispanic families out for Sunday dinner, maybe even an adventurous celiac in search of something really special as well as gluten-free. They come for the yucca fries, the ceviche, and this luscious Peruvian dish with ancho chile cream. In winter, I serve this with roasted pork tenderloin, avocado salad, and a simple dessert of minted fresh fruit and almond paste cookies. This really is food for the *alma*.

Quinoa Potato Gratin with Ancho Chili Cream

Ancho chilis, quinoa, *queso fresco*, and Spanish paprika can be found in almost any Hispanic market, but just as often these specialty foods are turning up, albeit a bit pricier, in places like Whole Foods Market and other gourmet emporiums. For the best-tasting quinoa, it's important to rinse the grains in several changes of fresh water until there is no bitterness left in the water.

Serves 6

1½ cups quinoa
 1 pound small waxy potatoes, such as fingerlings or new potatoes
 2 ancho chilis slit open, stems and seeds removed
 1 tablespoon canola oil
 ½ onion, chopped
 4 cloves garlic, smashed and peeled
 ¾ pound plum tomatoes, halved, seeded, and coarsely chopped
 1 teaspoon toasted ground cumin*
 1 teaspoon mild Spanish paprika
 2 cups heavy cream
 2 cups milk
    Salt
 ⅓ pound *queso fresco* (fresh Mexican cheese), sliced ¼-inch thick,
      then cut into thick matchsticks

1. Rinse the quinoa under cold running water several times. Bring a large pot of salted water to a boil over high heat. Add the quinoa and boil until tender and fully plumped, about 10 minutes. Drain and let cool.

2. Put the potatoes in a saucepan and cover generously with cold salted water. Bring to a boil, then simmer gently until a knife slips in easily. Drain and cool.

3. Toast the ancho chilis in a dry skillet over moderate heat until they are pliable and fragrant, about 2 minutes.

4. Heat the canola oil in a saucepan over moderate heat. Add the onion and garlic and sauté for about 3 minutes to release their fragrance. Add the chilis and stir for about 1 minute, Then add the tomatoes. Stir briskly for about 2 to 3 minutes to soften the tomatoes and release some of their juices. Add the cumin and paprika and cook 1 minute to bring out their fragrance. Then add the cream and milk. Adjust the heat to maintain a gentle simmer and cook until mixture is reduced to 3 cups, about 30 minutes.

5. Strain through a sieve, pressing on the solids. Season with salt.

6. Preheat the oven to 350 degrees. In a large bowl, combine the quinoa with the ancho chili cream. Divide the mixture among six 8-ounce gratin dishes or one large 6-cup gratin dish, spreading it evenly. Slice and salt the potatoes, then bury the slices halfway in the quinoa. Top with pieces of *queso fresco*.

7. Bake until the cheese has melted and the quinoa is hot throughout, about 20 minutes.

8. Let rest 5 minutes before serving.

*Note: Toast whole cumin seeds in a small, dry skillet over moderate heat until fragrant and beginning to color. Cool, then grind in a mortar or spice grinder.

Rebecca Bunting

Rebecca Bunting is a serious goldsmith, which takes an extraordinary amount of creative energy to begin with. She is also a celiac and one of the brightest stars on the gluten-free horizon. On a visit to Philadelphia's annual jewelry show, Rebecca phoned to introduce herself and ask if she could pop in with a few goodies that she had brought all the way from Guilford, Connecticut, her way of saying thank you for *Against the Grain*. I was drawn to her energy the minute I heard her voice and said, "Yes, come." One bite of her Linzer torte with its buttery shortbread told me I had encountered a rare talent.

Her forthcoming cookbook, *Sumptuous and Savory without Gluten or Wheat*, with more than 500 recipes, is a paean to a lifetime of tasting, experiment, and determination not to settle for second best in anything. Especially the tender, tricky, flaky piecrusts she grew up watching her mother turn out with apples, strawberries, blueberries, and rhubarb, even squash, from her father's beloved garden. Pie was a part of life, an unalienable American right. In Rebecca's family, it is what love tastes like.

Rock & Roll Piecrust

Many of you think making a piecrust from scratch is difficult. This is a myth. While pie making may be messier than other kitchen jobs, it's really quite simple. A food processor, a pastry blender, an old-fashioned rolling pin, and a nice flat surface (there are marble slabs made for just this purpose) will make the job much easier, but they are not necessary. Once you master the technique, pie and all its sweet and savory varieties are a permanent part of your repertoire. Rebecca Bunting gives us one crust and three variations—Apple Pie, Chicken Pot Pie, and Red Pepper Lobster Quiche, printed here with permission from this dazzling new star.

Makes 2 crusts

⅔ cup brown rice flour
⅔ cup tapioca flour
⅔ cup potato starch
3 tablespoons cornstarch
1 tablespoon xanthan gum
1½ teaspoons salt
10 tablespoons cold butter, cut into chunks
2 eggs, beaten

Food Processor

1. Place dry ingredients in food processor with metal blade, mixing to combine.

2. Add cold butter chunks and pulse until mixture resembles coarse cornmeal.

3. Add beaten eggs in steady stream through feed tube with machine running. Process until mixture forms a ball.

By Hand

1. Place dry ingredients in mixing bowl. Stir to combine.

2. Add cold butter chunks and cut into flour mixture with pastry blender, fork, or knife, until mixture resembles coarse cornmeal.

3. With wooden spoon, stir in beaten eggs until mixture holds together in a ball.

To Form Dough

1. Divide dough in half and form into two flattened balls.

2. Place one ball on an 18-inch sheet of plastic wrap, dusting lightly with cornstarch.

3. Place a second sheet of plastic wrap on top of dough and roll out with rolling pin into 12-inch disc.

4. Remove top layer of wrap and invert dough over pie plate, centering and easing dough into plate. Gently peel off remaining plastic wrap.

5. If using single crust, flute edges decoratively and use according to recipe. Otherwise, add desired filling and repeat process for top crust, and form decorative edging. Cut slots in top crust for steam holes with a sharp knife, in desired design.

Apple Pie

Select firm tart apples, such as Cortlands, Macouns, or Jonathans.

One 9-inch pie

⅔ cup sugar
2 teaspoons cinnamon
¼ teaspoon ground cardamom
5 to 7 cups peeled, cored and sliced apples

1. Preheat oven to 425 degrees. In large mixing bowl, combine sugar and spices.

2. Add apples and stir until slices are coated with sugar mixture.

3. Place bottom crust in a 9-inch pie plate and fill with apple mixture, forming an even mound.

4. Cover apples with top crust, sealing the edges and fluting decoratively. With a sharp knife cut a few slits in the top.

5. Place pie on baking sheet to catch drips, and bake for 45 to 50 minutes.

6. Serve with a scoop of gluten-free vanilla ice cream or a slice of good cheddar cheese.

Chicken Pot Pie

This is pure comfort food. It can also be made with leftover turkey or beef, which is probably how it was invented in the first place. You can make it with the crust on the bottom and top, or use only a top crust. If you choose the latter, you can half the crust recipe or make two and freeze half for the quiche recipe that follows. If ever there was a perfect winter Sunday supper, this is it.

One 9-inch pie

- 1 large onion, diced
- 1 tablespoon olive oil
- 2 large carrots, diced
- ½ yellow turnip, ½-inch cubes or smaller
- 2½ cups and ½ cup gluten-free chicken broth
- 2 medium potatoes, cubed
- 3 stalks celery, finely sliced
- 1 cup frozen peas
- 3 tablespoons GF flour mix
- 1 cup frozen peas
- 2 cups cooked chicken bits
- ⅓ cup minced fresh parsley
- 1 teaspoon dried herb mixture: thyme, marjoram, sage, rosemary— your choice

  Salt and pepper to taste

1. Preheat oven to 425 degrees.

2. For pie with top crust only, choose an oven-proof skillet or casserole that can be used on the top of the stove. For two crusts, prepare filling in any large saucepan. Sauté onion in oil over low heat until softened.

3. Add carrot and turnip and cook 2 to 3 minutes. Add 2½ cups GF chicken broth with potatoes and celery. Bring to a boil and simmer, covered, 8 to 10 minutes, just until vegetables are tender. Take care not to overcook them.

4. In small bowl, whisk together flour mix and remaining ½ cup broth until smooth. Add to vegetable mixture, along with the frozen peas, chicken, parsley, and herb mixture. Simmer, stirring occasionally, until heated through and thickened. If using canned broth, you may not need any salt.

5. If using one crust, roll out dough roughly to shape of pot, pressing lightly into place on top of filling. Peel off top layer and invert dough over pot, pressing lightly into place on top of filling. Let the edges meet the sides of the dish or not—it's appealing in rustic form. Cut a few slits with a sharp knife. Bake 20 minutes, or until crust is lightly browned.

6. If using two crusts, use a 3-quart casserole dish and line with piecrust. Add filling and top with crust as above. Bake 25 to 30 minutes, or until crust is lightly browned.

Red Pepper Lobster Quiche

We can thank the venerable Julia Child and her landmark *Mastering the Art of French Cooking* for introducing America to the classic quiche Lorraine. But nowadays there are as many variations on this rich bacon, cream, and Gruyère theme as there are kinds of pizzas. Herbs are wonderful in quiche, especially dill with spinach and mushroom. Experiment with whatever is fresh and in season. When using chunky vegetables, steam or sauté them briefly first. Rebecca Bunting's recipe is as glorious a combination as you can imagine with fresh tarragon, succulent lobster, a mild Jarlsberg or Gouda, and the peppery spark of cayenne.

One 9-inch quiche

1   unbaked pie shell
1   tablespoon Dijon mustard
1   cup diced onion
1   tablespoon butter
1   cup lobster meat, cut into bite-sized pieces
3   eggs
1   cup milk
½   cup light cream or half-and-half
1   teaspoon salt
1   tablespoon fresh tarragon, chopped
½   cup mild cheese, such as Jarlsberg or Gouda, cut into chunks
¾   cup thinly sliced roasted red pepper
⅛   teaspoon freshly grated nutmeg
    Sprinkling of cayenne pepper to taste

1. Preheat oven to 325 degrees. Bake pie shell 7 to 10 minutes, until dry but not brown. If crust puffs up at all, pierce it with a fork and lightly flatten. With pastry brush, spread mustard inside crust.

2. Raise oven temperature to 425 degrees. In small skillet, sauté onion in butter until softened. Add lobster and heat another minute. Take off heat and set aside.

3. In mixing bowl, whisk together eggs, milk, cream, salt, tarragon, lobster, and onion. Place pie dish on baking sheet, and pour filling into shell. Add chunks of cheese and arrange slices of red pepper on top. Sprinkle with nutmeg and cayenne.

4. Bake for 10 minutes at 425 degrees, then reduce heat to 350 degrees and bake for an additional 20 to 30 minutes, until knife inserted in custard comes out clean. Cool on rack 5 minutes before serving.

Betty Lou Davis

Few of us are born with an instinct for food as highly developed as New Yorker Betty Lou Davis. Accomplished cook, gardener, artist, and muse (the late Andy Warhol was among the enchanted, as well as a concert pianist or two), she celebrates the ripeness of each season with simple earthy food as only a lover of nature can do.

Simplicity and exactitude are the keys to Davis's remarkable talent. Whether it's tiny tender asparagus from the village farm stand, artisan cheeses, fiery Indian chickpea crackers warmed to just blistering to bring out their spice, ketchup that can only be found at New York's Oyster Bar, or vegetables grown by her own labor, no detail is overlooked. In her hands, simple pasta con aioli (gluten-free, of course) sends a shiver down a celiac's spine; her chestnut torte is a dream come true. She does this not with a showboater's tricks, but with ease and generosity, the marks of the truly gifted.

With this decidedly cloudlike concoction, Davis proves there is no food so humble, or healthy that it can't be seduced into greatness. Those of us lucky enough to find ourselves in her lavender and rosemary–scented sphere gasp with pleasure whenever she enters the kitchen. There are rumors of a cookbook, but until such time we can only hope we will be invited back.

Warm Rosemary Ricotta Mousse

Deceptively rich but oh-so-easy on the figure, this savory baked mousse will soothe and delight the most sophisticated celiac tastes without ever calling attention to its virtues. The secret to its ethereal quality is beating the eggs and ricotta separately. Fresh rosemary and grated lemon zest gives it its zing. Served with tossed spring greens, this is an exquisite light supper or lunch or the perfect beginning for a dinner party. Spread the leftovers (if there are any) on toasted gluten-free bread with a little jam and you've got a breakfast that will have you lingering a bit more than usual.

Serves 4 to 6

2½ cups ricotta cheese
1 tablespoon of finely snipped fresh rosemary
   Finely grated zest of 1 lemon
2 large egg whites
   Salt and freshly ground black pepper to taste
   Olive oil for greasing pan

1. Heat oven to 350 degrees.
2. Lightly oil an 8- or 9-inch springform baking pan.
3. In a mixing bowl, combine ricotta, rosemary, lemon zest, and salt and pepper and set aside. In a separate bowl, beat egg whites to form stiff peaks. Using same beaters, beat ricotta mixture until light and fluffy. Gently combine ricotta mixture and beaten egg whites and pour into a greased springform pan.
4. Bake until ricotta is lightly colored on top, about 30 minutes. It will have risen slightly. Allow to cool slightly and release from pan. Cut into wedges, and serve warm with toasted chickpea crackers or *socca* (see page 238 for recipe).

Variation: Fresh thyme, oregano, or chives may be substituted for rosemary.

Bobby Flay

Bolo, New York

Culinary Institute of America-trained Bobby Flay is a culinary rock star. Darling of the Food Network's *Hot Off the Grill with Bobby Flay*, this cheeky, flame-haired chef is a major force in the way we eat. Before he was thirty, he was voted the James Beard Foundation's Rising Star and sealed his reputation for his unique interpretation of southwestern American sizzle with the now landmark Manhattan restaurant, Mesa Grill, a place I will always hold in special affection as it was the scene of my editor's unveiling of the cover of *Against the Grain*. Bolo, his wildly innovative new kitchen, is dedicated to exploring Spanish cuisine. When he's not dazzling TV viewers with his grill technique, he's autographing his bestselling cookbook, *Boy Meets Grill*, or working on his latest, *Boy Gets Grill.*

It's a wonder he's had time to tempt us with these glamorous and totally gluten-free risotto cakes. A wonder indeed.

Saffron Risotto Cakes with Shrimp, Chili Oil, and Chive Oil

Tapas, or small plates, are a *pasión* of Spaniards who dine at nine or ten and prefer this sophisticated grazing to a heavy meal. It's no surprise these savory dishes have caught on over here in such a big way. These glorious gluten-free saffron rice cakes are one of the many wildly popular *tapas* dishes at Flay's restaurant Bolo. But they can just as easily serve as a spectacular first course or a light lunch. Look for *chilis de arbol* in Latin American markets and some supermarkets.

Makes 24 tapas

- 4½ cups (or more) low-salt, gluten-free chicken broth
- ⅛ teaspoon (generous) crumbled saffron threads
- 2 tablespoons olive oil
- 1½ cups chopped onion
- 1½ cups arborio rice, about 10 ounces
- ½ cup dry white wine
  Nonstick vegetable oil spray
- 1 cup white rice flour
- 4 plus 2 tablespoons canola oil, divided
- 24 large uncooked shrimp, peeled, deveined, and butterflied
  Red Chili Oil and Olive Oil, see recipes below

1. Combine 4½ cups broth and saffron in medium saucepan; bring to boil. Remove from heat; cover to keep warm.

2. Heat olive oil in another medium saucepan over medium heat. Add onion and sauté until tender, about 6 minutes. Add rice; stir 1 minute. Add wine; stir until absorbed, about 1 minute. Add ½ cup saffron broth; stir until absorbed, about 4 minutes. Continue adding broth, ½ cup at a time, until rice is just tender, allowing each addition to be absorbed before adding more and stirring frequently, about 20 minutes total. Season risotto with salt and pepper.

3. Spray rimmed baking sheet with nonstick spray. Spread risotto on prepared sheet, forming irregular 13 × 9-inch rectangle. Cover with plastic wrap; refrigerate until cold and firm, about 2 hours. (Can be made 1 day ahead. Keep chilled.)

4. Preheat oven to 300 degrees. Place rice flour in medium bowl. Season with salt and pepper. Using 2-inch diameter cookie cutter, cut out 24 rounds from risotto. Dredge risotto cakes in rice flour; place on clean baking sheet. Heat 4 tablespoons canola oil in large nonstick skillet over medium heat. Working in batches, add risotto cakes to skillet and cook until golden brown, about 2 minutes per side. Transfer risotto cakes to another baking sheet; place in oven to keep warm.

5. Sprinkle shrimp with salt and pepper. Heat remaining 2 tablespoons canola oil in another large skillet over high heat. Add shrimp and sauté until just opaque in center, about 2 minutes per side.

6. Top each risotto cake with 1 shrimp. Drizzle shrimp with Red Chili Oil and Chive Oil and serve.

Red Chili Oil

About ⅓ cup

4 chilis de arbol
½ cup olive oil

1. Place chilis in small bowl. Add enough hot water to cover; let stand until chiles soften slightly, about 1 hour. Drain.

2. Coarsely chop chilis. Combine chilis and oil in blender and blend until smooth.

3. Season chili oil to taste with salt and pepper. (*Can be made 3 days ahead. Cover and chill. Bring to room temperature before using.*)

Chive Oil
About ½ cup

½ cup olive oil
⅓ cup chopped fresh chives

1. Blend oil and chives in blender until smooth. Strain into small bowl. Discard solids in strainer.

2. Season chive oil to taste with salt and pepper. (*Can be prepared 3 days ahead. Cover and refrigerate. Bring to room temperature before using.*)

Beth Hillson

With her days judging pie-baking contests over, Beth's response to her own diagnosis of celiac disease was to rush off to culinary school. If she was going to cook gluten-free, it was going to be the best gluten-free cooking anybody ever tasted. Twenty years later, the Gluten-Free Pantry stands as a tribute to what can be accomplished when you see the plate as half full. Whenever I must have something gooey and sinfully chocolate (when nothing else will do), I bake a batch of Beth's Chocolate Truffle Brownies. I cut them up and squirrel them away at the back of the freezer to fool myself into not eating the whole pan, but I dream about them and, well, you know the rest. Nowadays, I make sure I've got friends around to share when I make these intensely rich brownies or bake her Danielle's Decadent Chocolate Cake (named for football star Rich Gannon's daughter, Danielle). It's a clever way to see people *and* guarantee no tempting leftovers. Breads made from Beth's white bread mix, straight from the oven and still warm, are the yeasty, chewy real thing as far as I'm concerned. I don't bother with a bread machine. I mix the dough by hand and use the opportunity to work on my muscle tone, changing hands to keep things even. And, of course, there are all kinds of muffins, cookies, breads. Beth Hillson is not only one of the most gifted chefs the celiac world has ever seen, she is one of its most attentive angels. The Gluten-Free Pantry quietly supports research, awareness, lobbying efforts, and all kinds of celiac-friendly causes, its founder and president being one of our most generous boosters.

Chicken Crepes

This is one of those dishes you thought you'd never enjoy again. Savory and rich, with a velvety chicken filling, these crepes are easier than you think. The secret is quick cooking, two 6-inch crepe pans or heavy frying pans and making sure the batter isn't spread too thickly. For an impressive dinner party centerpiece, double the recipe. Once you get your technique down, add sugar to the basic recipe and fill with berries and cream, ice cream and chocolate, and you've got a spectacular dessert.

Serves 4 to 6

CREPES
- 2 eggs
- ¾ cup rice flour
- ¼ cup tapioca starch
- ½ teaspoon salt
- ¼ teaspoon xanthan gum
- 1 tablespoon sugar (if used for dessert)
- ¼ cups milk

1. Whisk together eggs. Combine rice flour, tapioca starch, salt, xanthan gum, and sugar (if used). Whisk into the eggs just to moisten. Mixture will be very thick and gloppy.

2. Add milk, a little at a time, stirring vigorously until mixture is smooth and the consistency of heavy cream. Chill for at least 1 hour and up to 24 hours.

3. Lightly oil one or two 6-inch crepe pans or heavy frying pans and set over medium heat. Pour about 2 tablespoons of batter into each pan and swirl until pan is coated. Pour off excess batter and cook crepes until the edges look very dry, about 1 minute. With a sharp knife, loosen the edges of the pancake. Use fingers to grab the edges and flip the crepe. Cook another 30 seconds and remove each crepe to a platter. Repeat until all batter is used. Wipe pans with oiled paper towel if crepes begin to stick.

CHICKEN FILLING
- 1 tablespoon butter
- 1 medium onion, chopped
- 1 green pepper, seeded and chopped
- 3 cups cooked chicken, chopped
- 1 tablespoon capers

1 teaspoon Dijon mustard

Juice of 1 lemon

2 cups gluten-free chicken broth

2 tablespoons cornstarch mixed with 2 tablespoons water

½ cup heavy cream (or milk)

½ cup grated Parmesan cheese

1. Preheat oven to 350 degrees.

2. Melt butter and sauté onion and pepper until soft. Add chicken, capers, mustard, and lemon juice and stir to combine.

3. In a small saucepan, bring the chicken broth to a boil. Stir in cornstarch mixture and stir until broth thickens. Simmer 1 minute and remove from heat. Add the cream. Spoon ½ cup of this mixture into the chicken mixture.

4. Spoon ¼ cup of the filling into the center of each crepe and roll the crepes. Set snugly into a large, buttered casserole. Top with remaining sauce and sprinkle with cheese. Cover with a sheet of buttered aluminum foil. Bake until bubbly, about 20 minutes.

Shola Olunoyo

An unprepossessing house near the University of Pennsylvania, just like any other in the row of aging Victorians, is headquarters to one of the most talented, well-traveled, and widely experienced chefs in the world. Nigerian-born Shola Olunoyo waits at the top of the steep steps leading to his Studio Kitchen where he cooks for groups like us, caters special events, and gives cooking lessons to professional chefs-in-training. He is the color of good melting chocolate, tall and lean, and movie-star handsome, and we have been told to expect the meal of our lives. The stairs are lined with photographs, gleaming copper sauciers, whisks, bowls, and his tools of the trade, or *batterie de cuisine*. The studio itself is a tribute to his globe-trotting—with mementos of his education at the Cordon Bleu and apprenticeships in the most famous kitchens in the world, such as those of legendary teachers Paul Bocuse and Fernand Point. There is much cooking gossip (where to buy the sweetest scallops—Philadelphia's Reading Terminal Market—how to roast pork overnight so that it's fork tender—slowly in a low oven—whose reputation is undeserved and whose is not—I really can't say), all of it served up with humor and charm and food none of us will ever forget.

Least of all me. The friend who has arranged this special evening has explained to Shola that this meal must be gluten-free, not just for yours truly, but for everyone. Shola tells me he has tried the cheese soufflé he is serving as our first course with three different gluten-free flours before deciding it was potato starch that rose to his standards. I am amazed that he has gone to so much trouble, and he gently reminds me that it's not just my diet in question, it's *his* reputation, too. He knows there is no such thing as too much of a good thing when you have not tasted such delights for many years. Dessert is a puffed-up, intensely chocolate version of our first course, served with homemade pistachio ice cream. When it arrives, I am close to tears.

As I was again when Shola gladly gave me permission to share these treats with you.

Classic Cheese Soufflé

This savory concoction can be a spectacular first course or it can be the centerpiece of a simple supper or Sunday lunch. Accompanied by a robust salad of arugula and grilled mushrooms, a smoky merlot, and grilled fresh figs drizzled with some leftover wine—be still my gentle heart! As with all uncomplicated foods, the secret is not stinting on the ingredients. Buy the best, and freshest eggs and herbs and Gruyere you can find, and make sure you fold the egg whites into the béchamel and cheese mixture with a gentle hand. Imagine you are mixing clouds. Remember that a soufflé waits for no one. The minute it comes out of the oven, take it, triumphant, to the table.

Serves 8

8   eight-ounce ramekins
    Melted butter or cooking spray
    Gluten-free flour for dusting ramekins
4   tablespoons butter
3   tablespoons potato starch
2   cups half-and-half
    Salt, pepper, and nutmeg
2   egg yolks
    Fresh thyme
1   cup Gruyère cheese, grated, plus extra to sprinkle over the soufflés
5   egg whites

1. Preheat oven to 375 degrees.
2. Prepare the ramekins—spray with a nonstick cooking spray or brush with melted butter. Add some gluten-free flour and coat the bottom and sides evenly. Refrigerate to chill and set.

3. To prepare a béchamel sauce, melt butter on low heat. Add the potato starch and whisk until well blended. Add all the half-and-half at once, and whisk to blend. Raise the heat and whisk frequently, paying particular attention to scraping the bottom of the pan so it doesn't burn.

4. When the mixture thickens, lower the heat and season with salt, pepper, and nutmeg. Pass through a fine strainer to remove any lumps. Cool on a bowl of ice. (Béchamel can be made a day ahead and refrigerated.)

5. When cool, whisk the egg yolks, thyme, and cheese into the béchamel sauce.

6. In a mixer or with a handheld electric whisk, whisk the egg whites until they form firm peaks. Fold the whites into the béchamel and cheese mixture, a third at a time, with a rubber spatula. Fold gently until well combined, without losing too much volume on the egg whites.

7. Spoon combined batter into ramekins just below the rim. Sprinkle the top with the additional cheese. Soufflés can be chilled in the refrigerator for about 1 hour or baked immediately.

8. Bake for about 15 to 20 minutes until the top is puffed and golden. Serve immediately.

Dark Chocolate Soufflé

Dessert doesn't get much better than this. Good chocolate and cocoa, butter, eggs, and sugar is a fitting finale to a special meal. I like my chocolate soufflé unadorned, but a dollop of freshly whipped cream couldn't hurt. It bears repeating: a soufflé will not wait. Bake while clearing the dishes. Let people chat for a minute. Serve coffee. Then make an entrance.

Serves 8

8   eight-ounce ramekins (ceramic or foil)
    Melted butter for coating ramekins
    Cocoa powder for dusting ramekins
½   pound semisweet chocolate, chopped into small chunks
1   stick or 8 tablespoons butter
5   whole eggs
½   cup sugar
1   teaspoon gluten-free vanilla extract
3   tablespoons rice flour, sifted

1. Preheat oven to 375 degrees.

2. Brush the ramekins with melted butter and coat with cocoa powder (foil ramekins should be well coated). Chill in the refrigerator.

3. In a large bowl, melt chocolate and butter together over simmering water. Stir together with a rubber spatula until smooth. Let the mixture cool slightly.

4. In the bowl of a mixer, whisk whole eggs, sugar, and vanilla at high speed until tripled in volume. Fold ⅓ of egg/sugar mixture into chocolate/butter mixture. Add the rice flour. Fold in the rest of the egg/sugar mixture carefully.

5. Fill ramekins to just below the rim. Soufflés can be held in the refrigerator at this point for up to 24 hours.

6. Bake for about 12 to 15 minutes or until soufflés have risen and are slightly liquid in the middle. Serve straight from the ramekin or unmold onto a plate.

Christina Pirello

Christina Perillo really *did* save her own life and eat happily ever after. The first time we met, I understood exactly how transforming eating the right foods can be. From her glowing good looks to her vibrant energy, she is a living tribute to the benefits of eating a vegetarian diet featuring nonprocessed whole foods that are alive and bursting with health. Emmy Award–winning host of public television's *Christina Cooks*, Christina is the author of four cookbooks, including *Glow*, delicious proof that beauty is not what you put *on*, it's what you put *in*. A graduate of and teacher at the Kushi Institute, Christina combines ancient Chinese principles with her Mediterranean passion for food and puts noncarnivorous eating on the culinary map. There are foods for warmth, vitality, vibrancy, and balance; there are foods that are *yin* and others that are *yang*. Ask and Christina will explain. Or, she will simply teach you to cook first-class vegetarian fare, food with a global conscience as well as the ability to impress your family and friends. With a bit of adaptation and resourcefulness, any celiac can eat like someone who knows health is something you need to keep feeding.

This gorgeous paella comes from *Everything You Wanted to Know about Whole Foods but Were Afraid to Ask* (HP Books) and is proof that vegetarian pleasures can be gluten-free.

Spring Vegetable Paella

This vegan version of the Spanish classic is gloriously gluten- and lactose-free. Saffron and fennel give it its exotic flavor, while fresh vegetables and garlic give it its zing. The idea here is texture and multilayered tastes.

Serves 5 to 6

1	small fennel bulb, cut into 1-inch chunks and 2 tablespoons minced fronds
2 to 3	bunches baby carrots, left whole and tops minced
3 to 4	spring turnips, cut into large dice
3 to 4	new potatoes, cut into large dice
1	tablespoon extra-virgin olive oil, plus extra for drizzling
6 or 7	sprigs fresh flat-leaf parsley
3 to 4	cloves fresh garlic, finely minced
1	tablespoon sweet paprika
1	teaspoon saffron threads
	Sea salt
1	yellow onion, diced
4	ripe plum tomatoes, diced (do not peel or seed)
2	cups brown arborio rice
4	cups spring or filtered water
¾	cup dry white wine
10 to 12	asparagus spears, tough ends snapped off and stalks cut into 1-inch pieces
1	cup cooked chickpeas

1. Preheat the oven to 450 degrees. Place the fennel bulbs, whole carrots, turnips, and potatoes in a mixing bowl. Drizzle with olive oil and toss to coat. Transfer to a shallow baking dish and bake, uncovered, about 1 hour, until tender and lightly browned.

2. Take about 5 sprigs of the parsley and finely mince. Mix with the garlic, paprika, saffron, and about 1 teaspoon salt. Stir well to combine and set aside.

3. Place 1 tablespoon oil and the onion in a deep skillet over medium heat. When the onion begins to sizzle, add a pinch of salt and sauté for 1 minute. Stir in the tomatoes, rice, and the parsley mixture. Add the water and wine, cover, and bring to a boil. Reduce the heat to low and simmer for about 15 minutes. Stir in the asparagus, chickpeas, and roasted vegetables. Increase heat to medium, cover, and cook until liquid has been absorbed into the rice mixture, stirring often, about 20 minutes.

4. Season lightly with salt and stir in the fennel leaves and carrot tops. Serve garnished with remaining parsley sprigs.

Bryan Sikora and Aimee Olexy

Django, Philadelphia

Once upon a time, a talented Culinary Institute of America–trained young chef and his lovely, equally food-obsessed bride decided to quit their restaurant jobs in Denver, move back to Philadelphia where she was from, and open the kind of restaurant they had always dreamed of. It would be a place that indulged her dedication to fresh, local ingredients, artisan cheeses from small area farms and producers, and it would be homey and as unpretentious as she. He envisioned a kitchen that would feature the highly personal and improvisational cuisine that would spring from his classical culinary training. If food is memory, his dishes would live just on the tip of the tongue, evoking their Spanish, Italian, Northern European, and Gypsy roots, familiar yet indefinable, jazzy and deeply satisfying. They would fill this place with local art, handmade linens, wild flowers, music, and the sounds of neighbor greeting neighbor. And they would never get so big that they would lose sight of all the small but telling details.

The result is a tiny Philadelphia BYOB named for Django Reinhart, the Gypsy guitarist who was the toast of Paris in the 1940s. Django has been featured in the *New York Times, Gourmet Magazine, Los Angeles Times, Travel & Leisure, USA Today*, and was named by *Organic Style Magazine* as one of the top 20 "green restaurants" in the country. There isn't enough room to hang up all their stars. Has it gone to their heads? No.

Bryan pens little hearts next to dishes that are safe for me to eat. Aimee gladly tells me where to find the best local farm-raised trout, greens, goat cheese. And this is the heavenly cheesecake I dream about days before dining with this extraordinary young couple. For those of you who can't stroll in and order your own . . .

Goat Cheese Cake with Nut Crust
and Lemon Curd

This glorious cheesecake isn't as sweet and heavy as the typical cream cheese varieties. Its secret is a good goat cheese—a nice chèvre or Montrachet—spiked with the tartness of lemon curd, the crunch of roasted pine nuts and almonds, and the merest drizzle of ruby port syrup. This is a showstopper which can be baked in 4 individual 4-inch springform pans or one 8-inch springform pan.

Serves four to six

BATTER

- 10 ounces goat cheese
- 6 ounces cream cheese
- ½ cup sugar
- 3 large eggs
- Zest of one lemon

CRUST

- ½ cup pine nuts, roasted*
- ½ cup almonds, roasted*
- ⅛ cup brown sugar
- 2 tablespoons diced cold butter
- Dash of salt

*Note: To roast nuts, coarsely chop and arrange on a baking sheet in one layer Roast at 300 degrees for 10 minutes or until slightly golden in color.

Assembling

1. Preheat oven to 325 degrees.

2. Allow all batter ingredients to come to room temperature. Mix by hand or in mixer until batter is smooth—a few lumps are okay. Set aside. In a food processor, coarsely grind roasted almonds and pine nuts.

3. Add the rest of crust ingredients—brown sugar, butter, and salt to nuts—and pulse in food processor. Crust should resemble the consistency of graham cracker crust. Press crust in pans and bake for 7 minutes.

4. Pour batter into baked crust. Set baking pans in a bowl with a little bit of water and place on a baking sheet to ensure cakes bake evenly.

5. Bake until top is set and lightly colored, approximately 30 to 35 minutes for large pan; 20 to 25 minutes for individual pans.

LEMON CURD
    5 egg yolks
    ½ cup confectioners' sugar
    ¼ cup fresh lemon juice
    ⅛ pound sweet butter
    1 tablespoon cold water

1. Whisk together egg yolks, sugar, and lemon juice over double boiler until thick and slightly glossy.
2. Take off heat and whisk in butter and water. Set aside.

RUBY PORT SYRUP
    1 cup of Ruby port

1. Pour port into a saucepan over medium heat until glossy and reduced to about a ¼ of a cup, approximately 45 minutes.
2. Serve each slice of cheesecake with a dollop of lemon curd and a drizzle of warm port syrup. Expect requests for seconds.

Lee Tobin

They call him "gluten-free Lee." Life was good for this Whole Foods Market kitchen wizard from North Carolina until a diagnosis of celiac disease made for the ultimate cruelty—a chef who can't taste his own food. Depression set in, followed by one failed experiment after another. But Lee persevered, figuring that one day he'd get up one more time than he fell down. After convincing his company to let him do the unheard of—scrub down their huge commercial kitchen for any possible cross contamination and start again—he succeeded. He developed recipes for orange cranberry scones, chocolate chip cookies, blueberry muffins, then pizza crusts and cream biscuits. Next came bread. An edible version took a whole year to develop. Several more months later, he delivered the real McCoy—not the kind that's pre-sliced, frozen solid, and shipped out in the mail, but fresh, fragrant loaves of the caliber most of us had given up on ever tasting again. After that, Lee and his growing team started baking wedding cakes, from a tiny two-tiered miniature to a full-sized traditional French *croquembouche*, with over 300 gluten-free cream puffs. The rest is history. Customers flock to the Chapel Hill Whole Foods Market from as far away as South Carolina and Virginia. One customer ships a supply to a daughter in Alaska. Now Lee has opened the new Whole Foods Market Gluten-Free Bakehouse that will ship to all stores between Atlanta and Philadelphia. After that, the entire East Coast. Who knows where this will end?

The moral of the story: adversity makes us shine in ways we never dreamed.

Roasted Vegetable Lasagna

There is nothing like the fragrance of roasting vegetables or the taste of fresh pasta made from scratch with bubbly cheese and fire-roasted tomatoes. This classic vegetarian lasagna is the gluten-free real thing and it can make even the most carnivorous among us forget we are meat eaters. This dish takes time, especially, if you are going for the brass ring and making the pasta dough yourself. (Don't feel guilty if you don't have the time. Tinkyada lasagna sheets work beautifully here.) Put on some Puccini, chop, roast, stir, assemble, and bake, then phone around until you have enough friends to supply the bravos. With thanks to Lee Tobin and Whole Foods Market, this will be the best lasagna you've ever eaten.

Serves 8 to 10

THE VEGETABLES

2 medium onions, diced
2 green peppers, diced
1 yellow pepper, diced
12 ounces button mushrooms, quartered
1 small eggplant, diced
8 cloves garlic, peeled
2 tablespoons olive oil

THE MARINADE

½ cup olive oil
⅓ cup balsamic vinegar
1 teaspoon salt
½ teaspoon ground pepper

THE SAUCE
- 2 28-ounce cans fire-roasted diced tomatoes
- 1 tablespoon oregano
- 2 tablespoons fresh basil
- 1 teaspoon salt
- ½ teaspoon ground pepper

THE FILLING
- 2 cups ricotta cheese
- 2 teaspoons fresh basil
- 1 beaten egg

THE CHEESE MIXTURE
- 2 cups mozzarella, shredded
- ½ cup smoked mozzarella, shredded
- ½ cup freshly grated Parmesan

THE FRESH PASTA
- ½ cup cornstarch
- ½ cup tapioca starch
- ⅓ cup potato starch
- ⅓ cup rice flour
- 2 tablespoons xanthan gum
- 4 large eggs
- 2 tablespoons olive oil

Preparing the Ingredients

1. Preheat oven to 350 degrees.
2. Line 4 baking pans with parchment.
3. Toss the onions with ¼ of the marinade and spread in a single layer in one pan.
4. Repeat with the peppers, mushrooms, and eggplant, each in its own pan.
5. Roast the vegetables for about 30 minutes, or until they are caramelized and have given up much of their moisture. (You may need to roast 2 pans at a time if your oven cannot accommodate all 4 at once.)
6. Toss the garlic with 2 tablespoons of olive oil and roast it in a small metal bowl, covered with aluminum foil, for about 20 minutes, or until soft.

Preparing the Pasta

1. Mix the dry pasta ingredients well in an electric stand mixer with the paddle attachment. Add the eggs and olive oil, beating on high speed for 3 minutes. Turn the dough onto a rice-floured board, and divide it into 9 portions. A pasta machine is helpful at this point, but generations of Italian cooks have rolled dough by hand.

2. Crank or hand-roll each portion of dough onto a sheet approximately 3 × 5 inches. Mix the roasted garlic and vegetables into the sauce ingredients.

3. In separate bowl, mix the filling ingredients and cheese mixture.

Assembly

1. Grease the bottom and sides of a 9 × 15-inch baking dish with 2 tablespoons olive oil and layer the lasagna as follows:

¼ of the sauce
3 pasta sheets
½ of the ricotta filling (spread carefully to avoid tearing pasta)
¼ of the cheese mixture
¼ of the sauce
3 more pasta sheets
Remaining ½ of the ricotta filling
¼ of the cheese mixture
¼ of the sauce
Final 3 pasta sheets
Remaining ¼ of the sauce
Remaining ½ of the cheese mixture

2. Bake uncovered in a 325-degree oven for about 40 minutes, or until cheese starts to brown nicely. Let the lasagna rest for 10 minutes before serving (if you can stand it!). Garnish with chopped fresh herbs or parsley.

Bill Wavrin

There are so many reasons to go to a spa like Rancho La Puerta in Tecate, Mexico. My first visit was to heal after years of being sick, another time was to lose a few pounds along with some stress. Still another was to begin a new life as a novelist and to release my long pent-up creative energy in the shadow of Mount Kuchima. Sometimes we need to get away to take fitness to a new level, or maybe to think about what's next in our lives, to rededicate ourselves to an old path or to find a new one. One woman I know goes on her birthday every year and signs up for a program of meditation, yoga, and gentle contemplative walks called The Inner Journey.

One compelling reason to go back to Rancho year after year was Bill Wavrin, executive chef, now of Arizona's Miraval Resort. When I told him I wanted to see if I could survive the all-day mountain hike, he packed my backpack the night before with a celiac-friendly lunch and marked it with my initials. When I worried there was nothing for me to eat on his day off, he marched into the kitchen and made me a plate of spicy chili and tortillas, a favorite of the local ranch workers. It was so good, the other guests at my table wanted some, too. Every morning he made sure I had my quinoa porridge or rice cereal, gluten-free bread, and tortillas. He did it all with a big, broad smile and glad heart that let you know he really gets a kick out of pleasing people on special diets.

Herewith, a very special Mexican polenta from the author of the award-winning *Rancho La Puerta Spa Cookbook*.

Roasted Chili Polenta with Shiitake Tomatillo Sauce

With its silky sauce, this savory polenta is a masterpiece of texture, flavor, and heat without the usual calories and fat one would expect from such a rich dish. The trick is fresh Anaheim or Ortego chilis and roasting the peppers over an open flame to give them their smoky flavor. This is a great party dish or company casserole and can be assembled in advance.

Serves 8 to 10

- 1 onion, diced
- 1 rib celery, diced
- 1 red bell pepper, diced
- ½ teaspoon olive oil
- 3 cloves garlic, minced
- 1 teaspoon cumin
- ¼ teaspoon chili flakes
- 2 cups corn kernels, fresh, if possible
- ¼ cup polenta
- 2 carrots, shredded
- 2 tablespoons fresh oregano, chopped

  1 cup gluten-free nonfat yogurt
20 ounces Parmesan cheese, grated
20 ounces Monterey Jack cheese, grated
    Pinch of black pepper
    Gluten-free, low-sodium soy sauce to taste
  6 egg whites, lightly beaten
    Anaheim or Ortego chilis, washed, roasted, peeled, and seeded.
  2 cups gluten-free vegetable stock or water

1. Preheat oven to 375 degrees. In a sauté pan over medium heat, sauté the onion, celery, and red bell pepper in olive oil until onion is golden. Add garlic, cumin, and chili flakes and cook an additional 2 to 3 minutes.

2. Place mixture in a large mixing bowl, add 1 cup of corn, the polenta, carrot, oregano, yogurt, the cheeses, pepper, soy sauce, egg whites, and set aside.

3. Place the stock or water and 1 cup of corn in a blender and purée until smooth. Add to the mixture. Blend well. Adjust seasoning to taste with soy sauce.

4. Coat an ovenproof casserole with olive oil or cooking spray. Layer the chilis on the bottom of the pan and pour the mixture carefully into the casserole, smoothing with a spoon to even out the top.

5. Cover with foil and bake for approximately 1 hour and 15 minutes. Allow casserole to rest 15 minutes before serving. Top each serving with Shiitake Tomatillo Sauce.

SHIITAKE TOMATILLO SAUCE
  ¼ teaspoon olive oil
  1 onion, peeled and julienned
  1 leek, julienned, white section only
  2 shiitake mushrooms, stems removed and julienned
  4 cloves garlic, peeled and minced
  2 tablespoons fresh oregano, stemmed and chopped
  2 tomatillos, husked (you can substitute green tomatoes)
  2 cups gluten-free vegetable or chicken stock
  2 red bell peppers, stemmed, seeded, and roasted
    Salt and pepper to taste

1. In a saucepan over medium heat, sauté the onion and leek in olive oil until the onions are very brown (take care not to burn). Add mushrooms, ½ the garlic and oregano, and sauté 5 minutes more or until the mushrooms are soft. Set aside in a mixing bowl.

2. In a separate saucepan, combine the tomatillos, stock, and remaining garlic. Simmer over medium heat for 15 minutes. Strain the tomatillos from the stock, reserving the stock.

3. Place tomatillos in a blender with the bell peppers, adding a little stock and blend to purée (take special care blending as the tomatillos are hot).

4. Mix with the onion mushroom mixture. Adjust seasoning.

5. Place in a saucepan and bring to a simmer for 1 to 2 minutes. Serve hot over roasted chili polenta or other rice dishes.

PART III

You Need to Get Out More

etiquette for the allergic

Some years ago, my husband and I had the good fortune to attend a dinner party for which the hostess had planned months in advance. We found ourselves at an impeccable table full of flowers, candles, gorgeous food, exquisite wine, and the perfect mix of people, the seating of whom had been considered with great care and with a certain mischief. Conversation virtually crackled with good cheer and interesting stories until someone at the other end of the gleaming, mile-long mahogany table, too far away for the subtlety of a whispered reply, asked my husband if it was true, as the man's dinner companion had pointed out, that he had recently undergone brain surgery.

It was, unfortunately, true. My husband had had surgery several months earlier to remove a tumor that would certainly have killed him if it had not been discovered. In fact, his jocular presence at that very dinner table was nothing short of a miracle. I had been hoping this festive evening would help both of us to begin to forget our ordeal. I was not unaware of the frisson of tension that quickly took hold.

All conversation ceased. The guests waited. Soup spoons hung in midair. The hostess stared down at her plate and steeled herself for the pall that would surely settle over her lovely party along with the grisly details that would inevitably follow an affirmative answer. Sensing this and understanding that he held the success of our friend's evening in his power, my husband said nothing, merely smiled. He appeared to be considering the path that would lead him out of the discomfort that had become palpable.

Finally, and with the perfect timing of a stand-up comic, he paused, gave the gathering his most wicked look, winked at our hostess who was growing paler by second, and said, "Brain surgery? Yes, indeed. I've just had one installed."

The room exhaled, the guests once again broke up into conversation groups, our relieved hostess smiled broadly, and we exchanged the look between husband and wife that says, "Well done."

Someone, I believe it may have been Miss Manners, once said, "Etiquette is what you do for other people to make yourself feel better." Certainly, knowing what to do in any given situation involves a great deal of empathy. No doubt most social sins are committed not out of malice, ignorance, dim-wittedness, thwarted toilet training, or any number of failings on the parts of our parents, but out of sheer self-centeredness and the misguided belief that everyone around us will be fascinated by the minutiae of our suffering.

My husband saved that evening not because he is the world's greatest wit, but because he knew that as soon as the question was asked, the evening needed saving. Rather than point out his fellow guest's rudeness at asking in the first place, causing a different kind of discomfort, or mutter a long-suffering response meant to elicit pity for what was surely one of the most traumatic episodes of his life, he chose to save the man, and his own privacy. Most important, he rescued the spirit of joie de vivre our friend had worked so hard to achieve. He simply understood the situation from another's point of view and gave the answer our hostess was praying for. He empathized.

It is said that Abraham Lincoln did this when the White House butler dropped the Thanksgiving turkey in full view of the distinguished guests. With a sly look at his guests, he spared the poor man. "Why don't we just serve the other one?" the president said.

King George I was said to have abandoned his napkin and lifted his finger bowl to his lips when his guest, a chieftain from an African tribe, dined at court, showing all the snickering lords and ladies to be the snobs they really were (rumor has it the word snob comes from the French sans nobilité, meaning "without nobility"), thus proving that the greater the man, the greater his courtesy. Good manners always include, never exclude.

A diet as restrictive as ours is not without its social cost, but I find the harder I work at helping others become comfortable with my restrictions, the more comfortable they, in turn, attempt to make me. The old saws were never truer: "To be loved, one must love; to receive, give; to have a friend, be a friend." I might add, "To be well hosted, host often and well."

So how do you prevent your presence at the dinner table from causing an allergic reaction all its own?

We are told manners today are meant to be flexible. Forget it. The following rules apply to any situation where you are not among members of your own family, or very close friends who should know better.

Rule No. 1

Always, always, always let your host know about your diet ahead of time.

This includes weddings, bar mitzvahs, showers, parties, suppers, lunches, barbecues, picnics—any meal prepared for you by someone else. There are no exceptions. Even if the person is a casual acquaintance and you are included in a large party, ask what is being served, either personally or through a closer friend. Always explain why you need to know and, if necessary, offer to supply a dish that's safe for you. Nine times out of ten the hostess will surprise you with something gluten-free.

While it's perfectly acceptable to phone the bride and ask what is being served at a small reception at home, I'm not suggesting that you rush to the nearest phone if a large wedding is planned. Even if the bride is a brilliant surgeon, most likely she will be temporarily insane, living on a cloud of tulle, arguing the fine points of the seating plan, ushers, flowers, music, or last-minute fittings that will make your call seem hopelessly selfish and badly timed. You have a choice here: either eat first and nibble carefully at the reception, or treat it like any other large party.

When invited to a large party held in a restaurant, hotel, or catering establishment, phone the banquet office and ask to speak to the person in charge of the event. These people know the dinner down to the last radish rose. You can't change the menu, and it's extremely rude to try, but once you know what will be served, you will know how much to eat beforehand or if slipping a few extras into your purse or pocket would make sense.

At smaller dinner parties that are catered in the home, it is perfectly acceptable to walk into the kitchen and ask the caterer what's in the dishes being served. The hostess probably doesn't know the answers to your questions anyway, and she will be too busy being gracious to be bothered with them unless you seize up and topple into the pool. Who better than the cook to steer you in the right direction? In my experience, caterers love talking to guests, not only because they want to help, but because it's a great way to get more business. They certainly don't want you to get sick and mention their company's name.

A word of caution. Always be sensitive to the caterer's responsibilities before asking your questions—the moment before twenty individual chocolate soufflés exit the oven is not an ideal one if you want a serious answer. It is not polite, nor is it attractive, to ruin everyone else's dessert just because you can't eat it.

It's perfectly okay and, in fact, polite to let your hosts know that you have checked with the caterer. They will be relieved that you will not go hungry at their party, and you will be seen as supremely considerate, a quality worthy of many repeat invitations. You may even find the next time there is something special ordered for you.

Many celiacs say nothing because they don't want to create extra work or be any trouble. The truth is, it's rude not to explain your diet. There's nothing worse than finding out too late that one of your guests can't eat what you've taken the trouble to prepare. A party is a gift. Imagine how terrible you'd feel if yours sat in front of the recipient unopened.

Rule No. 2

Never, under any circumstances, embarrass the host or hostess by announcing that you can't eat something he or she is serving.

If the offending substance finds its way onto your plate, say nothing. Simply slide it to one side, move it around, hide it in a pile of potatoes or under a nice big soup spoon. If all else fails, give it to the dog. Think about how creative you were disposing of Brussel sprouts as a kid and do the same thing. It shouldn't be hard, given that you are not regarded with as much suspicion as you were then. Understand that no one but your dry cleaner will ever see the insides of your pockets.

If these and other diversionary tactics fail and you get caught anyway, try to be diplomatic. Try something like "It's my fault, I really didn't make myself clear." Or, "How could you have known, it took me years to figure out what gluten was." Or, "I'm perfectly fine, I had an enormous lunch"—then change the subject. "Speaking of pasta, how was your trip to Italy? . . . You know, these dumplings remind me of the twins. How are those darling chubby babies [insert grandchildren, godchildren, nieces, nephews, pets] of yours?" You get the idea.

When you phone the next day to thank the host (you always do that, don't you?), make it a point to say how sorry you are that you didn't explain your problem clearly enough. He or she may be too embarrassed to mention it, but this doesn't mean it is forgotten. By confronting your faux pas in the most gracious way possible, you'll be nipping any resentment in the bud. Unless the person is made of cement, you will be ensuring it won't happen to you again because you are providing an opening for the person to ask exactly what you can eat for next time.

It's never easy being a good guest, and it's even harder in your case.

Rule No. 3

Never, under penalty of death-by-pasta, answer the question, "What happens when you have a little?" with the truth.

In this case, it is not a sin to tell a lie. If "You don't want to know" or "After this beautiful lunch [dinner, brunch, whatever], I don't think [name of host or hostess] would appreciate hearing about this right now" isn't enough to change the subject and stop any further questions cold, make an answer up.

Say that when you have the tiniest bit of gluten, you are overcome with the urge to fondle warm rolls. Tell them that you cannot control your compulsion to lick plates, that you are overcome by "gluteny." Make up a story about catching cold from the wheat germs or a tale about a cereal killer. Say anything but the truth and all its gastrointestinal detail. No amount of coaxing or encouragement should delude you into thinking people really want to hear about it. They don't.

If the comment is funny enough, your inquisitor will soon forget the question, like you a whole lot better for the reply, and move on to another topic. This is not because the person has forgotten the question so easily, it's because most people really don't want to know the details. Questions like these are usually asked out of some odd social obligation to express interest in what they really don't care about. Most people expect the other person to play by the rules and keep the answer as short and as interesting as possible.

If you're not sure this is true, remember the time someone asked you how you were feeling after that hernia operation and you told him in excruciating detail. You'll see that same frozen smile if you talk about your gastrointestinal tract at the dinner table.

Of course, you never know. You may run into a gastroenterologist or a baker interested in developing a gluten-free tart or the government person in charge of food labeling, or, as I really did once, the inventor of Beano. While this conversation may be fascinating to the two of you, it's best to continue the discussion somewhere less public.

Remember that this rule only applies to social situations. If a waiter asks you what happens if you get a little gluten, the appropriate answer is "I'll get sick and die in this chair and my children will own this restaurant."

There are exceptions even to my rules. What if you are invited time after time to a family or friend's table where your special diet is never acknowledged? You know this because (1) they never liked you in the first place; and (2) make fun of your food at every turn. I say don't wait for the question that will never come. Wait until everyone is seated and warming to their favorite subjects, then let them have it. Describe in every lurid detail what happens to you, "just in case anybody is interested." The truth can be wonderful vehicle for venting hostility.

Rule No. 4

Always eat a little something before going out to eat.

The comedian Elaine Boozler does a wildly funny routine about women who eat entire quarts of ice cream, then pick at salads in front of their dates. Scarlett O'Hara made a career of this. While antebellum society felt it was unseemly for a woman of healthy appetites to be seen chowing down at a plantation picnic, your reason for doing the same should be obvious.

It's tough to be polite on an empty stomach. In fact, there's a strong potential for cheating if you arrive at a party and find there's nothing for you to eat. Your ability to hold a conversation and be an interesting and lively guest really takes a nosedive when your stomach is growling.

Even if you think you know what is being served, an evening out can hold some nasty surprises for people whose food is as restricted as ours. Spending an evening in a constant state of starvation is a rough way to find out. I once went to a traditional Italian Christmas Eve "Feast of the Seven Fishes" party thinking fish was a food I could eat, only to discover that absolutely everything was battered and fried. There were many guests, people who obviously looked forward to this menu all year. Good manners dictated that I keep my mouth shut and the items on my plate moving. Fortunately, the dinner was served buffet-style, so I was not in the glare of attention. My dinner consisted of cheese, nuts, chocolate, and many cups of espresso (I was up until New Year's). When I got home, I ate everything in my refrigerator, including the baking soda and the spare batteries.

Think of it this way: If you've eaten already and there is nothing for you, you'll survive without being tempted to cheat or punch a newly papered wall. If you're semi-full and there's plenty for you, your willpower and self-possession in the face of mega-calories and fat will become the envy of all present. Who knows? You may even end up being the topic of the next day's post-party gossip. Look for the silver lining. With a reputation for restraint to uphold, it won't be difficult to lose those last five pounds.

No matter how you look at it, if your stomach is full, you can't lose. If it's empty, you can't win.

Rule No. 5

Never forget to say thank you.

This should go without saying. But it's amazing how few people say thank you anymore.

Whether it's a chef who has prepared your special pasta, a pal who has remembered your favorite gluten-free crackers for the cocktail party, the weekend hostess who combed the health food store and found gluten-free English muffins so you could enjoy eggs Benedict with everybody, or, the ultimate demonstration of love, the person who made you scones from gluten-free scratch, never forget to accept these gifts—and make no mistake, they are gifts—without conveying your gratitude.

I don't mean the immediate reflex of saying thank you, which goes without saying, sincere and heartfelt at the time. I'm talking about a follow-up note, fax, e-mail, phone call, card, flowers, or even a gift, depending on your budget and the extent of your gratitude. I always send a note of thanks to a chef who has gone out of his or her way for me. (Phone calls are not always welcome in chaotic restaurant kitchens.) I do this not merely because it is a gracious thing to do, something my mother taught me always to do no matter how small the gift, but because in these times of moving fast and forgetting one's manners, it virtually ensures that I will enjoy more of that special treatment.

Here, too, there are no exceptions. Your note doesn't have to be formal, expensive, stylish, or even particularly well written, just sincere. My personal favorite note is a postcard really, usually a funny photograph from the forties or fifties involving food, such as classic diners and drive-in burger stands, vintage advertising, and old TV shows such as *I Love Lucy, Donna Reed*, or *The Honeymooners*. I collect them by the dozens.

When someone makes or buys something special for me, I flip through my collection and send the one that most fits the occasion. After a while, matching the postcard to the kindness becomes a game, and it has become my trademark thank you. You'll be surprised at how much food you can find on postcards.

This doesn't have to be expensive. Browse through the postcard tables at

flea markets. Look for food advertising and pictures of appliances, toaster assembly lines, cake mixes, refrigerators (especially good are ones that show
Betty Furness opening the door), ovens, muffin tins, and the like. If you have
as much fun saying thank you as you had enjoying the result of someone's effort, it is impossible to go wrong.

It doesn't matter what you send or how you send it, as long as you never
forget to do it. When you follow up with some tangible expression of thanks,
you salute the generosity of your friends and express your own graciousness,
which is refreshing behavior in these less than gentle times.

You may also be surprised that something as small as a note or a postcard
can open the door to a new friendship. Many years ago a stranger brought me
a gift of rice pasta when our visits to the home of our mutual friend coincided.
It was absolutely unnecessary and, as such, all the more appreciated, which is
exactly what my note said. If you make a habit of meeting every act of kindness, no matter how small, with the generosity of your own appreciation, you
will soon realize that the more you say thank you, the more reasons you will
have for doing so.

A person who says thank you is always welcome. Simple as that.

Rule No. 6

It is impolite to mistake a business breakfast, lunch, or dinner for a meal.

Business has it own etiquette or, perhaps more accurate, its own *non*etiquette.
To be brash and rude and ignorant of the basic pleasantries is to be considered dynamic, powerful, important, plugged-in, wired. Witness Martha Stewart, Jack Welsh, The Donald.

It is an unspoken rule that no one actually eats at a business meeting over
food, or, if so, eats as little as possible. I think this is to create the impression
that to be truly powerful, one must be beyond food, but willing and able to
foot the bill.

It seems that in business today, the very need to eat (or sleep, for that matter) seems to conjure images of weakness and corporate wishy-washiness.
Mistaking this ritual for a meal and tucking up to the corporate table can
arouse the predator in the meekest accountant. I would advise the upwardly
mobile celiac against it. I don't know why, but the amount of food left on one's
plate seems to correlate directly to one's position in the hierarchy—the more,
the higher. Wasteful. Selfish. And true. (For further study, read *Pigs at the
Trough* by Arianna Huffington.)

This can work to the benefit of those celiacs who must do business over a meal, not to mention the gluten-free wannabe. Eat a hearty breakfast at home—amaranth cereal, English muffin, jam, and gluten-free pancakes—and thus fortified, narrow your eyes, square your shoulders, and order a fruit salad or a small glass of orange juice with your coffee. Better still, drink mineral water with freshly squeezed lemon. Ditto for important lunch and dinner meetings. Have a gluten-free peanut butter sandwich at your desk, then nibble a salad or take two bites of an omelet with the boss or the client.

Whatever you do, don't discuss your diet over drinks. Bonding doesn't mean the same thing in business that it does in your real life. If you do, the next thing you know is you're being passed over for that beer account or the new pretzel business. Speaking of which, no one ever has to know you're not drinking, not because of the alcohol gluten issue, but because it simply isn't cool these days. Sip fizzy water or anything soft, and make sure you know what's in the cocktail mix before you grab a handful.

You say you haven't made it to the executive suite yet? Not to worry, politics affects those of us who share refrigerator space in the coffee room, too. What with downsizing, outsourcing, working weekends with no overtime pay, it's a wonder anybody has time to eat, much less eat safely *and* watch your back. I'm not suggesting everyone you work with is a cutthroat out for your job, and certainly many lifetime friendships have been known to bloom among coworkers, but in the shrinking ranks of today's job market, it's wise to be known for something other than your intolerance to certain foods.

Always keep snacks in your office or work space. This way, you won't succumb to the "we're ordering a pizza" mentality of most late nights. Whether you carry a briefcase or a backpack, make sure there's room for a bag of gluten-free pretzels or a few safe energy bars in a pinch. I work in my pajamas now, not far from my own stocked refrigerator, but when I worked for a large advertising agency fond of late-night pitches and working lunches in the conference room, I made a deal with the company steward. Whenever he saw my name on the luncheon list, he served me from the stock of bread, cookies, and muffins I supplied. No explanations necessary and no one was ever the wiser. No steward. Stash your lunch and snacks in the office kitchen. And don't forget to label everything. Long hours and lots of stress make pilferers of everybody.

Another strategy is to make a study of takeout places near the office that offer enough for you to eat. Keep their menus in your desk and pass them out to the designated order taker.

For larger office gatherings and morale-boosting events designed to make you forget you haven't had a raise in five years, such as picnics on the boss's lawn or taking over an entire bowling alley, eat first and wing it. When no one is looking, trade plates with your spouse, or, if you're single or this is an employee-only party, transfer small amounts of food (just enough to avoid arousing suspicion) into the plate of the person on your left. Keep doing this until yours is empty. If you get caught, say your throat closes up at these things. He or she will nod knowingly.

Bottom line: Be as gracious to business associates who go out of their way for you as you are to friends and try to make sure you have enough to eat at all times. The idea is never to make a big deal of your diet. If you're like most working people in business today, you've got quite a bit on your plate already.

Rule No. 7

In your case, it's okay to carry your own food where other food is served or sold.

This means restaurants, diners, snack bars, athletic stadiums, beach houses, cabins, cottages, mansions, apartments, lofts, church basements, picnics, pancake breakfasts, barbecues, lunches, brunches, boats, Greyhound buses, airplanes, trains, trolley cars, trailers, parlor cars, vans, sedans, SUVs, RVs, national parks, country clubs, swimming pools, sidewalk cafés, bistros, malls, movies, theaters . . . anywhere eating is allowed in the first place and as long as you do it with discretion and flair. That is, it is *not* polite to crack an egg on the back of a movie seat, but it is perfectly acceptable to slip a cookie or a gluten-free muffin out of a purse or pocket and nibble away.

It is perfectly acceptable to hand your bread to a waiter and ask that it be returned to you in form of French toast, eggs Benedict, or a Reuben sandwich, or a double cheeseburger as long as you make sure the grill is clean and there is no other gluten involved in the preparation.

It is *not* acceptable to do so without benefit of a plate. It's tacky to clutter the table where others are eating with plastic bags and napkins full of crumbs.

It is absolutely acceptable to transfer the contents of a ready-made sandwich to your bread in a public place, as long as you don't make a mess or call unnecessary attention to what you're doing, and provided there are no crumbs or ingredients to which gluten can stick involved in the maneuver. (Some very sensitive celiacs may want to pass on this one.)

When you've been invited to someone's home for the weekend, by all means arrive with a suitcase full of food. But don't expect to be waited on hand and foot. Just because you have a problem with grain doesn't mean you can't operate a toaster or a microwave oven.

Whenever you carry your own food, it's important to let those in charge know what you're doing ahead of time. Movie managers sometimes have rules about bringing food into their theaters where popcorn and other snacks are sold. Of course you're an exception, but if you don't want a scene with an usher and risk being treated like a criminal, which actually happened to me, mention that you will be doing this and why. With competition with home videos and DVDs as fierce as it is, what movie house in its right mind is going to rule against you?

While it is perfectly acceptable to eat your gluten-free corn muffin instead of the one served by the restaurant, remember it is rude to eat it before everyone else is served theirs. No matter how hungry you are, or how special you feel, you are not exempt from basic table manners. Comments such as "Boy, am I glad I have this roll" when others are starving are rude, mean, and totally insensitive.

Rule No. 8

It is acceptable to use your fingers when all else fails.

"All else fails" is the operative phrase here. If you are served a cracker on which there is a single, small piece of cheese or meat, it's fine to pick it up with your fingers and pop it into your mouth, provided, of course, the cracker is not crumbly, in which case no amount of scraping will render the topping harmless. Better, find yourself a plate, load up on the toppings and eat what you can with a fork or spoon. Never attempt to deconstruct a canapé with your fingers.

If you were smart enough to bring your own crackers, now is the time to fill up a plate and make the switch somewhere other than the buffet table in the center of the room. To get around the possibility of cross-contamination altogether, slip into the kitchen and ask for some toppings for your crackers (or, if you don't have any, ask for celery or cucumber slices). Never leave uneaten food lying around on a windowsill, next to someone's purse, or behind a photograph of the family dogs. Someone will find them eventually and know it was you. Dispose of them as neatly and as quickly as you can.

If you've come to this party with your own spoon, heap small amounts of safe items onto a cocktail plate, and enjoy the food from there. Never, under any circumstances, put your spoon directly into the serving dish. Always use the utensil from the table to serve yourself and use your spoon only to eat your portion. For dips, ask the host for a serving spoon and remember to serve yourself before the dish is tainted with cracker crumbs. If there is no powder room to rinse your spoon discreetly or guests in the kitchen are not encouraged, ask for a glass of water and use that, remembering not to leave that glass around either.

If you find yourself at a sit-down dinner, staring down a chicken that has been fried or otherwise coated with something inedible, don't panic. The trick here is making it look like you're eating. Don't cut up the chicken, otherwise you won't be able to eat your vegetables with the same utensils. Talk to the person next to you. Practice makes perfect.

Should an offending grain or a stray crouton find its way into your mouth, screaming and spitting it onto your plate is not a good social option. Use your napkin (pray it's paper) to dispose of the food, then dispose of the napkin immediately and have a nice big gulp of water. Attract as little attention to yourself in the process as you possibly can. I like to pretend I've dropped something, then duck under the table to empty my mouth in private. If you can complete this maneuver without laughing, you're doing well.

In summary: Your diet doesn't excuse you from applying all the basic rules of courtesy and social conduct and, in fact, requires that you learn some new ones, including tact and diplomacy. When in doubt, smile. If you are really in doubt, buy yourself a copy of Emily Post or Miss Manners. And never do anything in polite company involving food, gluten-free or otherwise, that you would not like to read about in the morning paper.

how to get a chef to eat out of your hand

You can get anything you want at Alice's Restaurant

—ARLO GUTHRIE

Frank Lloyd Wright once said, "Give me the luxuries of life and I shall gladly do without the necessities." Watching my French mother buy cheese, sniffing rinds, and sampling little slivers until she found the perfect Camembert or St. André, taught me all I needed to know about getting the best versus the most readily available. With her Gallic sense of frugality and inborn suspicion of anything shrink-wrapped or hermetically sealed, she disliked supermarkets and preferred small specialty shops where she was greeted warmly by the proprietor and applauded for her discerning ways. As I toddled behind, happily nibbling the slivers of cheese and pâté and cookies (who knew?) that rained down on me in her wake, she was my first and most shining example of exactitude. She shopped as though she had all day, and unlike most of us today, she did, stopping to share a joke here, a bit of gossip there, never above flirting with the butcher for the sake of the perfect lamb chop. She also taught me another iron-clad rule I follow to this day: never directly confront the butcher about a tough pork chop, a less-than-lean leg of lamb, or a fatty rib roast. If my mother got a bad cut of meat, she would smile sweetly and say, "I must not have cooked it properly." They both knew what she meant. Her tact in front of other customers guaranteed his tender best from then on.

Lesson: Social grace sometimes trumps self-assertion.

On those special occasions when we dined out as a family, we put on our good clothes and headed for one of a handful of local restaurants where my parents were well-known. My mother never ordered directly from a menu. Only after exchanging pleasantries with the cook, sweetened with a bit of neighborhood gossip, would the serious discussion of dinner begin. My mother would ask what was fresh that day, what would be fortifying for my father's heart or liver or my delicate stomach (after food, health was her consuming passion), and most important, what did the chef *feel* like cooking. She always listened carefully to what the chef thought would be a good choice for us that night and if there were any dismissive gestures regarding a particular dish she asked about, we understood this to be code for "not too fresh tonight." Only after all these details were discussed would we order. Wisely, most decisions went in the kitchen's direction and never without the chef's appreciation of my mother's discerning ways. As it turns out, life with my finicky mother was all I needed in the way of restaurant assertiveness training.

I know. The very idea of eating out in this glutenous world (the low-carb craze will be a distant memory before you can say, "cheeseburger, salad, no roll"), is terrifying to the newly diagnosed celiac. You cower before menus full of buffalo wings, fried mozzarella, meat loaf, and pannini. Brunch with its muffins and pancakes and Danish pastries is a particular kind of torture. Even your Bloody Mary may have come in contact with a croissant on the way in from the bar. What if the french fries are beer-battered? What if they're plunged into the same oil as the onion rings? And if that were not bad enough, you have to explain your diet to the waiter who must be sufficiently convinced that you are no mere faddist following the diet foolishness du jour, but a genuinely grain-challenged person whose health depends on that person taking you seriously, who, in turn, explains it to the chef, who hears it secondhand. You worry, justifiably so, that something will be lost in the translation.

Add to this the crash and clatter and kitchen acoustics of most restaurants and you wonder if you'll ever get out alive.

"The woman at table twenty can't eat wheat."

"What?"

"Wheat!"

"What, no heat?"

"No flour!"

"No flowers for table twenty!"

Not to worry. That's what I'm here for.

Negotiating with the Kitchen

These simple rules will have you sallying forth in no time at all with confidence and the anticipation one should bring to an evening out. You'll be making reservations without having any of your own. You'll be sweet-talking the waiter, standing up to the surly ones, as well as for your rights as a customer. In no time you'll be ordering fearlessly and well, eating like a pro. Some nights we just don't feel like cooking. I say why march into your own kitchen when you can march into someone else's? Herewith, how to get a chef to eat out of your hand.

And remember, less is more. Choose a few local restaurants and go there often, often enough for them to know exactly what you need and, even better, what you like.

Familiarity Breeds Content

The key to dining out well—not to be confused with grazing or frequenting the kind of place where food is prepared according to corporate formula, something I will talk about a bit later—is educating and cultivating a relationship with the person who prepares your meal. If you do it right, you will have a friend who takes professional pride in pleasing you.

Reservations

For starters, always make the reservation yourself. If, in the division of labor, you're not the one in your circle (or family) to do this, now is the time to volunteer. Whoever makes the calls, calls the shots. It's that simple.

If possible, do this in person, so you can introduce yourself and discuss your needs. (Yes, I know you're busy, but if you delegate this important opportunity and end up with a bad meal, it's nobody's fault but your own.) This is usually accomplished in the afternoon, when the kitchen is prepping for dinner, or midmorning, when it's getting organized for lunch. Don't settle for whoever happens to greet you, but don't be insulted either if you are asked to come back at a more convenient time. Anything can happen at any moment in a professional kitchen, so the last thing you want to do is find yourself explaining the gluten-free diet to a chef whose dish washer just walked out in a huff or is nervous about an important party or, worse, a visiting reviewer. Offer to call, e-mail, or come back at a time when the chef isn't distracted. Then again, a chef may just pop out of the kitchen at the right moment and, before you know it, you're both planning your supper. Serendipity? The chef may think so.

First Impressions Count

When you do get your opportunity, start off on your best foot. Be deferential to the chef's greater skill and remember this is a request, not a confrontation. Asking for help always trumps making demands. Never be defensive. The idea is to appeal to the artist as well as to the businessperson. Do say how hard it is for you to find foods you can eat and that you would love to be able to really enjoy his or her cooking. Do say you are looking for a restaurant and a chef with whom you can enjoy a regular and frequent relationship. Do mention the rave review you read in the local newspaper, the friend who recommended the place highly. Remember my mother's advice: a little well-placed flattery will get you everywhere. At this point, the chef will most likely rise to the challenge and say, "Don't worry, I'll make anything you like. Just let me know what you can eat and when you come in." With more and more restaurants aware of celiac disease and the gluten-free diet, you may find the chef is way ahead of you.

Leaving something behind for the chef to read later on is always a plus. I'm talking about simple things like a list of forbidden ingredients, information on why it's important to clean off the grill before cooking your meal or start a fresh pot of boiling water for the pasta you supply, although neither should be a substitute for conversation. One idea is to leave a printed dining card for reference. (Use the English version of the foreign-language dining cards in Appendix A or order one of the many variations offered by the different support groups listed in chapter 21.) Be careful, though, that what you leave behind doesn't come back to bite you. We live in litigious times. An effective card strikes a balance between conveying enough information without scaring the cook into thinking you'll sue if he so much as carries a loaf of bread past the pot with your food in it. Don't forget to jot down your phone number or e-mail address on the back of the card for any follow-up questions the chef may have.

By all means, share your likes and dislikes as well as your restrictions, but try to resist dictating the menu. The idea is for the chef to know the parameters so that he or she can improvise. If the meal doesn't work for the chef, it's not going to work for you.

Case in point, my visit to California's Napa Valley last spring. After much discussion, the owner/chef of the fabulous Terra in St. Helena decided that in my honor he would do his haricot vert tempura with rice flour. After tasting my green beans and comparing their lighter sweeter flavor and texture to his usual wheat flour version, he realized that rice flour made for a much more interesting tempura batter. My rice flour tempura is now a permanent part of a four-star menu. Not only did I negotiate a wonderful meal for myself, I left behind a great dish for other celiacs to discover.

If enduring the hard labor that comes with cooking for a living has any point at all, it's rising to a culinary challenge and seeing in the customer's delight proof of success.

Some Assembly May Be Necessary

If you want the chef to use a special ingredient, ask ahead of time if you may bring it along. Never just show up with it. Make the request during the week, when the kitchen is less chaotic. It's just plain bad manners to ask a well-timed, flawlessly choreographed kitchen to add an unplanned pot on a Friday or Saturday night.

It helps to supply cooking instructions, if needed. For instance, most gluten-free pasta takes longer to cook than semolina and can ruin a chef's timing if that information is not given up front. The first time I brought my spaghetti to one of my favorite restaurants, the owner stirred and tasted, stirred and tasted, and stirred and tasted some more, and held the rest of our party's meals too long waiting for mine to cook. We all had a good laugh that night, but now all I have to do is show my face, hand over the pasta, and a fresh pot of water is started.

In another local eatery, I am given a special menu with hearts drawn by the chef next to items that are safe for me. I am steered gently to selections that not only take into account my needs, but my food preferences as well. Small pleasures arrive unbidden—a Parmesan tuile, a soft chickpea crepe to dip in olive oil, and a little plate of crisped chickpea *socca* for spreading the meal's finale, a gorgeous sampling of cheeses drizzled with honey and pine nuts. (For those of you who cannot come to Philadelphia, the recipe for this restaurant's spectacular goat cheese cake is on page 141.) This kind of devotion to one's enjoyment doesn't happen overnight. It evolves over time, the way a friendship does, with mutual appreciation and a genuine desire to please. Small mishaps become something to laugh about together.

Special Treatment Doesn't Have to Be Expensive Treatment

We all know those places where knowledge of the Heimlich maneuver is a prerequisite for delivering the check. While it is always nice to have in reserve a special restaurant that knows how to cook for you, you don't have to spend more to get more. Whether you choose a modest family restaurant, the little café around the corner, the new BYOB everybody's talking about, or even the local pizza palace, the key word is *habit*.

One celiac friend endures an arduous three-hour daily commute. Some nights, mustering the strength to take that final step off the train is all she can handle. Forget about cooking dinner. Twice a week, the family meets at the village diner, an unprepossessing place where waitresses still tease their hair and wear handkerchiefs fanned in their pockets, seniors come in for the early-bird special, and locals gather for the town news with a piece of homemade pie. Here everyone knows to clean off the griddle and wipe down the slicer for my friend's simple meals of eggs, sandwiches (with supplied bread), ordered with a side of fresh hot french fries from the dedicated fryer. They happily wash the ice-cream scoop lest cookie dough or some other glutenous flavor cling to my friend's all-time favorite dessert—a double dish of Breyer's chocolate and coffee ice cream. Last year, on her birthday, they bought a gluten-free cake mix and surprised her with an old-fashioned layer cake (the leftovers were boxed for her to take home).

Another grain-challenged pal furnishes gluten-free pizza shells to the local pizza parlor and enjoys "vegging out" at home with a cheese and anchovy pizza and salad and a rented movie at least once a week. The checks don't add up to much, but the experience is priceless. The point is, a good gluten-free meal prepared by a professional does not have to send you into sticker shock.

Make a game of finding your favorite sauce or preparation that can be rendered gluten-free by your favorite restaurant chef. Why not a gratin made with your gluten-free bread crumbs, a delicate batter made of rice flour, a cutlet à la Milanese using cornmeal, lasagna made with corn tortillas, or gluten-free lasagna noodles, an ice-cream shell or tuile made with rice flour and coconut or focaccia made with your manioc flour? Anything is possible in a good relationship.

Your Compliments to the Chef

There is nothing more satisfying during a long, bruising night behind a hot stove than the sight of a happy and well-satisfied customer. If the meal has been truly extraordinary, by all means, take pen to paper. Equally effective is popping in to the kitchen to say a quick thanks. *Quick* is the operative word here. Never spend more than a few minutes thanking a chef, unless it's the end of the night and he or she has come out of the kitchen. If the kitchen is too small or chaotic to do the quick "pop," tap on the window and blow a kiss, tip a hat, place a hand over your heart, press palms together in the Buddhist "namaste" or peace gesture. Or simply touch fingers to the lips in the universal gesture of gustatory bliss. I once drew a heart on a Post-it, wrote "I am yours forever!" addressed it to the chef, and stuck it on my clean plate. Do anything but leave the restaurant without conveying your compliments to the chef.

In a world that has forgotten its manners, no chef will ever forget you if you remember this simple and endangered courtesy.

There's Always One Bad Apple

For the rare chef who gives you a bad time, the pen can be mightier than the fork. A few succinct words like, "I would love to have a birthday party for 200 at your restaurant, but alas, you weren't willing to make the effort," will have the desired effect. If hyperbole is not your style, summon the manager and calmly register your disappointment. Seldom have I had to resort to tactics like this. People who cook for people are, by nature, nurturing types.

Often the problem is not with the chef at all, but with the manager, receptionist, or waitstaff who take it upon themselves to present their "back-of-the-house" rules to you. This happens more and more these days, with the emphasis shifting away from customer service and toward customer compliance. (Are we consumers or are we sheep?) I can't tell you how many times I have had to say to a clerk or a store manager, "I am not interested in your rules, I am interested in returning this book. You are the clerk and I am the customer. Figure it out."

At a neighborhood restaurant that shall remain forever nameless, a waiter told my husband we couldn't bring our own wine after the owner told us we could. Turns out the waiter took it upon himself to make sure we were tipping on a bill that included wine. Any conversation with a waiter that starts with "You can't . . ." should be a red flag to call the owner.

If you are not able to speak with the owner personally, by all means, drop a note registering your disappointment at not being able to enjoy the establishment because you were not made to feel welcome. Be specific about your experience and why you feel you cannot come back. Chances are the owner or chef has no idea what's going on, as in the case of our greedy waiter who is no longer telling people what they can and can't do in that particular establishment. We, on the other hand, continue to enjoy bringing our own wine *and* my gluten-free pasta.

A Word about Waiters

Despite the fact that waiting tables is one of the most exhausting, stressful, and deafening jobs, the majority of waiters are hardworking and professional people, who honestly want to make your experience a good one.

Just because a good waiter knows to serve from the left and can bone a whole fish and operate a fancy corkscrew, doesn't mean he or she has any understanding of your special diet. A good way to get the waiter in your corner, or to your table, to be more precise, is to warn him or her that some extra trips to the kitchen on your behalf might be necessary. It's hard to resent extra work you can plan for. Empathy. There's nothing like it for getting what you want.

As soon as you arrive, just after the menus are handed out and the initial seating chatter dies down, draw the waiter aside for a private word. If you have had an earlier conversation with the chef, now is the time to ask that your arrival be announced to the kitchen. If you have brought some of your own food to fill in—a dinner roll, a portion of pasta, individual pizza crust— this is a good time to hand it over and ask that it be brought to you as similar items are brought to the others in your party. (You don't want your roll warmed and delivered before the bread and butter arrives for the rest of the table.) If you have brought your own pasta, hand it over immediately, say the chef is expecting it, and ask the waiter to remind the kitchen to start a fresh pot of water.

If you have not previously explained your problem, do so now. Explain that you are going to need help ordering and that it may be necessary to ask the chef some important questions. Whenever possible, appeal to the person, not to the job description. Language like, "I really need your help with this" or "You know so much more about how the chef works than I" is much more effective than rude demands, suspicion, or hostility.

I've heard celiacs say things like, "You had better not give me anything with flour in it or else." Would you want to wait on someone like that? Given some of the books out there about what really goes on in a restaurant kitchen, a waiter with a grudge might see to it you get a whole lot more than crumbs in your food.

While visiting with a celiac family during one of my speaking tours, I was taken out to dinner. When the dessert arrived, a plate of ice cream with one of those "cigarette" cookies stuck on top, my host turned purple and screamed "Contamination!" at the top of his voice. The poor server was mortified. The other diners stared at us as if we were consumptives out on leave from the sanitarium. It could have been handled with a "I know you meant well, but we can't have a cookie in our ice cream. Would you mind bringing us fresh dishes?" Instead it was a scene. With the shocked looks of the other customers boring into us, I can't remember enjoying ice cream less.

The moral is this. Do not assume anyone is plotting to keep you sick. People make honest mistakes and, if the restaurant is worthy of it, give them a chance to make it up to you. With obese Americans suing fast food restaurants for making them fat, the last thing a restaurant wants to do is encourage a gluten reaction.

Always try to involve the waiter in solving the problem. Try to begin a sentences with "What if . . .":

"What if the chef used rice flour (cornmeal, ground nuts) to dust the soft-shell crabs, coat the flounder, or thicken the sauce (if it is not pre-made)?

"What if the chef put this sauce on my pasta instead of that one?"

"What if the chef pan seared my lamb chops instead of using the grill?"

"What if I ordered the dish without the orzo?"

"What if the chef put the polenta from that dish on the chicken I'm considering?"

"What if I asked for a side dish of risotto with my grilled steak?"

You get the idea.

Gratuities

With the exception of four-star restaurant waiters who earn more than some new doctors, the average server earns a meager salary supplemented by tips, so their reasons for encouraging you to enjoy yourself are not entirely altruistic. I firmly believe that extra service deserves extra consideration, so if you have been given special treatment, you really should find it in your heart *and* your pocketbook to leave a fair and generous tip.

I'm not talking lavish or excessive here. If a normal tip is 15 percent, making it 18 to 20 percent for extra special service should be the rule. If you budget for a dinner out, factor in the tip. Spending more than you planned is easy in a good restaurant, but stiffing the waiter is not the solution. It is one of the worst restaurant sins, and it all but guarantees a really bad experience the next time. Can you say gratuitous violence?

Do read the small print on the menu, though. Many restaurants will tell you (usually in the teeniest mouse type) that parties of six or eight or more will have a hefty service charge (18 to 20 percent) added automatically to their bill. This is not information a waiter will freely mention if he or she is smart. If this is the case, never tip on top of this. All or part of the service charge will be given to your waiter.

Okay. You're the most solicitous customer ever born, but this is not a perfect world. You will occasionally run into trouble. This is inevitable, so you may as well be prepared.

The Rude (and Otherwise Difficult) Waiter

You know the type. Remember *Seinfeld*'s Soup Nazi? This creature arches his or her eyebrows, speaks in a condescending tone, is inattentive, steers you to the most expensive items on the menu, interrupts your conversation to recite the specials (doesn't he or she know a waiter is supposed to wait?), or even worse, talks right over one of your guests to introduce himself or herself, delivers a raw chicken then tells you the chef cooks it that way, and never fails to clear the plates before everyone is finished. This is the kind of person who makes global pronouncements ("No Substitutions!"), and after being told politely that you can eat no gluten and need to know the exact ingredients of each dish you are considering, sneers, "Is this some kind of new diet?"

If reason and good manners fail to make an impression on this person, you have my permission to say, "Yes. It's the if-I-get-so-much-as-a-speck-of-wheat-I'll-own-this-restaurant diet."

If a story you are telling with perfect timing is interrupted with, "I'm Richard and I'll be your waiter this evening," it is perfectly acceptable to reply, "I'm so-and-so and I'll be responsible for your tip this evening, so you'd better wait until I'm finished talking to make your announcements."

The waiter is tapping his foot and letting his attention stray to another table as you ask about the ingredients in a particular dish you are thinking of ordering. You sense he hasn't heard a word you said and when your dinner arrives inedible that confirms it. When you ask that the food be taken back, you get a roll of the eyes and a look of undisguised annoyance. "It's only a little flour," he says with a bored shrug.

This is your cue to say, "In that case, I'll only sue you a little."

Or, if confrontation isn't your thing, simply ignore the waiter's rudeness and order something else. But don't forget to ask to see the manager to have the offending item removed from your check. Never, ever, pay for what you didn't eat. That is simply adding insult to injury.

You've been through all the desserts on the menu and every one of them is made with flour. You ask if there is sorbet or fresh fruit and get a flat no, and no offer from the kitchen to fix something special. Like the relative who tries to get off the hook by putting you on it, the difficult waiter will try to sell you an expensive dessert by suggesting that you "just eat the middle."

This is your cue to say, "Why don't I just pay just for the middle, too?"

Sometimes, the person you assume will be a bad waiter isn't. Recently, a big party of us, with tots in tow, wandered into a fairly good restaurant without a reservation. Remembering our manners and in consideration of the other diners, we asked politely if the establishment served children. (Remember that consideration goes both ways.)

"We do," said the man who greeted us, "but I find I can never finish a whole one."

We didn't know whether to laugh or walk out the door.

Turns out, this fellow was quite solicitous of our needs and my gluten-free diet, but as first impressions go, his odd sense of humor put us all off balance. Sometimes you just have to resist comment and wait someone out before you make assumptions.

I realize some of you may not be comfortable saying things as dramatic, jaw-dropping, and conversation-stopping as the things I've uttered. (Practice does help. Rent the classic *When Harry Met Sally* and watch it until you are no longer uncomfortable with how Meg Ryan orders food.) You may not want to engage the difficult waiter at all, which is perfectly fine. You may want to ask to see the manager, instead. Explain the problem and request that another waiter be assigned to your table. If even this is more confrontation than you are able to handle, supply the script and ask someone in your party to do the dirty work for you. As long as the restaurant knows why it has failed you, it doesn't really matter who tells them.

I would, however, resolve to work on why you can't demand what you need when you're paying the bill. On a diet as restrictive as this one, this problem is going to come up time after time; you may as well settle it now. More often than not the inability to assert one's requirements comes from being taught that making "a fuss" or calling undue attention to one's needs is selfish or unseemly. Women are especially uncomfortable for all the obvious cultural reasons. Try to see self-assertion not as a negative trait, but as a healthy way of honoring the self without being selfish. Think of it as an example for your children to follow. By standing up for yourself (not only in restaurants, but in life as well) you are teaching them an invaluable lesson; that they, too, are important enough and worthy enough to ask for special treatment.

Of course, if reason and all else fails, you have the ultimate weapon—a sarcastic "thanks" scrawled across a bill with a nickel tip says it all.

Do your restaurant assertiveness skills need a little fine tuning? Or are you reservations ready? Take this simple multiple choice quiz and find out.

Restaurant Assertiveness Quiz

1. You phone a hot new restaurant and a bored-sounding hostess says they won't be able to fit you in for at least six weeks. You . . .
   a. reserve a table anyway, knowing it will be even harder to get in once the place is reviewed.
   b. ask if they could possibly fit you in sooner.
   c. explain that you won't be hungry by then and make a reservation someplace friendlier.

2. You order a bowl of onion soup and discover a hunk of bread lurking under the melted cheese topping. You . . .
   a. ask the waiter to remove the bread and return the bowl to you.
   b. accept it as is and fish out the soggy bread yourself.
   c. find out what kind of cheese is used and ask that a fresh bowl be made *sans* bread if it is a safe cheese.

3. You ask for a side dish of rice instead of the spaghetti that comes with the meal and the waiter says, "No substitutions." You . . .
   a. get huffy and leave.
   b. order something you don't like and resolve not to patronize the establishment again.
   c. explain your problem and ask if the management is willing to make an exception for you.

4. You are considering a dish that derives its sauce from something called a *roux*. You . . .
   a. don't want to expose your lack of culinary sophistication and order the dish anyway, assuming the sauce involves red wine.
   b. decide not to take any chances and order something less complicated.
   c. make a joke about not being accustomed to rouge in your food and ask the waiter what it is.

5. Your friends decide on the local Italian restaurant for the Friday night get-together. You . . .
   a. decide you are outnumbered and agree, figuring you'll have a good lunch and nibble on a salad for dinner.
   b. tell them you'd love to come, but you really have to sort out that pesky sock drawer of yours.
   c. explain that if they really would like your company, they'll have to choose someplace less difficult for you.

ANSWERS:
1. (c) That old saw about first impressions has never been truer. If a restaurant employee is rude on the phone, just wait till you ask for special treatment from the kitchen. Bad manners can cool a hot restaurant faster than a deep freeze.
2. (c) The bread may seem like the obvious culprit, but the cheese could be processed as well. Never pick your food apart or let a waiter do it for you. Not only is there a good chance you'll get some unwanted crumbs, not asking about the cheese and starting over sends the wrong message back to the kitchen. If you don't take your diet seriously, why should the restaurant?
3. (c) Shooting from the hip is never a good idea, especially when you're hungry. Understand that the waiter is simply stating the restaurant's policy. The idea is to keep the conversation going until you get past no or it becomes apparent that you are the exception to this general rule. If this doesn't work, you have my permission to skip to answer (a).
4. (c) It doesn't matter how you ask, just do it, even if you think you know what a menu term means. You'll "roux" the day you don't.
5. (c) It's so easy to go along with the crowd. Do it often enough and you'll end up resenting your friends. Lie and they'll end up resenting you. How can you ask a restaurant for special treatment if you can't ask your friends?

This is one time when being a C student pays off. You don't need me to tell you how to eat out. Let's do lunch some time. If you answered with some A's and B's, you are either too hotheaded, which gets you nowhere, or too worried about what people think. Study the menu terms below, practice going out with people you trust to be supportive, or do a little role-playing with friends before your big night out.

The Menu: A Crash Course

We all like to think we are well-informed, sophisticated, well-traveled, witty, and urbane, even if we are not. Nobody likes to be viewed as ignorant, even if the information at hand is obscure, esoteric, or even downright arcane. Is there a soul among us who hasn't committed the sin of pretending to have read a classic or to have seen a film in order to hide what we consider a gaping hole in our education or cultural blind spot? Haven't we all skimmed the latest issue of *Time* magazine only to find ourselves pretending to have read thoroughly the article that's under discussion?

Truth time: How many of us can say we have never skipped lightly over our ignorance of Pilates, bronzino (the fish, not the sunless tanner), Tivo, or Dr. Phil? We do it because we all have memories of the time the worst happened—when we ordered our steak *tartare* medium rare, when we mistook tuna *carpaccio* for an Italian opera, *bordelaise* for a good French wine, etc., etc. Who doesn't remember the time everyone laughed as our cheeks burned?

Fear of exposure is a powerful force. However, when we pretend to understand a menu term, we are indulging in a particularly pernicious form of dietary Russian roulette. We literally swallow our pride.

I've designed the following glossary to help you sharpen your knowledge of cooking techniques commonly and not so commonly found on restaurant menus. Your newfound knowledge may amaze your friends, but it will keep you blissfully gluten-free. Herewith, defining our culinary terms . . .

Roux and Other Flour Sources

According to *Larousse Gastronomique*, a *roux* is a mixture of flour and a fatty substance, most commonly butter, which is cooked and used as a thickening element for sauces and soups, most notably gumbos and bisques. A *roux* can be white, blond, or brown, depending on how it is prepared. No matter what color, it is to be avoided like the plague it is for celiac plumbing.

Many popular French sauces are based on this technique. Because of this, most are not gluten-free unless the chef specifically tells you the *roux* has been omitted or has been prepared with gluten-free flour. Many modern chefs have omitted this classic and artery-clogging step in the name of modern cuisine and now rely on vegetable reductions for the intensity of their sauces. That said, you'll never go wrong asking for specific ingredients whenever you see the following sauces listed on the menu:

Africaine, Albert, Alboni, Allemande, Americaine, Anglais, Béchamel, Béarnaise, Bigarade, Bordelaise, Bourguignonne, Butter, Cardinal, Chateaubriand, Chaud-froid or Brown Sauce, Chausseur or Hunter, Diable, Lyonnaise, Madeira, Maître d'hotel, Moutarde, Mornay, Nantua, Provençal, Ravigote, Robert, Supreme, Soubise, Veron, Velouté, and plain old American White Sauce.

Sauces

Classic demi-glacé sauces or reductions are usually not made with flour and form the basis for many other sauces, including tomato coulis and Espagnole sauce, which can be made with fish or meat stock. Since many chefs pride themselves on the liberties they take with the classics, it is always better to be safe than sorry. For those of you who wish to avoid vinegar and mustard, watch out for mayonnaise-based rémoulade, which also contains mustard, and vinaigrette, which is based on vinegar and can be made with mustard as well.

Breads and Cakes

In the words of the famously politically incorrect Marie Antoinette, "Let them eat . . . baba, baguette, beignet, brioche, bûche de Noël, charlotte, crepe, croissant, croquette, croustade, éclair, flan, fritters, galantine, galette, gâteau, genoise, gougere, gnocchi, kugelhopf, kulich, macaroon, mazarin, neapolitan, napoleon, nougatine, pain, pain anglais, panettone, pannequet, pâté, pavé, petits fours, pirogie, praline, profiterole, quenelle, quiche, roti, roulé, savarin, St. Honoré, strudel, tarte, terrine, torte, vacherin, vol-au-vent, zuppa inglese, and, oh, *yes* . . . cake." No matter what you call this sweet mix of butter, sugar, and flour, you can't.

Pasta

And don't forget, wheat pasta by any other name . . .

bucatini, capelli d'angelo (angel hair), cannelloni, cappellacci, cappelletti, conchiglie, fettuccine, fusilli, gargarelli, lasagna, maccheroncini, maltagliatti, manfrigual, orecchiette, pappardelle, penne, pizoccheri, quadrucci, ravioli, raviolini, rigatoni, spaghetti, spaghettini, striccheti, tagliatelle, tagliolini, tonnarelli, tortelli, tortellini, tortelloni, vermicelli, ziti

is just as dangerous.

Lots of don'ts. But do memorize the following handy glossary of culinary foods terms and techniques. Not only will you be smarter about what always contains gluten and what doesn't, but your knowledge will be as impressive as your confidence.

Safe in Any Language

Acaraje: Brazilian black-eyed pea fritters made with pure chickpea flour.

Dal: The gluten-free lentil puree of India.

Dosa: The rolled, usually gluten-free pancake of India. Do ask before ordering.

Edamame: Japanese soybeans boiled in the pod.

Fagioli: Italian for beans.

Flagelot: French for beans.

Finocchio: Not a puppet with a penchant for stretching the truth, but the Italian word for fennel, a green related to the licorice-like anise, but milder. As are all vegetables in their natural state, finocchio is gluten-free.

Frittata: A flat Italian omelet that is dryer than its French cousin and is never folded. It can be filled with almost anything except flour, which is never used in a frittata.

Fungee: Also called *coo coo*, and made with pure cornmeal, this is the Caribbean's answer to polenta.

Gravlax: Swedish marinated salmon.

Masa harina: Finely ground Mexican corn flour. Perfectly safe.

Meringue: A dessert made with egg whites and sugar. No fat. No flour.

Raita: The cool cucumber, yogurt, and watercress sauce from India. Dip your papadum, but not your nan.

Seviche: Raw shrimp, scallops, lobster, or other fish marinated in fresh limes and hot chilis for at least six hours. Gluten-free.

Tandoori: A mildly spiced style of cooking meats, vegetables, or fish that's been marinated in lemon, garlic, and ginger and cooked in a hot *tandoor*, or Indian oven.

Zabaglione: A frothy Italian dessert made with whipped egg yolks, sugar, Marsala wine, and, some say, clouds. Have this with an almond cookie for a totally gluten-free dessert.

Usually Safe, but Ask Anyway

Enchilada: A Mexican dish made with fish, chicken or beef, sauced and rolled in a corn tortilla served with melted cheese and sour cream. Freshly made enchiladas are almost always gluten-free. In chain or fast-food restaurants, the tortilla is often *wheat* and bears no resemblance to the real thing. The sauce is often thickened with *flour*.

Macaroon: A dessert cookie made of almond paste, sugar, and egg whites. Some macaroons contain a small amount of *flour*. Others do not. Ask.

Pakoras: Spicy Indian vegetable fritters that may contain gluten. Ask.

Polenta: A white or yellow, fine-grained or coarse cornmeal that is stirred until it reaches a creamy consistency. Mixed with butter and cheese or allowed to harden, it is then fried and served as an entrée or an accompaniment. This northern Italian specialty is wheat and gluten-free unless the chef gets fancy and mixes in another grain. Safe 99 percent of the time. Ask.

Risotto: This Italian classic is made with wine and a short-grain creamy rice called arborio. The pasta of Venice, there are hundred of varieties of this rich, satisfying dish—vegetables, cheeses, mushrooms, shellfish, and meats—and unless the chef has decided to guild a lily, it is always gluten-free.

Torte: A flourless cake usually made with finely ground almonds or chestnuts. Some modern chefs mix in tiny bit of cake flour, but most don't. Ask. Or risk missing out on one of the all-time classic desserts.

Absolutely Not

Albondigas: Mexican fried meat cakes that usually contain *wheat flour*.

Americaine: A tomato sauce once based on lobster coral but now commonly thickened with the more plentiful *wheat flour*.

Arlesienne: A dish or garnish composed of fried eggplants and fried onion rings dredged in *wheat flour*.

Au gratin: Translation: floury cheese sauce and *bread crumbs*.

Beef Wellington: This dish is always served "en croute" or in a *wheat pastry* crust that has been slathered with pâté. Forget it.

Beignet: A dessert fritter made with *wheat flour* popular in Lousiana and restaurants specializing in Cajun cuisine.

Blanquette: A veal or chicken ragoût or stew based on a white *roux*.

Bisque: A thick soup or purée commonly thickened with *wheat flour*.

Bouchée: Any bite-size puff *pastry* that is filled with sweet or savory ingredients as a dessert or hors d'oeuvre.

Bourguignonne: A stew containing Burgundy wine and *roux*.

Cellophane noodle: The flat rice noodle of Shanghai.

Couscous: A North African specialty usually made of crushed *durham wheat* or millet flour, chick peas, or rice, and steamed with spices and lamb, mutton, or chicken.

Crepinette: A small, fat sausage encased in *bread crumbs*.

Croque Monsieur: A grilled *sandwich*, usually ham and Gruyere cheese.

Crouton: A small, buttered cube of dried *bread* usually served in salads and soups, often invisible until it ends up in your mouth.

Escabeche: A Spanish dish consisting of *floured* and fried smelts, mackerels, whiting and red mullets.

Focaccia: You don't care how it's made. It's *bread*.

Fricassée: Stew consisting of *flour*-thickened white sauce and cut-up poultry.

Fritto misto: A traditional Italian dish of foods fried in *flour* and egg batter.

Gnocchi: Italian potato dumplings, which always contain a small amount of *flour*.

Goulash: A *roux*-based Hungarian stew flavored with paprika.

Matelote: Any fish stew made with red or white wine and thickened with *flour*.

Milanaise or Milanese: An Italian method of preparation usually involving veal or chicken cutlets dipped in egg and *bread crumbs* mixed with cheese and fried in butter or olive oil.

Moussaka: A thick Greek eggplant casserole that is thickened with a *flour*-based béchamel sauce.

Navarin: A ragoût or stew of mutton or lamb that has been thickened with *roux*.

Paninni: An Italian grilled *sandwich*.

Pasticcio: Any dish that is a mixture of meat, vegetables, or pasta and bound by eggs, béchamel sauce, and topped with *bread crumbs*.

Polonaise: A popular method of preparing cauliflower involving *bread crumbs*.

Posole: Mexican corn stew studded with bits of pork. Ask if it has been thickened with *flour*.

Quiche: A savory tart bound with eggs, cream, Gruyère, and, alas, *pastry* crust.

Semolina: A fancy name for *wheat flour*.

Soufflé: Any sweet or savory dish that consists of puréed ingredi
thickened with egg yolks and stiffly beaten egg whites carefully folde
in and baked, frozen, or refrigerated in a high-sided soufflé dish. If the
baked version did not contain a tiny bit of *flour*, it could not rise to
such dizzying culinary heights, but frozen soufflés most likely do not.
Ask, if it does or risk missing out on the mother of all French desserts.

Spelt: A form of *wheat* considered more digestible than the standard. But
not for celiacs.

Stroganoff: A ragoût of beef containing sour cream, thickened with a dark
roux, and most commonly served over egg noodles.

Shall we review?

The Ten Rules of Order

1. Discuss. Don't dictate.
2. Never allow another person (even someone who loves you) to explain
   your diet.
3. Become a regular. Familiarity breeds content.
4. Always give advance warning when asking for special treatment on
   weekends.
5. Show your appreciation often and well.
6. Never discuss your requirements with a waiter unless you have his or
   her complete and undivided attention.
7. Never pretend you understand a menu term or method of preparation
   if you don't. Ask.
8. Never pay for what you can't eat. Even if it's no one's fault, send it back
   and tell the waiter why.
9. Be prepared to leave any establishment in which you are denied the attention and consideration you request and deserve.
10. Never accept anyone's best guess, however sincere. Insist on verifica-
    tion that what you are putting into your mouth is gluten-free. If it can't
    be proven, don't order it.

There Are Exceptions, Even to My Rules

Recently, some friends and I were the recipients of a surprise Valentine's Day
dinner hosted by our husbands. All the men would say is my diet would be
taken care of. Keeping secrets from someone who needs a bit more control

...ts and sly grins is never a good idea. But there is the odd ...er to say nothing and have a snack beforehand than ...s of someone who loves you. You can always get an- ...lways a second chance to mend feelings.

...e, the men trotted us off to a local restaurant school ...quires of its patrons a kind of culinary trust. I adore adventures, but that night as the fledgling waitstaff served course after course, polishing their tableside manners and blushing over minor faux pas, it became clear I would be disappointed. The onion soup was watery without its floating island of Gruyère, my lamb pallid next to its crumbed cousins. The entire meal was gluten-free, not by substitution, but by elimination. This is what airlines do, not fine restaurants.

I couldn't very well complain without offending my husband who grinned like a schoolboy that he had managed to pull it off. So I smiled sweetly, pushed my food around, and pretended to eat. However, when the school's director came to our table to ask how his students did, I took him aside, introduced myself as the author of *Against the Grain*, and offered to instruct them on how to make a memorable gluten-free meal. In short, I seized the opportunity to enlighten a dozen newly minted chefs on the notion that the creative preparation of food for people with special diets can provide an important edge in the dog-eat-dog world of professional cooking.

Granted, most people don't get an opportunity to educate the next generation of chefs or restaurateurs, nor would they want it. But the moral is this: If you've had a bad experience, never slink away complaining when you could be explaining and fixing it for the next celiac. This is what awareness is—one person at a time lighting the way for the next.

Eating High on the Food Chain

Chain restaurants are another story altogether. All aspects of the dining experience are routinized, formularized, standardized, and franchised. They are "eating theme parks" right down to the tablecloths, waitstaff uniforms, and clowns at the front door whose very greeting is lifted from a big fat operating manual employees are expected to memorize. Not a lot of room for improvisation. Or getting special attention. There is also reluctance to disclose ingredients (or should I say formulas?) to customers. Almost as covert as drug companies in their operations, many of these corporations are more worried about intra-restaurant espionage than your plumbing. They are also worried about getting sued, which is why when you are told about an item that may be gluten-free (operative word: *may*), you get with it a disclaimer about possible

cross-contamination. This doesn't mean it isn't safe for you to eat. It m
they are giving you a legal answer. Rarely will you be told something is a
solutely, 100 percent gluten-free. Understand this and order accordingly.

Conformity, however, it not all bad. It can work in your favor because once you discover a menu item you can eat, you can be pretty sure (I said *pretty* sure, not *completely* sure) you can trust that it will be presented, prepared, packaged, boxed, bagged, and served the same way from location to location. If you have teenagers, you know this is because the average adolescent waiting on you cannot be expected to discover independent thought for at least another decade. I happen not to like the chains, not because a gluten-free meal cannot be gotten (they can, and many even have GF menus), but because these establishments typically lard so much fat and sugar into the average serving, which is getting obscenely bigger by the minute, they may as well call it heart attack on a plate.

High-fat meals are literally a strategy to keep people coming back. It seems greasy food has a high satiation factor and these corporations use fat the way grocery stores use price-off coupons. It's satisfying and feels good in your mouth (the industry calls this "mouth feel"). The average meal in one of these places contains more calories than an active adult male should consume in an entire day. The children's menu, while offering gluten-free items, is no better. Given the fact that kids are sitting in front of computers, Game Boys, and television sets when they're not sitting at a school desk or being driven from place to place, it's no wonder we have an explosion of childhood obesity and diabetes in this country. In my view, these places should come with a warning like the one on a pack of cigarettes:

> Frequent high-fat meals can cause heart disease, diabetes, obesity, and stroke!

Isn't the point of following the gluten-free diet to regain maximal health and avoid the toll our peculiar genes may take on us? Okay, end of lecture.

Proceed with caution and don't make a habit of any chain restaurant unless you are comfortable ordering from the healthier portion of the menu. Here are just a few examples of what you can expect from "theme park eating."

Bonefish Grill

The advertising says, "Fresh fish, what a concept." And in today's world of frozen, partially frozen, flash frozen, rock solid frozen, this is refreshing information.

183

eans

Omelet Alert

. . . .

nts, most notably IHOP, add pancake batter to their
...... them fluffier. Always ask that yours be made with
EGGS ONLY, or risk puffing up in a way you hadn't counted on.

Everything's fishy here. Grilled fish. Yes, you can get beef and pork and chicken dishes, too. But why? Meat is not the point of this place. The theme is sleek, modern, and polished, right down to the metal mangroves and original fish rubbings. There is an open kitchen where the occasional flame-up gets the adrenaline flowing.

With ten locations and growing (Alabama, Florida, Indiana, Kentucky, North Carolina, Ohio, South Carolina, Tennessee, Virginia, and Washington), this chain, which opened in 2003, offers a gluten-free menu to download and study before dropping anchor.

With fresh grilled fish, only a bonehead would pass this up. For information, phone (866) 880-2226, www.bonefishgrill.com.

Boston Market

When *Against the Grain* first appeared, these people flatly refused to disclose their ingredients. This time a call to their customer service department netted a list of gluten-free menu items. Not a huge selection, mind you, but you won't go hungry either. It's nice to report progress.

Feel free to order the rotisserie chicken or turkey breast (no gravy), plain grilled chicken breast, garlic and dill new potatoes, butternut squash, whole kernel corn, cranberry relish, creamed spinach, green beans, hot cinnamon apples, fruit salad, and Jumpin' Juice squares.

For locations and further question, phone (800) 365-7000, or www.boston market.com.

Carrabba's Italian Grill

Working with Cynthia Kupper, R.D., and president of the Gluten Intolerance Group (GIG), this folksy Old Country Italian chain has not only designed a gluten-free menu, it guides and reminds the celiac to request that no pasta be added and make sure garlic toast is left off the order. This, of course, is to ensure that the server does not forget. And right there in black and white (or should I say red, white, and green) is an exhortation to request no croutons be mixed with your salad and that your greens be tossed in a clean bowl. A friendly reminder tells us to order all grilled specialties to be cooked with no grill baste.

Those legal caveats aside, the gluten-free antipasti include shrimp scampi, sausage and peppers, and fresh Canadian Cove mussels steamed in white wine, basil, lemon butter, and Pernod.

Gluten-free soups are lentil and sausage and Mama Mandola's Sicilian chicken. Salads or *insalata* include house, Italian, Caesar, and chicken Caesar, Fiorucci (mixed greens, artichoke hearts, roasted red bell peppers, and grilled eggplant in vinaigrette, topped with a medallion of hazelnut Caprino cheese), Carrabba (mixed green with mozzarella and Romano cheese, black olives, tomatoes, and red onions in vinaigrette, topped with grilled chicken), and Johnny Rocco (greens with grilled shrimp and scallops, roasted red peppers, olives, and ricotta cheese in vinaigrette)

For dinner, there is fresh, grilled fish of the day, and two steaks, a center-cut tenderloin steak called Filet Fiorentina or Sirloin Marsala, a center cut topped with mushrooms, proscuitto, and Marsala wine sauce. Chicken Gratella is grilled with herbs and olive oil and served with garlic mashed potatoes. And there is Chicken Marsala, Chicken Bryan with Caprino cheese, sun-dried tomatoes, and a basil lemon butter sauce or chicken Rosa Maria with fontina cheese and prosciutto, topped with mushrooms and a basil lemon butter sauce.

Dolci (or dessert) is a concoction called John Cole, which is gluten-free vanilla ice cream with caramel sauce and roasted cinnamon rum pecans. See www.carrabbas.com.

Outback Steakhouse

This chain of Aussie-inspired eateries has spread across the country faster than you can say "G'day!" With menu items like Shrimp on the Barbie, Kookaburra Wings, Bonzer salads, and other Down Under-isms, why bother to book a flight to Sydney? Given the above disclaimer, you'll be happy to know this fast-growing chain offers a gluten-free menu for adults and for kids. Remember, I didn't say healthy, I said gluten-free.

Talk about legal disclaimers! The Outback Web site clearly disavows any responsibility for items labeled gluten-free and declares itself not culpable for any damages incurred as a consequence of eating something that may contain gluten. It further states that Cynthia Kupper, a registered dietician, president of the Gluten Intolerance Group, and someone I would trust with my food any day, prepared the information for their gluten-free menu. This does not mean their food is unsafe. It means, in our litigious society, they figured out how to pass the buck and protect themselves from any wandering croutons. Kudos anyway.

The company slogan is "No Rules. Just Right." But as a celiac, you must follow a few simple rules to ensure that your meal is entirely gluten-free.

Never order Aussie Chips. They are not gluten-free. Avoid the seasoned rice as well.

According to the menu, most salads are gluten-free, as long as you remember to request no croutons and that your salad be mixed in a clean bowl. Ditto for barbecue sauce, pickles, and honey mustard sauce. A good gluten-free and reasonably healthy choice is Grilled Shrimp on the Barbie (as long as you ask that the shrimp not be served on bread slices and no garlic toast). Ripper Shrimp, as advertised, are a half-pound of you-peel-it, gluten-free shrimp with cocktail sauce. Most burgers are gluten-free, as long as you are careful about the bread.

Interesting menu note about bread: The company states that some states will allow you to bring your own bread (which ones do not?) and never to send it to the kitchen. Simply order your sandwich without bread and build your own sandwich at the table. Good advice in a chain restaurant where anything can happen between toaster and table (cross-contamination, most likely), so make sure the bread you take along tastes good untoasted. If you want toast, make it at home and let the bread dry completely before packing it. You don't want it soggy, do you?

If you've been good and are willing to run a few laps before dinner, this is the place that offers sinfully rich gluten-free desserts. Chocolate Thunder from Down Under is a gluten-free brownie and vanilla ice cream with chocolate sauce and chocolate shavings. Sydney's Sinful Sundae is GF vanilla ice cream rolled in toasted coconut and slathered with chocolate sauce and whipped cream.

I would download their printer-friendly GF menu and have it with me when I went to an Outback Steakhouse. This way, everybody is on the same page, and you can figure out what you want beforehand. Do I have to tell you not to wear tight clothing to this place?

For information and locations, call Outback Steak House at (813) 282-1225, or www.outbacksteakhouse.com.

P. F. Chang's China Bistro

As a love of all things Asian sweeps across America's fickle heart, the fare in this 30-state empire is remarkably light (for chain eating, that is) and not as fat and calorie dense (I didn't say low-calorie) as many other similar places.

The theme is described as "a harmonious balance of the Chinese principals of fan and t'sai—fan foods include rice, noodles and grains and t'sai foods are vegetables, meat, poultry and seafood." Southeast Asian cuisine is fused with traditional Chinese dishes as well as modern Chinese cuisine. When viewed from a dramatic exhibition kitchen, the Mandarin-style wok cooking becomes an entertaining diversion while waiting for your order. You can also see what they're doing to your food.

No "crouching crouton, hidden gluten" here.

There is a full and satisfying gluten-free menu, which features Shanghai cucumbers with wheat-free soy sauce, oriental chicken salad without wonton strips, and ginger chicken with steamed broccoli in gluten-free sauce. The Cantonese shrimp or scallops can be made with gluten-free sauce, as can the steamed fish of the day. The chow fun noodles and the Singapore noodles are 100 percent rice and all of the marinades are thickened with cornstarch. For something really light, ask that your lettuce wrap be made with any of the gluten-free fillings.

For gluten-free and the ability to avoid consuming as much fat as in other similar establishments, this one is near the top of the corporate food chain. For information and locations, call headquarters at (866)-PFCHANGS, or www.pfchangs.com.

Tony Roma's

As the story goes, one weekend in the seventies, down in Miami, chef David Smith and Tony Roma took a weekend off and threw some baby back ribs on the grill, using Tony Roma's secret barbecue sauce. The plan was to go back to grilling burgers and steaks on Monday. Well, the rest, as they say, is corporate history. With 225 locations on five continents, including Dallas, San Francisco, Orlando, Vancouver, Las Vegas, Tokyo, and Madrid, this is truly a worldwide operation. That's a long way to go for "down home" cooking.

They advertise a gluten-free menu at every Tony Roma's restaurant and make it available by mail or online, downloadable for serious study.

If you like beef ribs and barbecued chicken, this is the place for you. Some items declared free of gluten: corn tortilla chips, spinach artichoke dip, potato skins appetizer, all salad dressings (remember the croutons!), cole slaw, and, of course, ribs and chicken with original, Carolina Honey, Blue Ridge Smokies, or Red Hot barbecue sauce.

Better to surf the Web for them, the corporate office is in Port of Spain, Trinidad. Phone: (868) 627-RIBS, or www.tonyromastt.com.

Wildfire Restaurants

With restaurants in Chicago and Minneapolis, this savvy chain began to see an uptick in requests for gluten-free meals and decided to do something more about it than advising celiacs to skip the bread basket. The result is a full gluten-free menu that includes White Cheddar Au Gratin Potatoes and Flourless Chocolate Cake. Back in the kitchen, there's a system of checks and balances that prevents cross-contamination, complete with an Ingredient Alert Form which triggers actions like cleaning the grill, mixing salads by hand, and checking every special order at each step along the way to your table. Talk about market responsive. For locations and current menus, visit www.wildfire restaurant.com.

Fast-Food Nation

Sooner or later you are going to head to the mall and shop till you drop. Your stomach will growl so loudly, you won't be able to hear the announcement of a one-hour sale on designer drawer organizers. And before you know it, you will find yourself surrounded by strange and exotic foods like chicken-on-a-stick, gyro, wraps, smoothies, gooey soups, and potatoes stuffed with things nature never intended. The tabloid headline will read "Celiac Sentenced to Starvation in Food Court."

The faster the food, the slower the torture. It is not only possible, but also entirely likely, that you will go hungry in the land of plenty.

The idea is always, always, always eat before going out and getting stuck in a situation like this. Ditto for long drives on roads with nothing but fast-food restaurants. Fill a baggie with protein-packed mixed nuts, or nuts and raisins and other dried fruits, and nibble to your heart's content. Stick a banana or an apple or a pear in your purse or in the car, maybe a gluten-free muffin or one of the gluten-free energy bars. Try not to get crumbs all over the place.

If you've remembered to bring two slices of gluten-free bread (never, never, never go shopping without doing this), head for the nearest deli or sandwich counter and ask them to make a plain roast turkey or roast beef sandwich. You will make sure the meat has not been marinated and the server wipes the slicer before he or she makes your sandwich, won't you?

Again, remember to pack bread you enjoy untoasted. A toaster isn't a common sight in a food court, but you should always ask. With counter and prep space at such a premium, chances are there's one in the back. If you can arrange a grilled sandwich, make sure the grill is scraped clean before your bread is put on. Another trick is to carry a gluten-free wrap like Don Pancho and ask for a roll-up. Condiments are usually in individual packets. Read the label before you squeeze.

Okay, you forgot. Now what?

Go to the nearest Mexican takeout and ask if you can buy a corn tortilla (remember that most premade wraps are made with wheat flour), then order the sandwich you want as a platter and do the rolling yourself. If you're really desperate, buy a big box of plain, unbuttered popcorn, and avoid any flavored varieties.

Salad bars are no-nos, not only for gluten-contamination but also for basic hygiene. *Put down that olive, you never know where it's been.* Smoothies are dicey as well, what with all that energy-inducing protein powder around. If you can see a list of ingredients and can coerce the teenager behind the counter to wash out the blender, be my guest.

As for hamburger and other fast-food chains, I am not a fan of going to a place where I have to munch a green salad and a gray meat patty while everybody else chows down double cheeseburgers. Let's just say I like to have things "my way." The thought of getting a burger without its plump padded roll isn't my idea of lunch. However, we've all found ourselves with no hamburger buns in our purses, suddenly starving and with no other acceptable options in sight. If you have to eat something right now or you'll explode, order a plain meat patty or a chicken breast and resolve to do better next time.

A nice cup of Starbucks coffee is an option, or chai with a little piece of pure chocolate to fight the four o'clock blahs. Avoid the blended drinks and Frappuccino, though.

The Japanese sushi takeout bar is another fairly safe option, a good place for a plain salad or a steaming cup of miso soup as long as you know what's in the soup.

When all else fails, think ice cream and frozen yogurt. While some of these confections are not exactly stingy with the butterfat, others are fat-free and many are quite safe. If you really can't afford the calories, console yourself with the idea that you're having dessert for lunch.

Here's the scoop on what to expect in our "fast-food nation."

Baskin-Robbins

Chocolate, Chocolate Chip, Chocolate Fudge, Jamoca, Jamoca Almond Fudge, Mint Chocolate Chip, Pistachio Almond, Old-Fashioned Butter Pecan, Peanut Butter 'N Chocolate, Pralines 'N Cream, Rocky Road, Very Berry

Strawberry, World Class Chocolate, Banana Strawberry, Black Walnut, Baseball Nut, Cherries Jubilee, Chocolate Almond, Chocolate Mousse Royale, Chocolate Raspberry Truffle, English Toffee, Chunky Heath Bar, Rum Raisin, Winter White Chocolate, Oregon Blackberry—all drippingly, indulgently gluten-free.

Ditto for Chocolate and Vanilla Twist nonfat ice cream and low-fat Espresso 'N Cream. Gluten-free No Sugar Added flavors are Call Me Nuts, Cherry Cordial, Chocolate Rassmatazz, Mad About Chocolate, Pineapple Coconut, and Thin Mint. Gluten-free FroZone kids' flavors include Eerie I Scream, Neon Sour Apple, Ice Polar Paws, Pink Bubblegum, Skullicious, and Watermelon Ice.

Safe sorbet? Black Tie Bubbly, Mixed Berry Lemonade, and Pink Raspberry Lemon. So what if you spoil your appetite for dinner? www.baskin robbins.com.

Ben & Jerry's

While we hear the founders are licking winter in Florida, this quirky company is still quirky. They actually suggest that you examine the labels on their ice cream in stores and on their Web site and make it easy for you to do so. They say it's because flavors and their gluten-free status change too often to risk publishing a reliable list. It worries them that someone might read an old list and accidentally eat something they shouldn't. Go to the Web site listed below and click on nutritional information. There you will find an easy-to-read chart with every flavor they make, fully disclosing every calorie, carb, and fat gram, complete with a little window to click on the ingredients printed on the label. We've heard this company is socially conscious. This proves it. For starters, Organic Strawberry, Organic Vanilla (this contains vanilla extract for those of you who still avoid it), Butter Pecan, Chocolate, Pistachio, Original Strawberry, Original Vanilla, Vanilla Swiss Almond, and Uncanny Cashew all look to be gluten-free. Forget Chubby Hubby and Chocolate Carb Karma. There is no gluten in the latter, but there is enough Sorbitol and chemicals to keep you in the bathroom for a week. You're done with that, aren't you? www.benandjerrys.com.

Burger King

According to the downloadable list of items containing wheat (mind you, there is no gluten-free list) from Burger King, you can safely enjoy a "side garden salad" with Kraft Creamy Caesar Salad Dressing, any of their soft drinks and juices, water, milk, Kraft Ranch Dipping Sauce or Honey Dipping Sauce. At this writing, french fries were advertised as being cooked in a dedicated fryer, but alas are no longer. Vanilla and chocolate shakes are listed as free of wheat with syrup added. (I must confess I get the shakes thinking about the chemicals in these things.) While a separate nutritional brochure lists the Whopper® burger as 100 percent USDA-inspected beef, the allergen list includes the roll and therefore calls the burger off-limits. A plain burger dipped in honey sauce, soft drink, and a garden salad—all things considered, it could be worse. www.burgerking.com.

Carvel

When I was a kid growing up in New York I loved their Flying Saucers, vanilla ice cream swirled between dark chocolate sandwich cakes. As a teenager, no date for the movies or drive home from the beach was complete without a stop at Carvel. We are told by Carvel customer service that the icing and the gel that is used to personalize their cakes is gluten-free, as are vanilla, chocolate, fat-free vanilla and chocolate, and sugar-free vanilla ice cream. The company lists flavors and ingredients like Carvella flavoring, coffee, butter, maple, pistachio, rum, mint, lemon, orange and lime sherbet, cheesecake flavor, simple syrup, whipped topping, cocoa, strawberry, black raspberry, eggnog, pumpkin purée, caramel fudge topping, chocolate syrup, bittersweet fudge, butterscotch topping, caramel topping, peanut butter topping, chocolate chips, mini M&Ms, marshmallow topping, and praline pecans as gluten-free.

With all due respect to Thomas Wolfe, maybe we *can* go home again. www.carvel.com.

Dairy Queen

Things are pretty basic here. The perennial favorites, Chocolate and Vanilla Soft Serve, are gluten-free—without the cone of course. It's a good idea to verify the mix at each store. Just in case. www.dairyqueen.com.

Denny's

These people have come a long way since their first appearance in *Against the Grain*. Their gluten-free list includes eggs and omelets, and, of course, hamburgers without the bun. Here you can ask for plain tuna if you aren't comfortable eating tuna mixed with mayonnaise and pickles, which both

And the "Corporate Obfuscation Award" Goes to . . .

Friendly's. In response to a consumer request for a list of their gluten-free flavors, their public affairs person supplied a really long list of flavors that *do* contain gluten. Once you have memorized all their flavors and can fill in the blanks, this should be easy to figure out.

Not terribly friendly, are they?

Too much ice cream in the world to worry about theirs.

contain vinegar. French fries and hash browns are safe as long as you can verify a dedicated fryer has been used—this may vary from restaurant to restaurant. Side dishes considered by this company to be safe are apple-sauce, cottage cheese, fresh fruit, salsa, baked potato, and grits. There's oat-meal for those celiacs who are comfortable with oats, but I wouldn't bet my life on these being whole Irish oats. This isn't the place to conduct the great oat experiment. Here we are invited to ask store personnel for information before we order. And it isn't a problem if you insist on seeing a questionable product's label. Kudos for customer service. www.dennys.com.

Häagen-Dazs

This company, as I do, cautions you to avoid any flavor or ice-cream bar using the word cookie, cheesecake, dough, brownie, or burst. Alas, the company says, *dulce de leche* is not gluten-free. However, soft-serve vanilla, chocolate, banana, and coffee frozen yogurts is. Sorbet, too.

And there is ice cream, the glorious full-fat variety. Belgian Chocolate, Chocolate, Butter Pecan, Chocolate, Chocolate Chip, Chocolate Peanut Butter, Macadamia Brittle, Macadamia Nut, Pralines & Cream, Rum Raisin, Strawberry, Swiss Chocolate Almond, Vanilla, Vanilla Fudge, and Vanilla Swiss Almond.

Who cares about the cone. www.haagendazs.com.

McDonald's

We're grateful to these folks for downsizing their portions, but you may want to go back for seconds on the french fries, which are gluten-free, prepared in a dedicated fryer, and in my humble opinion the *ne plus ultra* of fast-food fries. Other options include grilled chicken bacon ranch salad, Caesar salad without the chicken, honey and hot mustard sauce, Newman's Own Cobb Dressing, Low-Fat Balsamic Vinaigrette, or Ranch Dressing. For breakfast McDonald's says the sausage, scrambled eggs, and hash browns are gluten-free. For dessert, choose a Fruit 'n Yogurt Parfait, strawberry or chocolate sundae or hot fudge sundae with nuts, unless of course you're allergic to them. They say their chocolate, strawberry, or vanilla Triple Thick Shake are gluten-free as well, but may contain small amounts of other unsafe shake flavors served at their restaurants. This, of course, is a legal fudge in case any of their workers get sloppy. Use common sense and see for yourself. www.mcdonalds.com.

TCBY

According to the company, all frozen yogurt flavors but Cheesecake, Chocolate Malt, and Cookies 'N Cream are gluten-free. Nonfat and no-sugar added flavors are also safe as their flavorings are derived from corn. How refreshing. www.tcby.com.

Wendy's

Surprise, surprise. A fast-food chain that supplies an easy-to-read list of gluten-free products. Here you can have a plain side or Caesar side salad, or a spring mix salad minus the dressing or pecans. The burgers are gluten-free, without the bun, of course. According to their Web site, Wendy's baked potatoes with broccoli and cheese, chili and cheese, bacon and cheese, chives, liquid margarine, sour cream, or Country Crock spread are considered gluten-free. Ditto for the chili, Frosty, soft drinks, Taco Supremo Salad without salsa, and taco chips are also advertised as gluten-free. Okay condiments are American cheese, bacon, lettuce, tomato, and onion.

With the usual disclaimer, Wendy's states this list is effective as of August 2003. I would check from time to time for updates. Never assume menu items considered gluten-free now will remain so forever. Wendy's gets high marks for this service to celiacs. www.wendys.com.

A final word. Always, always, always check in periodically with the fast-food company that makes your favorite ice cream or favorite anything, for that matter. Menu items and flavors go out of style just like fashion, and it pays to touch base from time to time. The new labeling law (see chapter 19, "How Many Celiacs Does It Take to Change a Label?") makes it mandatory to list wheat, as well as other common allergens. Once the FDA standardizes a label for gluten content, things will be even easier. But until then, and especially in franchised operations, it pays to be up to date and well-informed.

Learn More

Check periodically with other favorite companies for gluten-free items.

Arby's
1000 Corporate Drive
Ft. Lauderdale, FL 33334
(800) 487-2729
www.arbys.com

Hardee's
505 North 7th Street, Suite 200
St. Louis, Missouri 63101
(877) 799-STAR
www.hardees.com

IHOP
450 North Brand Boulevard
7th Floor
Glendale, CA 91203
(818) 240-6055
www.ihop.com

Olive Garden
P.O. Box 592037
Orlando, FL 32859
(800) 331-2729
www.olivegarden.com

Red Lobster
5900 Lake Ellenor Drive
Orlando, FL 32809
(800) LOBSTER
www.redlobster.com

Shoney's
171 Elm Hill Pike
Nashville, TN 3702
(615) 391-5395
www.shoneys.com

Sizzler
12655 West Jefferson Boulevard
Los Angeles, CA 90066
(818) 662-9900
www.sizzler.com

Subway
325 Bic Drive
Milford, CT 06460
(800) 888-4848
www.subway.com

Taco Bell
1701 von Karman
Irvine, CA 92714
(800) 822-6235
www.tacobell.com

Starbucks
(866) 355-3780
www.starbucks.com

TGI Friday's
4201 Marsh Lane
Carrollton, TX 75007
(800) 374-3297
www.Fridays.com

a map of the gluten-free world

Only those who go too far
find out how far one can go.

—T. S. ELIOT

Armed with a suitcase full of rice cakes and enough French phrases to buy the fabulous pair of riding boots I prize today, I prepared for my first gluten-free April in Paris by penning the forerunner of the language cards that first appeared in *Against the Grain*. Written in the most stilted and ridiculous schoolgirl French (I hold the record for the most beginner classes ever taken by one person at the Alliance Française), this first card announced, basically, that "if I have any *farine*, I'll have a disease in my chair." I was ready for the city that a young and starving Hemingway once called "a moveable feast."

Upon reading my explanation of what I could and could not eat, inconsolable that someone should come to Paris and not be able to sop up his *pistou* or eat his *coq au vin* with a heel of bread, the manager of Le Petit Zinc gave me a wonderful bottle of Brouilly.

Despite my protestations that it did not bother me at all, he refused to roll the pastry cart to our table, raising a warning eyebrow at my husband who was definitely entertaining the idea of something flaky. Cheese it was. Only a beast would ogle a tart in front of his *farine*-challenged wife.

One look at my silly little card and chefs fussed, concierges accommodated, maître'd's melted and even the snootiest waiters marched into kitchens to investigate the *pommes frites* for the slightest soupçon of offense. One night, in a sidewalk café in the shadow of St. Sulpice in a tiny street near the Boulevard St. Germain, a party broke out because of my "*petite carte.*" When the owner of the place asked to keep it among other souvenirs tacked up behind the bar, I graciously handed it over, knowing I had several copies back in the room for just this eventuality. The man pressed it to his heart, gave a wicked grin, and showed it to a table full of regulars. One by one, they peered at it, pointing at us and smiling, as intent on my husband as they were on the woman who could "*ne mange pas farine.*"

Finally, one of them approached our table, a jovial Brit who exclaimed that my husband, a jovial Brit himself who sports an impressive handlebar mustache, looked exactly like Capitaine Haddock, the blustery English naval officer in the popular French cartoon strip, *TinTin*. I reminded them of the hapless princess locked in a tower, or, in my case, a patisserie. Tables were joined, introductions made, glasses of wine all around. In the soft spring air, dogs barked, lovely French voices rose and fell, and a gnarled old couple passing by stopped to dance to music drifting down from an open window. An unforgettable evening in Paris, all because of my special diet.

The point is, laughter doesn't always mean someone is making fun of you or your diet. My little card is in tatters now, at the bottom of a chest full of postcards, photos, and an official-looking letter I received while in Paris from the Royal Society of Blokes informing me that I was the first American female ever to achieve that honorary status. (My husband sent it, of course, with the help of an accomplice.) The card stays among these cherished things because it reminds me that a good life is something you invent as you go, that laughter is the great healer and that strangers are just friends you haven't met yet.

Of course, at times all of France seems like one long baguette, so there is great irony in the fact that the English word for *pain* is the French word for bread. (Even more so if your relatives are called Petitpain.) Like poor young Hemingway who did it out of poverty, especially on those moody days when the wind is blowing a certain way, sometimes it's better to avoid passing the patisseries that dot every Parisian street. We do what we must.

Yes, you wish you could leave your diet in another time zone. It won't wait patiently at home while you take a little vacation, but there is absolutely no reason to let being a celiac ground you. With ample notice, some preparation, a willingness to try new foods, and with the exception of the obvious danger zones, there's no place in the world that's off-limits.

Having said that . . . somewhere, sometime, no matter how carefully you've planned, especially in exotic locations, you may find yourself miles away from a safe meal and struggling to make that chocolate bar or emergency bag of nuts and raisins last all day. I look at it this way: I haven't come this far for the food. The truth is, for most Americans, especially those of us fortunate enough to have the means to travel, there's no such thing as truly going hungry. It may be a while, but there will always be another meal. Many of the world's people cannot say that.

If you do find yourself in that rare situation, suck in your newly flat stomach and realize that what you may never get is another chance to drink in the beauty of an Alpine lake, hear the church bells pealing on the Piazza San Marco, breathe in the saffron-scented air of a bazaar, or see Kilimanjaro at sunrise. Travel is food for the soul.

Besides, in the presence of such wonders, who can swallow?

Taking Flight

It's ironic that as more and more restaurants and shops cater to special diets, airlines seem to be dispensing with food altogether. Nowadays, a bag of nuts is a meal on most domestic flights and many carriers have stretched airborne time not requiring food to four hours. (I'd like to see a planeload of airline executives try that some time.) I never fly without a couple of bottles of water, a packet of gluten-free crackers, some nuts and raisins, or a muffin or an energy bar. This not only comes in handy in the air but it's a lifesaver when the plane is stuck on the runway for hours. As often as not, I'm the only one with food. You can't imagine what people will do for half of a banana or a bite of a Bumble Bar.

On longer flights, many airlines do offer gluten-free meals, but the definition of what constitutes said meal varies with each airline. Comparison shopping is tricky on most, unless you make a reservation. Talk about a catch-22. I would insist, though. These are competitive times. Unhappily, too many carriers consider anything served with a rice cake a meal worth advertising, while others really do make the effort. At thirty thousand feet, mistakes cannot be rectified. I usually request a fruit and cheese plate to accompany the roll or crackers in my carry-on—far preferable to pallid chicken and undercooked rice pellets.

Once upon a time, when the skies were friendlier to Americans, I carried a set of portable camping utensils (these come in handy in outposts where the cutlery seems, well, less than clean), but security issues have put the kibosh on that. Personally, I would rather feel safe on a plane than have my creature comforts. Still, eating with one's hands is messy, so it's wise to pack moist towels as well. Whatever you do, don't wrap bread in tinfoil and stick in your suitcase. By the time bomb-sniffing dogs stop drooling on it and the security people X-ray it and poke it with sticks, scaring people and wasting their time, it will have lost its appeal. More about the serious issue of security later on. It's never been easier to buy gluten-free products when you get where you're going, so travel light.

There are exceptions, of course. If you are heading for Africa or Chile or the Brazilian rain forest or some other spot off the beaten path where gluten-free food is unheard of, it's wise to send a shipment well ahead of your arrival. It if seems unlikely that the package will coincide with your stay, put these items in a separate bag with a letter from your doctor stating your need to travel with these foods for medical reasons (this expedites clearing customs on the other end). Carry these products in their original packages and call your carrier to ask what security regulations apply. It's chancy, but if you take extra care to prove the legitimacy of your packages, they just might make it to your destination with you.

Reservation requirements vary for special meals, some carriers require as much as three days' notice and others as little as six hours'. Most cannot confirm what will be served on your flight, but if you pin them down, they will give you the details of a meal that "might" be served to you. There are some notable exceptions, Aer Lingus and British Airways, among others.

Aer Lingus, (800) 223-6537, www.aerlingus.com
Aer Lingus requires at least 24-hours' notice for gluten-free meal requests, but suggests you give as much warning as possible to ensure that your food is aboard your flight as well as on each leg of your journey.

Air Canada, (800) 247-2262, www.aircanada.com
Gluten-free meals are available on the flights that serve food. Ask before you book and carry a snack in case.

Air France, (800) 237-2747, www.airfrance.com
With 48-hours' notice, Air France offers gluten-free meals on all transatlantic flights.

Air India, (800) 223-7776, www.airindia.com
This carrier assures the traveler that any special meals, including gluten-free, will be made available with 48-hours' notice at no additional charge.

Air Jamaica, (800) 523-5585, www.airjamaica.com
Gluten-free meals are available, and it is suggested that you reserve your special meal at least 48 hours prior to takeoff.

Air New Zealand, (800) 262-1234, www.airnewzealand.com

With 72-hours' notice, this airline will serve you a proper gluten-free meal. I'd give them even more notice and ask for confirmation in writing. It's a long way to go without food.

Alaska Airlines, (800) 426-0333, www.alaskaair.com

Diabetic, salt-free, kosher, low-fat, low-cholesterol, everything but gluten-free. It's Alaska, not Mars.

Alitalia, (800) 223-5730, www.alitalia.com

With a week's notice, this airline will serve you a gluten-free meal.

American Airlines, (800) 433-7300, www.aa.com

On any flight of four hours or more, either domestic or international, with six hours' notice (I'd give more), you can expect to be served a gluten-free meal.

Avianca, (800) 284-2622, www.avianca.com

With three days' notice you'll be flying down to Rio with a gluten-free meal.

American Trans Air, (800) 435-9282, www.ata.com

You'll get whatever is on board on this food-for-sale operation, except on the Hawaii flight. With 72-hours' notice, you'll get a gluten-free meal.

British Airways, (800) 247-9297, www.britishairways.com

These people know their stuff. Put in your request for a gluten-free meal *prior* to 24 hours before flight time.

China Airlines, (800) 227-5118, www.china-airlines.com

When you book your ticket (at least 48 hours ahead), request a GFML (gluten-free meal).

Continental Airlines, (800) 525-0280, www.continental.com

Not all flights serve food. And only some food service flights provide gluten-free meals. Ask before you book.

Delta, (800) 221-1212, www.delta.com

While Delta claims to have gluten-free meals on certain flights, I am told this "cannot be assured."

El Al Israel Airlines, (800) 223-6700, www.elal.com

With 24-hours' notice you will get a gluten-free version of a kosher meal on all El Al flights.

Finnair, (800) 950-5000, www.finnair.com/us
You can enjoy a gluten-free meal on this carrier as long as you order it 48 hours ahead of time.

Iberia Airlines, (800) 772-4642 www.iberia.com
Ask for a meal *sin* gluten and give as much notice as you can and you may end up with gluten-free bread and corn tortillas with your dinner. *Muchas gracias.*

Japan Airlines, (800) 525-3663, www.japanair.com
If you're traveling first class, it's a good idea to carry your own wheat-free tamari or soy sauce for the sushi appetizers. Otherwise let them know at least 48 hours in advance and you'll get a standard gluten-free meal.

KLM Royal Dutch Airlines, (800) 374-7747, www.klm.com
Ask the booking agent to call the catering manager when you book your ticket and an individual gluten-free meal will be created and put on board. The more notice you give, the better.

Korean Air, (800) 438-5000, www.koreanair.com
Sorry, no gluten-free meals.

Lan Chile Airlines, (866) 435-9526, www.lan.com
You can have low-calorie, low-fat, low-sodium, low-protein, non-dairy, just fish or vegetarian, anything but gluten-free. A chilly reception for celiacs.

Lufthansa German Airlines, (800) 645-3880, www.lufthansa-usa.com
Gluten-free meals are served with safe breads as long as you have given at least 72-hours' notice.

Mexicana Airlines, (800) 531-7921, www.mexicana.com
No gluten-free meals on this airline, but I am told there are always corn tortillas in the galley. Ask and yours shall be warmed.

Midwest Airlines, (800) 425-2022, www.midwestairlines.com
No special meals of any kind are available. There are bags of glutenous crunchy things as well as meals for purchase, also riddled with gluten.

Northwest Airlines, (800) 225-2525, www.nwa.com
Whether flying domestically or internationally, 24-hours' notice will get you a gluten-free meal on this airline.

Qantas, (800) 227-4500, www.qantasusa.com

With 24-hours' notice on all international flights, a gluten-free meal will accompany you Down Under. Within Australia and New Zealand, gluten-free is supplied as long as food is served.

Scandinavian Airlines, (800) 221-2350, www.scandanavian.net

The emphasis here is on as much notice as you can provide and a gluten-free itinerary will be made for you.

Singapore Airlines, (800) 742-3333, www.singaporeair.com

With 24-hours' notice you'll fly gluten-free.

Swissair, (877) 359-7947, www.swiss.com

Who cares about dinner when there's pure Swiss chocolate? A gluten-free meal is offered on all transatlantic flights with at least 48 hours' notice.

TAP Portugal Airlines, (800) 221-7370, www.tapusa.us

I am told "more than 24-hours' notice" will get you a gluten-free meal.

United Airlines, (800) 241-6522, www.united.com

Availability of special meals is determined by point of departure and destination. My best advice: call with specific plans and ask before you book.

US Airways, (800) 428-4322, www.usairways.com

On any flight that serves food (two hours or more flight time), either domestic or international, gluten-free meals are available with at least 24-hours' notice.

Varig Brazilian Airlines, (800) 468-2744, www.varigbrasil.com

With 72-hours' notice, you can fly down to Rio gluten-free.

Virgin Atlantic, (800) 862-8621, www.virginatlantic.com

With 24-hours' notice, Virgin will supply a gluten-free meal with allowable foods. They're English. They understand this.

Security Note

In our post–9/11 world, worse things than gluten can befall an American abroad. The first stop in any travel itinerary should be the State Department Web site (www.state.gov), which offers travel advisories and warnings for Americans around the world. Another good site to cruise before traveling is the Orwellian-sounding Department of Homeland Security at www.white

house.gov/homeland. This is sad, but it is a fact of life for the foreseeable future. We are told by the Transportation Security Administration (www.tsa .gov) to keep foods like chocolate, cheese, and fruitcake out of our checked luggage. This rule is not a plot against traveling celiacs, it is simply that the new detection systems cannot tell the difference in density between food and bombs or other explosives. If the alarm is sounded because you've got a nice fat loaf of gluten-free bread in your bag, it will undergo several more levels of bomb checking, often with the owner of said bag present. This is not how you want to start your vacation.

I have read posts from celiacs decrying this rule, and I must tell you I am not in favor of making an exception to the no-food-in-the-suitcase rule. There are many things more important than our diets, and traveling safely is one of them. I'd much rather buy food when I arrive and know I haven't gummed up the security process for everyone else. We don't live in a vacuum.

We've been living on Yellow/Elevated to Orange/High alerts these days, and it pays to know your colors—Red is Severe, Blue is Guarded, and Green is Low. Any change in the alert status will change the rules at the airport, so always check before you leave and allow plenty of time for clearing security.

For snacking on board, always carry your food (and your medicine) in clear plastic bags. Carry your film with you as well, as the new security machines are not kind. Don't lock your bags (bungee cords are good here) and never gift-wrap food packages to take to your celiac sister in Detroit. Pack the paper separately and wrap them when you arrive. If you're carrying books, don't stack them. Spread them out evenly in the bag. And forget that Swiss Army knife that comes in so handy for fruit and cheese. Always pack your shoes on top.

You don't have to be a celiac to remember to wear something you can slip off easily for security checks and to avoid lots of jewelry and other metals. (Some screeners are so sensitive, even underwire bras set them off.) Wear something simple, cozy, and travel under the radar. In foreign countries, do try to fit in. I know it's hard when you're asking for directions to the nearest *reformhaus* in halting German. If women wear skirts, wear one yourself. If men wear a coat and tie to dinner, do so yourself. Find out the local customs and never wear shorts or skimpy clothing to religious shrines, etc. This is no longer a courtesy. It is a safety precaution.

Celiacs Abroad

In London, where celiacs are as ubiquitous as the damp, Harrods and Marks & Spencer and other large department stores have impressive gluten-free sections in their food halls, as do most supermarkets, often in dedicated sections, but just as often alongside gluten-containing items in the relevant aisle. In fact, all over England you will find gluten-free foods, many not available here. From the health food store to the local pub and the tiny thatched bed and breakfast tucked away in the Cotswolds, just say the word *coeliac* and you won't go hungry.

In Ireland, too, where the condition is quite common, you will find great solidarity and understanding. From the lowly ploughman's lunch (cheese, fruit, and a hunk of gluten-free bread) to a posh Dublin tea, you'll find much to eat and the Irish eager to please.

In Paris, look for Valpiform and other gluten-free products in food chains like La Vie Claire and Monoprix or in stores like Rendezvous de la Nature in the 5th *arrondissement*. Ask for *produits sans gluten* (products without gluten) and you'll be in business.

All Italian pharmacies carry gluten-free foods. All you have to do is say *"senza glutino."* But never drink hotel coffee from a warming urn. It almost always contains barley. Have freshly brewed espresso or cappuccino instead. Risotto is a national treasure in this country, especially in the Po Valley, where arborio rice is grown. In Milan, look for the BeBop Café for amazing gluten-free pizza. The Italian celiac society offers a list of approved restaurants and the best gluten-free pastas are widely available (see their listing in the following section).

Sin means "without" in Spanish. *Sin* gluten is gluten-free. And remember that a Spanish pancake is not a pancake at all, but a thin potato omelet. Gluten-free brands like Singlu, Sanavi, and Proceli breads are found in pharmacies, and in El Corte Ingles department stores.

In German-speaking countries, the word *reformhaus* on health food stores means gluten-free products inside. You'll find them in Drogeries and Apothekes (pharmacies), too. Go to the Swiss group's home page and bone up on all the local brands.

Sweden, Finland, and Norway are celiac heaven, where every supermarket has a gluten-free section; even the Big Mac buns are gluten-free (not that you've come all that way for American fast food). Imagine popping in to a pizza joint and ordering a safe slice. Even the oats are grown in dedicated fields.

In the Netherlands, gluten-free foods are sold in health food stores called *reformwinkel* or *naturveodingswinkel*. If you don't see what you want, ask, gluten-free products are often kept frozen.

Slovenia's gluten-free products are sold in pharmacies, health food stores, and in some supermarkets like Merkator and Interspar.

There is a slight difference between the Spanish spoken in Spain and that of Latin America. For your purposes, this is too subtle to merit a separate card. In addition to your translation cards, always carry a pocket dictionary, so you can easily decipher what is written on a menu. In Mexico, corn is the staple food and it makes traveling here a pleasure for the gluten-free. Be careful, though, as it is customary to use bread crumbs to give *chiles rellenos* their crunch, as well as to stretch their ground meat stuffing. Always ask.

When traveling in remote locations, it's always a good idea to pack a doctor's note stating the requirements of your diet (especially if you are bringing in your own food), as well as several copies of one of the language cards from the appendix of this book.

In Ethiopia, the local flat bread is called *Injera*, made from a gluten-free grass called teff. You must always ask if wheat flour has been added to it.

In North Africa and the Middle East, couscous or cracked bulgur wheat is a common ingredient. Ground corn is an African staple with meat, fish, and vegetables. Very little food is manufactured here, so if someone tells you there's no flour in something, you can be pretty sure there isn't. Outside of cities, expect to see grilled goat, impala, warthog, and lamb.

Tribal customs prevail in many parts of Africa. In rural areas where there is no plumbing, the left hand has one use and one use alone. Never use your left hand to reach, touch, point, shake hands, or, God forbid, eat. Manners also dictate keeping hands in plain sight at all times and I am told smelling food cooking in a pot is not appropriate in these parts.

If you ever find yourself in Mozambique, a reader tells me there is a Pick 'n Pay grocery store in Nelspruit, on the South African side of the Mozambique border, that makes fresh gluten-free bread in their bakery. Pick some up on your way to Johannesburg.

International Celiac Organizations

A vacation isn't usually long enough to really understand how a place works. By the time you find the bakery that makes the best gluten-free bread or the restaurant that makes an amazing pizza out of safe flours, it's time to leave. Why not touch base with those insiders in each country before you leave or, at

Codex Alimentarius

Many Europeans follow Codex Alimentarius standards for gluten-free products that allow a form of wheat starch considered safe for celiacs but is not in keeping with stricter U.S. and Canadian standards. Bone up on the differences before you leave at www.celiac.com, and consult your doctor if you are considering a "when in Rome" strategy.

Rome Codex: www.codexalimentarius.net
Committee reports: www.codesalimentarius.net/reports.asp
Information about U.S. Codex activities:
www.fsis.usda.gov/oa/codex/index.htm

the very least, the minute you arrive? This way, you'll have the eating part taken care of, leaving you free to enjoy all the other pleasures.

Argentina
Asistencia al Celiaco de la Argentina, Buenos Aires
www.acela.org.ar

Australia
Coeliac Society of South Australia, Inc.
www.coeliac.org.au

Austria
Osterreichische Arbeitsgemeinschaft Zoliakie
www.go.to./zoeliakie/

Belgium
The Belgian Portal for Celiac
www.vcv.coeliakie.be

Bermuda
Coeliac Support Group of Bermuda
Ms. Elizabeth Boden
P.O. Box 1556
Hamilton HM FX, Bermuda
1-441-232-0264

Brazil
ACELBRA
http://www.acelbra.org.br

Canada
Canadian Celiac Association
www.celiac.ca

Foundation Québeçoise de la Maladie Coeliaque
www.fqmc.org

Chile
Club de Celiacos de la Universidad
Dr. Guillermo Benegas
Urrutia Manzano 330
Conception, Chile

Croatia
Hrvatsko Drustvo za Celijakiju
www.celiac.inet.hr

Cuba
Grupo de Celiacos de Cuba
Ms. Edith Gonzalez
Gamido 20708, Herarra y San
Antonio
Reparto Carolina, San Miquel del
Padron, Havana

Czech Republic
Czech Coeliac Society
www.coeliac.cz

Denmark
Danish Coeliac Society
www.coeliaki.dk

Finland
Finnish Coeliac Society
www.keliakia.org

France
Association Française des Intolerants
au Gluten
www.afdiag.com

Germany
Deutsche Zoliakie-Gesellschaft.e.V.
www.dzg-online.de

Hungary
Hungarian Celiac Society
www.liszterzekeny.hu

Iceland
Samtok Folks meo Glutenopol
Fannafold 231,
112 Reykjavik, Iceland
354-860-3328-560-3350
Magnus@esso.is

Ireland
Coeliac Society of Ireland
www.coeliac.ie

Israel
Israel Celiac Association
www.celiac.org.il

Italy
Associazione Italiano Celiachia
www.celiachia.it

Latvia
AML Children's Hospital
Riga, Latvia
amlbo@acad.latnet.lv

Lithuania
Lithuanian Celiac Society
Dr. Vaidotas Urbonas
122-720-429
uvaidas@altavista.net

Luxembourg
Association Luxembourgeoise des
Intolerants au Gluten
4A Rue de la Paix
Dudelange L-354, Luxembourg
352-52-02-79

Malta
Coeliac Association Malta
Lamut, Upper Gardens STJ 05, Malta

Mexico
Asociación de Celiacos de México
www.celiacosdemexico.com

Netherlands
Nederlandse Coeliakie Vereniging
www.coeliakievereniging.nl

New Zealand
Coeliac Society of New Zealand
www.coeliac.co.nz

Norway
Norsk Coliakiforning
www.ncf.no

Poland
Polish Coeliac Society
glutenO@polbox.com

Portugal
Clube dos Celiacos
www.7mares.terravista.pt/apdig

Romania
Aglutena Romania
Karin Kober
Avram Jancu no. 24
SIBIU RO-2400
69-21-76-22

Slovenia
Slovensko Drustvo za Celiakijo
www.drustvo-celiakija.si

South Africa
Gluten Intolerance/Celiac Support
Group
Lucille Cholerton
73 Old Mill Way
Durban North 4051
031-563-3109

Spain
Federación de Asociaciones de
Celiacos de España
www.celiacos.org

Sweden
Svenska Celiaki Forbundets
www.celiaki.se, kansli@celiaki.se
Swedish Celiac Youth Society
www.scuf.net

Switzerland
Association Suisse Romande de la
Coeliakie
www.coeliakie.ch

United Kingdom
Coeliac UK
www.coeliac.co.uk

Uruguay
Associación Celiaca del Uruguay
Montevideo
www.acelu.org

Cruisin'

Did you know the word *posh* comes from the era of steamship travel? To avoid the blazing sun at sea, well-heeled travelers crossing the Atlantic from Liverpool to New York paid dearly for cabins on the port side of the ship going out, on the starboard side going home. Port Out, Starboard Home; hence the term posh. Expensive, but worth it.

Ocean travel nowadays is no longer a floating exercise in class structure. Nor is it merely a means of getting from one place to another. Cruising is a destination unto itself, with ports of call here and there to lose one's sea legs. Some ships are small, others are floating cities. Some cruise lines offer land adventures, others provide leisurely shopping and touring, and still more offer ways to work off the buffet and get you home shipshape. Whether you are traveling in a first-class cabin or on a deck lower down, no amount of money or connections will get you something to eat beyond what's on board when you set sail.

Good planning and a willingness to work with the kitchen makes for smooth gluten-free sailing. With plenty of notice, upward of three weeks before you set sail, most cruise lines will accommodate any dietary need. Some will ask you to supply certain items and they will fill in the rest. Cruise-savvy celiacs say it's always a good idea to remind the kitchen of your next day's requests/needs the night before to avoid any snafu. And, of course, you'll remember to stash lots of gluten-free goodies in your stateroom.

Sightsee, practice yoga at sunrise, dance till dawn, shop till you drop. Do remember to wash your hands frequently. Whether you are gluten-free or not, cruise ships are love boats for microbes. To find the cruise that's right for you, do a little surfing on your own.

Above and Beyond Tours/Gay Celiacs, (800) 397-2681, www.above beyondtours.com
Bora Bora Cruises, (800) 828-6877, www.islandsinthesun.com
Carnival Cruise Lines, (888) 227-6482, www.carnival.com
Clipper Cruise Line, (800) 325-0010, www.clippercruise.com
Costa Cruise Lines, (800) 332-6782, www.costacruises.com
Cunard Line, (800) 728-6273, www.cunardline.com
Crystal Cruises, (800) 820-6663, www.crystalcruises.com
Delta Queen Steamboat Company, (800) 543-1949, www.deltaqueen.com
Disney Cruise Line, (800) 951-3532, www.disneycruise.com
Holland America Line, (877) 724-5425, www.hollandamerica.com
Norwegian Cruise Line, (800) 327-7030, www.ncl.com
Olivia Cruises and Resorts, (800) 631-6277, www.olivia.com

Take the Plunge

. . . .

If your idea of cruising is scuba diving to the bottom of the sea, Aqua Cat Cruises offers a luxury 102-foot catamaran for exploring the teeming coral reef in the Exumas, full-certification diving courses, underwater photography, and a chef who will do the gluten-free honors when you come up. (888) 327-9600, www.aquacatcruises.com

Princess Cruises, (800) 774-6237, www.princess.com
Radisson Seven Seas Cruises, (800) 285-1835, www.rssc.com
Royal Caribbean Cruises, (800) 327-6700, www.royalcaribbean.com
Royal Olympia Cruises, (800) 872-6400, www.roc.gr
Seabourn Cruise Line, (800) 929-9391, www.seabourn.com
Silversea Cruises, (800) 722-9955, www.silversea.com
Star Clippers, (800) 442-0551, www.starclippers.com
Swan Hellenic, (877) 800-7926, www.swanhellenic.com
Windstar Cruises, (800) 258-7245, www.windstarcruises.com

The Open Road

There's nothing like driving through the Painted Desert while little Tiffany plays the comb or getting lost in Brooklyn looking for that gluten-free kosher bakery you've only just heard about. Or letting the breeze whip through your hair as the map flies out the window.

Car trips allow the most flexibility and spontaneity for a gluten-free vacation, whether a romantic getaway or a family adventure. Who knows where the next turn will take you? There is much to be said for the road less traveled. Gas prices aside, it's the most economical way too. Always remember to change drivers every 200 miles, and to pack an emergency kit. After that you're on your own, free to roam the countryside, find a gluten-free restaurant, and picnic by a stream knowing you've got a trunk full of gluten-free road food and a radio that plays all your favorite traveling music.

If you're not the adventurous type and would like a bit of structure, make sure you've got your copy of *Viva's Healthy Dining Guide* to health food stores around the country. Or, for a guide to dozens of gluten-friendly restaurants around the country, go to www.goodhealthpublishing.com. New York's Westchester Celiac Sprue Support Group has a growing list of restaurants in

their Gluten-Free Restaurant Awareness Program at www.glutenfreerestaurants
.org, and it's always good to check in on the listserv before you leave town.
Why not plan a drive that includes a special treat like one of the restaurants
below? Here are just a few of the gluten-free pleasures awaiting your next
great American road trip.

ARIZONA

Los Sombreros, 2534 North Scottsdale Road, Scottsdale, (480) 994-1799,
specializes in "authentic" Mexican food and has a gluten-free menu.

Pugzie's Restaurant and Catering Company, 4700 North 16th Street,
Phoenix, (602) 279-3577, www.pugzies.com. Lynn Pugliano's son is a
celiac and she just happens to be a talented chef.

CALIFORNIA

Maurizio's Italian Restaurant, 135 North Maryland Avenue, Glendale,
(818) 247-5600. Call a day ahead and order the gluten-free pizza.

Pasta Pomodoro, a chain of restaurants in Northern California, offers
gluten-free pasta on the menu. For locations, www.pastapomodoro.com.

Pizzacotto, 11758 San Vicente Boulevard, Brentwood, (310) 442-7188.
These folks will prepare gluten-free pizza to order.

CONNECTICUT

Frascati Restaurant, 581 Newfield Avenue, Stamford, (203) 353-8900.
Gluten-free specials include pizza, bruschetta, pasta, and desserts.

ILLINOIS

Da Luciano, 8343 West Grand Avenue, River Grove, (708) 453-1000. Not
far from O'Hare Airport, this Italian restaurant boasts a four-page
gluten-free menu. Pasta, soups, veal dishes, even a separate oven for GF
pizzas. For dessert, homemade cannoli, tiramisu, biscotti, and almond
cookies. Reservations are advised.

Frontera Grill and Topolobampo, 445 North Clark Street, Chicago, (312)
661-434. This is authentic regional Mexican food as only the celebrated
Rick Bayless can do it (see page 242 for his Quesadillas Asadas). Frontera is casual, Topolobampo a bit more formal. Special diets are welcome in both places.

Stashu's Deli & Pizza, 4200 44th Avenue, Moline, (309) 797-9449. Gluten-
free pizza, calzones, and boli rolls. Call ahead to order and ask for
directions. Ask for Jim or Becki.

KENTUCKY

Ferd Grisanti Restaurant, 10212 Taylorsville Road, Louisville, (502) 267-0050, www.ferdgrisanti.com. This restaurant specializes in northern Italian cuisine and with a day or two's notice will make rice and corn pasta, as well as any special requests.

MASSACHUSETTS

Elephant Walk, 900 Beacon Street, Boston, and 2067 Massachusetts Avenue, Cambridge. You can be assured a gluten-friendly reception and Cambodian-French meal as part of the Gluten-Free Restaurant Awareness Program.

MICHIGAN

Celiac Specialty Bakery, 48411 Jefferson, Chesterfield, (586) 598-8180. Cruise by and fill up on muffins, cream puffs, and homemade donuts for the trip, www.celiacspecialties.com.

OREGON

Corbett Fish House, 5901 SW Corbett Avenue, Portland, (503) 246-4434. Nothing fishy here, except gluten-free rice flour–battered fish and chips.
Talarico's Mercado, 14559 Westlake Drive, Lake Oswego, (503) 620-7723. Absolutely glorious gluten-free pizza.

NEW YORK

Bruno King of Ravioli, 2204 Broadway, New York City, (212) 580-8150. If you're planning a trip to Manhattan, pick up a gluten-free pizza crust and ask the hotel or restaurant to top it and serve it to you.
Café Baldo, 2849 Jerusalem Avenue, Wantagh, Long Island, (516) 785-4780. Gluten-free pizza, ravioli, baked clams, and much more. This place is worth a trip from anywhere.
Mama's Restaurant, 1352 Montauk Highway, Oakdale, Long Island, (631) 567-0909. Gluten-free calamari, grilled shrimp, and chicken Parmagiana, veal marsala, ten kinds of pasta. Oh, mama.
Risotteria, 270 Bleecker Street, New York City, (212) 924-6664. Gluten-friendly Italian. Go to www.risotteria.com and peruse the gluten-free menu.
The Roycroft Inn, 40 South Grove Street, East Aurora, (716) 652-5552, www.Roycroftinn.com. Vegetarian, vegan, and gluten-free meals. Go for the flourless gâteau.

Sacred Chow, 522 Hudson Street, New York City, (212) 337-0863. Animal-free specialty foods and delicious gluten-free brownies and cookies, www.sacredchow.com.

Thai Basil, 20-02 Utopia Parkway, Bayside, (718) 352-8100. Gluten-friendly Asian fusion, Pad Thai, and other delights. No far from La Guardia Airport.

WASHINGTON

Kaili's Kitchen, Edmonds, (206) 542-1462. Remember when you ate from the bread basket? This Seattle gluten-free restaurant is home to many a GIG function. If you're heading that way, it's a must-stop. This growing restaurant is on the move. For new address, call or go to www.wheatless inseattle.com.

WASHINGTON, D.C.

Asia Nora, 2213 M Street N.W., (202) 797-4860 or www.noras.com. This organic Asian fusion restaurant in the Foggy Bottom neighborhood is a marvel of gluten-free delights. The night we visited, chef Haidar Karoum doted on us with five exquisite courses, including a spiced flourless cake topped with cardamon ice cream. Call well ahead to reserve and request the same special attention.

VERMONT

Hemmingway's, 4988 Route 4, Killington, (802) 422-3886, www.hem mingwaysrestaurant.com. This restaurant is pricey and deserving of its four stars. All produce is organic and there are no processed foods on the premises. Rice pasta and gluten-free bread are on hand and they are always glad to customize the menu for you.

CANADA

Casa du Spaghetti, 604 Principale, Granby, Quebec, (450) 372-3848. Not only will you find a gluten-free Italian dinner at this restaurant near Montreal, you will be able to order a nice cold glass of their gluten-free beer.

Café Pescara, 6752 Sherbrooke Est, Montreal, Quebec, (514) 253-2658, not only specializes in seafood with a French and Italian accent, it offers its guests a gluten-free menu.

Panne Rizo, 1939 Cornwall Avenue, Vancouver, (604) 736-0885. This bakery and casual café is owned by two wheat-challenged sisters. The result is a wonderful lunch and a bag full of goodies for the road.

If you ever find yourself in Milan . . .
Be Bop Ristorante & Pizza, V. Le Col di Lana 4, phone 02 8376972.

Or Australia . . .
Silly Yaks Bakery Café, 105 High Street, Northcote 3070, phone (03) 9482
3999, or www.sillyyak.com. This totally gluten-free restaurant, café, and bakery is a definite must for trips Down Under.

Celiac-Friendly Resorts, Ranches, Bed-and-Breakfasts, and Tour Companies

There's a reason why they call it the hospitality industry. Hoteliers, innkeepers, and the hosts of bed-and-breakfasts who open their homes to you are just that: hospitable. Once, at Garrick House, a rose-covered hotel high on the cliffs of St. Ives along England's North Sea, I fancied a nice gluten-free lobster for dinner. The owner said he was sorry, but there were none in the kitchen that night. The next afternoon as I lay snoozing on the lawn (overcome by the sea breezes and a healthy hike along a sizable stretch of the path that runs the whole length of England), my husband tapped my shoulder and pointed to a large orange creature in the grass next to my lawn chair. Our host had radioed his "mates" out on a fishing boat, put in my request, and drove down to meet them at the pier. They had delivered a lobster big enough for two dinners and lunch the next day. And what a lunch it was— chilled lobster dressed with a bit of mayonnaise and herbs from the garden. His smile, my delight, and the deluge of requests from other guests, made for a happy situation for everybody.

Advertising is nice, but word of mouth is what these good people rely on. Celiac-friendly is anyplace you are welcomed and happily accommodated. You may not find a lobster on the lawn, but with a little notice, you may discover bread baked, muffins served, backpack filled, even an entire menu redesigned just for you. A vacation is someplace you return from happier and better fed than when you left. Harbor no reservations about traveling. Ask and you shall receive. Here are a few ideas to get you started. Or you can search for a celiac-friendly bed-and-breakfast inn anywhere in the United States, Canada, and around the world at www.innseekers.com/gluten.cfm. For spas and health resorts, go to www.spafinder.com.

United States

Alaska

Glade House Bed and Breakfast, Anchorage. The owner of this modern style house tucked in among native birch and spruce trees is a celiac and has become quite proficient at gluten-free baking. Expect homemade goodies on weekdays and pancakes, waffles, or omelets on weekends and, if the urge to explore strikes early, ask that a breakfast bag be packed. For rates and booking information, go to www.customcpu.com/commercial/gladehousebnb.

Arizona

Canyon Ranch, Tucson. This wonderful spa has much to recommend it, including mountain hiking and just about every exercise and beauty service imaginable and a kitchen that bakes gluten-free muffins and bread every morning. The Lennox, Massachusetts, branch in the Berkshires is a horn's toot away from Tanglewood. For information, rates and packages, www.canyonranch.com.

Colorado

Damn Yankee Country Inn, Ouray. What is a doting innkeeper to do when their daughter is diagnosed with CD? Learn to cook for her and open the doors to everyone else. For rates, reservations, and information, www.damn yankeeinn.com.

Maine

Edgewater Farm Bed and Breakfast, Phippsburg. They say you can hear the sea from this lovely and pet-friendly inn not far from Bath. Gluten-free breakfast for those crisp Maine mornings. For directions and rates e-mail ewfbb @suscom-maine.net.

Maryland

Creekside Inn Bed & Breakfast, St. Mary's County. This romantic bed and breakfast in horse country is the perfect spring weekend getaway. The owner understands the basics of the gluten-free diet and accommodates her guests with gluten-free goodies. For rates, directions, and a peek at the lovely accommodations, www.creeksideinnmd.com.

Massachusetts

Treetops Suite, Maldon. This very private and spacious furnished duplex apartment (yes, literally in the treetops) in a fabulous architect-designed residence fifteen minutes away from Boston is the ultimate gluten-free hideaway.

With its own entrance, an exercise room, bath with skylight, two bedrooms, and a porch overlooking a lush garden, it can easily accommodate two couples or a family and is perfect for long stays and hibernations. For rates and information, contact owner Candace Julyan at (781) 321-2888 or see the place for yourself at www.treetopsboston.com.

NEW MEXICO

Rancho Magdalena, Magdalena. In a quiet corner of New Mexico this 1,000-acre ranch is home to horses, longhorn cattle, goats, dogs, and one high-strung rooster. The innkeepers treat guests like family and, with a little notice, will produce gluten-free miracles while you visit local artists in their studios. www.ranchomagdalena.com.

OHIO

Locust Grove Ranch Bed and Breakfast, Mt. Vernon. This celiac-friendly place will not only see to your diet, it will board your horse for the night. Phone (740) 392-6443.

PENNSYLVANIA

The Artist's Inn & Gallery, Terre Hill. Nestled among Amish Farms in Lancaster County, this is where you can hear the clip-clop of a bygone way of life. Whether you go for the antiques in nearby Adamstown, the local handmade quilts, or browse innkeeper Bruce Garrabrandt's lovely drawings, you will find this romantic inn charming, intimate, and completely celiac-friendly. www.artistinn.com.

TENNESSEE

Iron Mountain Inn, Butler. Deep in the Smoky Mountains and tucked away in a remote corner of northeast Tennessee is the perfect gluten-free getaway. The inn is rustic and the surrounding countryside serene. There are hiking trails of varying difficulties, including the challenging Damascus/Hampton leg of the Appalachian Trail nearby. Other sports include golf and fly fishing, swimming in Watauga Lake, and/or just rocking on the porch and drinking in the sweeping views. Phone ahead and let owner Vikki Woods know you're a celiac and she'll do the rest. (888) 781-2399, www.ironmountain.com.

VERMONT

The Inn at Ormsby Hill, Manchester. Chris and Ted Sprague will tell you how Ethan Allen hid in the house during the Revolutionary War, and no wonder: with Chris's gluten-free cranberry scones, who'd want to go back and fight the British? The Spragues cater to the dietary needs of all their guests and work closely with Nature's Harvest in the town center, on historic Route 7A, to make sure everyone's happy and fortified for snowmobiling, skiing, golf, or the two-day Orvis Fly Fishing School nearby. Children over 12 are welcomed. For rates and reservations, (800) 670-2841 or www.ormsbyhill.com.

Swift House Inn, Middlebury. Built in 1815 by Samuel Swift near Middlebury College, historic Swift House had been a private family residence until 1982 when it was transformed into a posh, four-star inn. With the help of chef Carrie Moody, new owners Dan and Michelle Brown have upheld its reputation for superb cuisine and taken it one step further—offering mouth-watering meals to guests with special dietary restrictions, like wheat, gluten, dairy, nuts, or eggs. For room rates, special weekend packages, call (802) 388-9925 or www.swifthouseinn.com.

Virginia

Edgewood Farm Bed and Breakfast, Standardsville. In the lush Blue Ridge Mountains and an easy run from Washington, D.C., Baltimore, Charlottesville, and Richmond, this historic farm was once part of a land grant made by King George to Catlett Conway, founder of the Virginia Humane Society. There is hiking, hot-air ballooning, wine tasting, antiqueing, outings to nearby Monticello, and with advance notice, a gluten-free breakfast made by the proprietors, Eleanor and Norman Schwartz. For room rates and directions, (800) 985-3782 or visit www.edgewoodfarmbandb.com.

Wyoming

Two Bars Seven Ranch. This 7,000-acre ranch in wide-open Wyoming is owned by celiacs and they know how to provide a great, worry-free vacation for the gluten-free. Near Laramie in a small town called Tie Siding, there is horseback riding, fishing, hiking, and dining in the great outdoors. (307) 742-6072, www.twobarssevenranch.com.

Mexico and Central America

Cala Luna Resort, Tamarindo, Costa Rica. Most 5-star hotels like this celiac-friendly paradise will bend over backwards to accommodate a gluten-free diet. All you have to do is contact the chef and be willing to work with them to create a menu and you will have the first, or second, honeymoon of a lifetime. www.calaluna.com.

Rancho La Puerta, Tecate, Mexico. This magnificent spa an hour or two from San Diego is a wonderful place for a celiac to unwind and get healthy (I have visited the place many times over the years). The Mexican spa kitchen is gluten-friendly, and with a little direction, a gluten-free backpack will be ready to accompany you on the all-day hike up Mount Kuchima. Produce is organically grown on the premises and there are as many classes and activities as you have the strength for. For rates, reservations, and information, www.rancholapuerta.com.

Pacific Rim

Turtle Island Resort, Fiji. Candlelit dinners on the beach. Sailing, snorkeling, dancing the night away, and yes, turtles. This eco-friendly resort will serve you just about anything with a little notice, including gluten-free meals. This South Pacific paradise is the place for an unforgettable honeymoon. (800) 255-4347, www.turtlefiji.com.

New Zealand

Cedar House Bed & Breakfast, Gisborne. Once the starchy St. Winifred's, a private school for girls, this gabled Edwardian mansion was originally built in 1909 for a prominent New Zealand family. Situated to catch the sea breezes from two verandas and just steps away from spectacular Pacific beaches, wilderness trekking, and exploring Maori culture, Cedar House has been lovingly restored with native Kuri, Rumu, Matai, and, of course, fragrant cedar timbers. With a little notice (who pops down to New Zealand?), this celiac-friendly outpost will be glad to serve you a fortifying gluten-free breakfast before you set off on a tour of this magical and rugged countryside. Quaint Gisborne is the first city in the world to see the sun each day. For rates and travel information, nzti.com/cedarhouse.

England and Ireland

Coulsworthy House, Combe Martin, North Devon, England. This charming country hotel with its thick stone walls and its pristine spring has been standing since 1600 and is now one of the loveliest hotels in Devon, itself a soft green landscape unrivaled in the world. There is the sea, crumbling castles, the vast mystery of Exmoor, with over 250 square miles of wild moor to walk and a kitchen that, with a bit of notice, will cook you up a real country breakfast. For reservations, rates, and directions from London, 01271-882813, or www.couls worthy.co.uk.

Coxtown Manor, Laghey, County Donegal, Ireland. Breathtaking views of Slieve League from some of the highest cliffs in the world. Hiking, of course, golf, antiques, and tea in the village, maybe a little snooping around church yards, if your ancestors are from here. In summer, dinner is served daily and lunch on Sundays only. Special diet accommodations are happily made with enough notice. (353) 7497-34575, www.coxtownmanor.com.

Cromleach Lodge Country House, Castlebaldwin, County Sligo, Ireland. While Irish bacon and eggs are still the world's best and sizzling fillets of John Dory indescribably fresh, you'll find this spectacular and award-winning country house kitchen, near Boyle in County Sligo, about as sophisticated as they come. With a little notice and some explanation of your needs, Christy and Moira Tighe will make sure you don't miss out on the spectacular mountain hiking and stunning views of Lough Arrow. For rates, travel information, and reservations, call (353) 7191-65155, or www.cromleach.com.

The Grand Tour

Sometimes we just want to let someone else worry about dinner reservations, hotel accommodations, language barriers, kitchen contamination, and all the obstacles that can occur away from home. If you like organized vacations, the following people are pros at marshalling kitchen staff, inspecting cooking conditions, ordering entrées, sending them back if necessary, and snacking en route. They'll even sing on the bus—"A hundred bottles of gluten-free beer on the wall"—as you tour Tuscany, Paris, the wine country. Take a Caribbean cruise, and head for other points exotic. As with any travel tour, ask about cancellation policies, taxes, insurance, and other fees, travel partners and connections, accommodations, and, depending on where you are going, security precautions.

Bob and Ruth's Dining and Travel Club

This peripatetic couple (celiacs themselves) has been everywhere—China, Italy, New Zealand, and Australia, St. Petersburg, Russia, even to the CIA (no, not the spy agency, the Culinary Institute of America) for gluten-free gourmet cooking by the chefs-in-training. For an annual membership fee, the emphasis is on the highly organized, all-inclusive package, whether for the grand tour or the mini getaway. For club prices and information about upcoming trips, contact Bob and Ruth Levy, 22 Breton Hill Road, Suite 18, Baltimore, MD 21208, (410) 486-0292 or www.bobandruths.com.

Glutenfreeda

This Seattle-based company takes small groups to the magnificent San Juan Islands. Included in the package are five days' lodging, kayaking, whale watching, horseback riding, sailing and gourmet breakfasts, lunches, and dinners. For information, prices, and schedules, call (804) 965-0014 or go to www.glutenfreeda.com.

Lotus Tours

New York–based Lotus Tours is a dream come true for those who believe special dietary needs should not preclude traveling in grand style. These people have created a series of truly spectacular and gluten-free touring vacations where everything is taken care of and every meal is memorable, as it should be. This year's destinations included Japan, China, and Hong Kong, and New Zealand and Australia. For details on upcoming excursions, contact Michael Kong, (212) 267-5414 or e-mail him at mk@lotustours.info for current itineraries.

Culinary Getaways

Not everybody is a born Bette Hagman or a Beth Hillson. Newcomers often complain that they have to learn to cook all over again to accommodate the gluten-free diet and veterans like myself get in a gluten-free rut. We all know interesting and great-tasting food is what keeps us on the straight and narrow, and it's what makes family meals a celebration rather than a restrictive chore. What better way to celebrate your new gluten-free life or take the old one to new pleasures than with a culinary course in the joys of gluten-free cooking?

Gluten-Free Baking with Anna Sobaski. Creator of the gluten-free bread mix, Manna from Anna, Anna gives her lessons in Iowa at the Coralville New Pioneer Co-operative, (319) 338-9441.

Glutenfreeda Cooking Classes. Seattle, Washington. For schedules and locations, call (804) 965-0014, or visit www.glutenfreeda.com.

The Gluten-Free Cooking School. Scottsdale, Arizona. For class schedule and locations, contact director LynnRae Ries at www.glutenfreecooking club.com.

Natural Gourmet School. New York, N.Y. Gluten-free baking classes in spring and fall. For information, www.naturalgourmetschool.com.

Linden Travel offers cooks' tours of Northern Italy. For approximately $1,400 per week, you can take a gluten-free cooking vacation on a farm in Il Fae in the Tuscan countryside. For details, contact their U.S. representative Margot Cushing at mcushing@lindentravel.com. My advice is to go in the fall when the vegetables are at their best.

Reading Terminal Market in Philadelphia, Pa. offers a full schedule of cooking classes, including one concentrating on GF cooking. Irina Smith organizes the classes and can be reached at www.readingterminalmarket.org/phil_class.htm.

The Ruby Range. Estes Park, Colorado. If you don't mind a cooking class with a sales slant (this company makes wonderful baking mixes using Native American mesquite flour and teff, an American-grown version of the Ethiopian staple), this is a great way to master the mixes. For a schedule of classes, go to www.therubyrange.com.

Torte Knox. Hawley, Pennsylvania. Sheelah Kay Stepkin has founded this aptly named "recreational" culinary school in a renovated bank. Now this majestic stone structure, complete with vaults, is home to the workshop kitchen featured on House & Garden TV (HGTV). Rebecca Reilly, star chef, school administrator, author, and gluten-free goddess is the magician in residence (see page 416 for her Thanksgiving stuffing). For class schedules, wine weekends, etc., go to www.torteknox.com.

Lost in Translation?

Few of us are multilingual, and even if we know enough French, Spanish, Italian, or Greek to get ourselves a room and a bar of soap, we're out of our league trying to get a safe meal in somebody else's language.

I've updated the original dining cards from *Against the Grain* in French, Spanish, Italian, German, Portuguese, Polish, Swedish, Danish, Hebrew, Russian, Greek, Japanese, and Chinese, and I've added new ones in Arabic, Thai, Dutch, and Swahili. All include oats on the list of forbidden grains. You don't want to confuse the cook with a discussion of the finer points of dedicated fields in a language not your own. This is entirely up to you in Ireland and other English-speaking places where you may feel comfortable experimenting.

Before you leave home, make enough copies (the translation cards can be found in the appendix, starting on page 483) for your purse, suit, pocket, fanny pack, passport case, and wallet. And don't forget to tuck one in your evening bag.

for The Big Night Out. If you want to make them last longer, laminate them and they'll survive messy kitchens, fingerprints, and hastily packed suitcases.

For resorts, cruises, and extended stays jot down your room or cabin number and give one to the restaurant and room service manager, and don't forget the concierge. This way, when a reservation is made on your behalf, the restaurant is not only prepared for your arrival but it has had the benefit of a native speaker explaining your needs. Make extra copies for the inevitable request for a souvenir. After you leave, they will speak of your visit as "The Night of the Curious American Who Could Not Eat Gluten."

A Word of Caution: While these cards have been professionally translated, they are only as good as the people reading them. If the waiter is not literate or chooses to translate the card as a joke at the tourist's expense (this actually happened to an unsuspecting celiac on a certain Greek island), or a tour translator overstates his or her abilities, I cannot vouch for their efficacy. There are variables, as well as bad apples, everywhere. Let common sense prevail, and don't forget how useful the cards can be right here at home in your local ethnic restaurant.

Do write me of the adventures you've had as a result of them. Like Blanche DuBois in Tennessee Williams's *A Streetcar Named Desire*, "I've always relied on the kindness of strangers."

F.Y.I.

The worldly celiac remembers where she's been and keeps track of little finds. After all, you never know when you'll be back. Besides, in the interest of awareness and supporting gluten-friendly businesses, you'll want to tell others. Why not keep them all in the same place?

My Discoveries:

_____

_____

_____

_____

_____

_____

_____

_____

_____

gluten-free goes global

The world is your rice noodle.

—JAX PETERS LOWELL
Against the Grain

If you've never been an adventurous eater, now is the time to break out of your shell. It doesn't take long before you realize that the standard American diet, with its reliance on starchy, thickened gravies and deep-fried everything, is just not going to cut it. We are faced with a choice: cling to what was and be forever hungry for what cannot be or expand your culinary horizon to friendlier cultures and eat your fill. Dare to look beyond what you know, and the world becomes your rice noodle, your risotto, your enchilada, your papadum. Saying bye-bye to American pie and hello to Pad Thai never tasted so good.

Following my own diagnosis (and a period of adjustment during which I resisted the urge to pen the ultimate history of the commode), a wise friend took me to dinner at a local Indian restaurant. After a consultation with the chef, who assured me my condition was common in his native Bombay, I discovered gluten-free heaven right here on earth. That night I enjoyed a spicy lamb dish called *Biryani,* made with lamb, saffron, fragrant basmati rice, and served with two traditional sauces—a lentil purée called *dal* and a cool cucumber, yogurt, and watercress sauce called *raita.* My host waved away a basket of traditional Indian breads and ordered a peppery crisp made with lentil flour called *papadum.*

I never looked back.

The next day, I stopped crying over spilt milk toast and headed for my library's international cooking section. There I discovered the Indian culinary principals of fiery hot quenched by soothing and cool, spice balanced by sweet. A quick trip to the blender with cucumber, watercress, and yogurt yielded a smooth *raita* worthy of a native. It wasn't long before I produced a silky and well-spiced dal. I learned to cook *pakoras*, spicy vegetable fritters held together with lentil flour, and *dosa*, a rice flour pancake rolled and filled with ground meats, potatoes, and spices. I experimented with curries ranging from mild to so hot the soles of my feet perspired. I fell in love with tandoori, a mildly spiced style of cooking in which meats, vegetables, and fish are marinated in lemon, garlic, ginger, and yogurt and cooked in a hot tandoor, or Indian oven (the American stove in my kitchen worked just fine).

It's hard to mourn for macaroni and cheese after food like this. In no time I was exploring my own corner of this great melting pot of ours, grateful for being able to count among my urban blessings a giant Asian market. There among the pickled eels, dried sea urchin, and star anise, I have unearthed rice crackers, rice sticks (*haw fun*), broken rice, sweet brown rice, cellophane noodles, rice vermicelli (*mi fen*), and the flat rice noodle of Shanghai called *ho fun*. I've learned to handle the fragile transparent rice wrappers seen in fancy Asian fusion restaurants, stuff them with shrimp and green onion and dip them in a fiery mix of hot chili oil and gluten-free fish sauce, soy sauce, or tamari. I have fallen in love with glutinous—sticky—rice balls, a sweet, deep-fried treat with a bean paste filling and sesame seeds that, contrary to their name, contain no gluten. Another love is a Malaysian cake called *tan kim hock*, made with coconut flower water, coconut milk, sugar, and glutinous rice.

The Asian market is where I stock up on dried shiitake mushrooms for miso soup and for sheets of nori, the crisp seaweed used to wrap sushi. Once you get the hang of making nori rolls, you can duplicate almost any dish in a Japanese restaurant. (Remember, when dining out it's always safer to order sashimi with plain rice on the side and bring your own gluten-free shoyu or soy sauce. Avoid, too, the imitation seafood so popular in Japan. Wheat fillers are what allows them to be molded into such real-looking shapes.) Dulse, another Japanese sea vegetable, crisps up nicely with a little sesame oil and serves as a salty substitute for artery-clogging bacon in my healthy "d.l.t. sandwiches," made with gluten-free bread, of course.

The housewares aisle is a real bonus. Teapots, sushi plates, shoyu cups and bowls in traditional blue or celadon cost a fraction of what they would elsewhere. Not to mention silk slippers, jade bracelets, and embroidered evening bags. Against the lovely cacophony of dozens of Asian dialects, I discover something new every time, stocking my pantry with crystallized ginger, edamane (protein rich soy beans to boil in their pods Japanese style), and all kinds of imported teas and wasabe mustards that cost a mint in specialty stores.

Across town, in the bodega, there are corn tortillas, ancho chilis, peppers to make your hair curl, masa harina soaked in lime and salsa fresca that bears little resemblance to the bland concoctions found on supermarket shelves.

Italian markets yield cheeses, *amaretti*—cookies made from pure almond paste—and the cured ham called prosciutto. There is short-grain arborio rice for risotto and ground corn for the satisfying porridge called polenta. Polenta can be served soft with tomato sauce and freshly grated Parmesan cheese or baked, sautéed, or fried in olive oil and served crisp as a side dish with grilled lamb chops or a savory roast. Polenta requires constant stirring, which is why Italian grandmothers have such fabulous and strong arms.

It helps to live in a large city or have access to one with multicultural neighborhoods and authentic restaurants. If you don't, there is always mail order; most good cookbooks list their sources for traditional ingredients.

Don't speak the language? Having trouble being understood? Aren't sure of the ingredients? Use your noodle and take along the travel cards in the appendix. Not only will they help others help you, they could make you some new friends in the bargain.

In uncertain times, eating ethnic right at home requires no long security lines, and involves no testy baggage handlers. The sad fact is, these days Americans abroad face bigger problems than a case of the screamers. When you get home with your new exotic ingredients, crank up the Rossini and stir up a risotto with the abandon of a born Venetian. Put on your mariachi hat and whip up some *chile rellenos, heuvos rancheros*, or the perfect winter stew—a silken concoction studded with bits of pork called *posole*. Forget crackers and cheese, nibble *dolma*, the grape leaves stuffed with rice the Greeks can't eat just one of, or slice rounds of cucumber to dip into the chickpea purée called *hummus*. Dream of the Aegean.

A note of caution—recipes vary from restaurant to restaurant, and every chef puts his or her personal stamp on even the most traditional of dishes. As with everything you buy or order, you must always ask how a food is prepared and what's in it before you consume it. The following suggestions are merely guidelines, but they should go a long way toward helping you negotiate an unfamiliar menu and decide which dishes to investigate further. In or out, eating ethnic is the gluten-free way to go.

Afghan

Once upon a time, few of us could say with certainty where on the map Afghanistan was exactly. Unhappily, that is no longer the case. Even worse, this magnificent mountainous country has fallen to the worst kind of devastation. All the more reason for those of us in urban areas to find and patronize pockets of Afghan cuisine like Philadelphia's Kabul. While we cannot break bread with these lovely people, we can offer our solidarity and sample the cuisine they have brought to our shores with their eternal memories of home.

Unlike its neighbors, India and Pakistan, where chefs fight the fiery climate with more heat in their curries, Afghanistan's cooking is milder, more subtle, cooler, like the temperatures at the country's higher elevations.

Exotic spices and flavors predominate—cardamom, saffron, orange peel, rose water, yogurt, and mint. Lamb and yogurt feature strongly, but dishes are surprisingly mild, despite their intricate seasonings.

Skip the appetizers, which are usually turnovers, dumplings, and deep-fried pastries, and move right along to the main course. Not all restaurants use the same ingredients, so remember to ask before you consider the following dishes.

Kabuli-palaw is a gorgeous combination of lamb, rice, carrots, raisins, almonds, and pistachios in a spiced tomato sauce. *Norenge-palaw* is a sweeter version of this dish with the addition of cardamom and orange peel soaked in rose water. *Badenjan-chalaw* combines lamb and eggplant, and *facilliya-chalaw* is a mixture of green beans and lamb.

Kabobs of chicken or lamb or ground beef are usually marinated in yogurt, spices, garlic, and lemon before cooking. In this land where meat is not as plentiful or as available as it is here, vegetables are made much of.

Buranee badenjan is sautéed eggplant with meat sauce and yogurt.

Sabzi is pureed spinach with onions, and *buranee kadu* is sautéed pumpkin with meat sauce and yogurt.

Afghan desserts tend to be sticky, sweet, and off-limits for celiacs, but *firnee*, a silky Afghan pudding sprinkled with pistachios and almonds, is usually thickened with cornstarch. Asking before ordering never hurts.

An Afghan meal is typically finished off with green tea or chai, a traditional tea. You haven't come this far for a cup of coffee.

African

In Swahili, *karamu* is the word for "feast." Unusual flavors come together in Africa because of the vast differences in climate, temperatures, and confluence of cultures. North African cuisine, featuring couscous, is heavily grain-based and therefore difficult for celiacs. Teff, an Ethiopian grain, is the smallest in the world and gluten-free.

Papaya and chile soup is a South African specialty mixing two unexpected flavors. Traditionally, cornstarch is used as thickener.

Tanzanian fruit and cashew salad with rum cream is worth searching for, and so is the beef and plantain cake from Kenya called *matoke*. Not a real cake, this is a casserole of highly spiced pieces of beef that have been folded into a plantain and spinach puree, then baked and garnished with shredded coconut.

Cachupa is an exotic vegetable stew of kale, corn, lima, and kidney beans, bananas, name (white yam), and calabaza (acorn squash), among other exotic ingredients from the Cape Verde Islands off the coast of West Africa. This traditional dish often contains chorizo (Spanish sausage), and it's important to find out how the sausage is made before ordering.

Beware of *bobotie*, a curried beef casserole from South Africa that contains bread crumbs.

Yassa is a spicy marinated chicken in onion sauce from Senegal that can be served over rice or couscous. Find out which one is used in your restaurant, then ask that yours be served over rice.

Doro wett is an Ethiopian chicken stew that should not be made with any wheat or gluten. It is typically served over injera, a flat bread made of teff, which is allowed only if it is made with no other flour. If there's any doubt, order this over rice and explain why, so as not to be perceived as rude or unconcerned about tradition.

Angolan shrimp are marinated in a spicy mixture that may turn up on the menu as *pilli-pilli*, or even *peri-peri*. There should be no glutenous ingredients in any of these versions, but ask anyway.

Tiebou dienne are Senegalese fish fillets stuffed with rice. If prepared properly, they should not contain bread crumbs.

Pass up *kotokyim*, the crab gratin from Ghana. Like gratins everywhere, this one contains bread crumbs.

Drink a cup of strong coffee, or soothing mint tea. Then make a *tamsbi la tutaonama* (farewell statement) in Swahili or just say thank you (see Swahili traveling card in appendix) and pay your bill.

Ghenet Ethiopian Injera

Injera, the flat, spongy, and slightly sour teff bread of Ethiopia, signifies the bonds of loyalty and friendship and is traditionally eaten with the fingers, a piece at a time torn off and wrapped around a mouthful of food. This recipe comes courtesy of Yeworkwoha "Workeye" Ephrem, owner of Ghenet Restaurant on Mulberry Street in New York's SoHo, and uses gluten-free teff flour from The Teff Company in Caldwell, Idaho. Dip it in *doro wett* or any other stews (Ethiopian or otherwise) in your repertoire. It's a great substitute for dumplings and makes for an interesting change of pace for pizzas and open sandwiches.

Makes approximately 15 *injera*

  2 tablespoons yeast
1½ pounds of teff (tef, t'ef) flour
6½ cups warm water

1. Dissolve yeast according to package instructions. In a large bowl, combine yeast, teff flour, and water, and mix until smooth. Cover with plastic wrap and let sit in a warm place for three days. (You read right, three days!)

2. On the third day, throw away the water that has risen to the top.

3. Add a small amount of fresh warm water until the dough is a little bit thinner than pancake batter. Cover for at least 30 minutes or until the batter rises.

4. Pour ½ cup batter onto a medium hot nonstick skillet or a griddle heated to 450 degrees, swirling the batter to coat the bottom of the pan. Cook for approximately 1½ minutes or until bubbles appear. Do not turn. Place the cooked *injera* on a clean towel or tablecloth to let cool. Repeat until batter is finished.

Brazilian

This is barbecue country. There is no place to hide gluten in a steak that comes straight from Brazil's ranches or from the pampas of its neighbor Argentina. If you like good beef, this the country of origin. And so far, the cows there are not even cranky. You will remember to ask about any sauce or marinade, won't you?

If you are not a carnivore, *bacalhau* is dried, salted codfish and very popular in Brazil. *Acaraje* are black-eyed pea fritters, which should be made from pure black-eyed pea flour.

Seviche is popular all over South and Central America. Whether it is shrimp, scallops, lobster, octopus, bass, or black conch, it is always raw fish that has been marinated in fresh lime or the juice of Seville oranges, peppers, tomatoes, chilies, onion, and other ingredients for at least six hours. The fish loses its translucence and fishy taste in the juice and needs no further cooking. Really.

Quibe is winter squash soup or, sometimes, West Indian pumpkin, but it does not require thickening except for vegetable purée. A true Bahian shrimp stew does not contain flour.

A good Brazilian restaurant will prepare salt cod (*bacalhau*) many ways: in chili and almond sauce or Bahia style with coconut milk and tomato, or with cabbage a la mineina, or with eggs.

Roupa velha means "old clothes" in Portuguese. It is also the name for a stew of shredded or leftover flank steak. Before you order it, ask the chef if it has been thickened with flour.

Feijoada completa is the national dish of Brazil. The recipe can include everything from dried salt pork, salted beef, pig's ears, tail, and feet; tongue; pork sausage; kielbasa; Brazilian sausage (*linguica*); and turtle beans. A major discussion is in order before you attempt to order this. There are too many variables here.

Brazilian chocolate mousse is usually made with cashews, and coconut blanc mange is typically thickened with anything but cornstarch. Remember, this is America, land of shortcuts. Ask the chef.

Cha is tea, and *guarana* is Brazil's favorite soft drink. A not-so-soft drink is the *caipirinha*, Brazil's national and extremely potent cocktail.

Caribbean

The flavors of Africa, Spain, France, and other European colonists predominate and mix with the island abundance of fresh fish and fruit, resulting in a few special dishes worth noting.

Ginger beer is not real beer. This West African import is made with fresh ginger, honey, and lemon. No malt. Sorrel tea is also a wonderful ginger-based refreshment from Jamaica. Not to mention Jamaican rum.

Fried plantain is a Caribbean staple. Just make sure they are not breaded and, if possible, find out what else is fried in the pan or deep fryer.

For years I would not order an odd-sounding dish called *fungee* or *fungi*, which is also called *coo coo* or *cou cou*, depending on whether you are in Trinidad, Antigua, or Barbados. This is really the Caribbean answer to polenta. *Jug jug* is the Barbadian version with chicken and peas and is gluten-free, but may contain millet if you're sensitive.

The conquistadores gave the Caribbean a dish called *cristiaos y moros* (Christians and Moors), which refers to the white rice and black beans that give it its stunning appearance.

There is always good fish on a Caribbean menu. The highly spiced "jerk" style of cooking refers to the distinctive Caribbean paste of scallion, chili, and allspice that is rubbed into the flesh before slow cooking over coals. It is wonderful, but don't order it unless you can determine the ingredients in the marinade.

Stay away from Caribbean stews unless you are positive they do not contain *roux*.

Chinese

In order to enjoy good Chinese cooking, you need to get on speaking terms with the chef. Since many Chinese chefs do not speak English well, or at all, and Mandarin isn't exactly a second language in most American neighborhoods, this may take a little doing. One way to break the language barrier is using your Chinese traveling card (see page 485). It's also important to find a really good Chinese restaurant, as much of what is found in the average Chinese takeout is just that, average. It is also loaded with soy sauce and MSG.

Chinese cuisine uses an enormous amount of soy sauce and other sauces that contain it. I love rice noodles (*bi-fun*), especially stir-fried with shrimp and pork curry or with vegetables, but they can't be ordered in just any Chinese restaurant. Nor can you order *guon fun*, rice roll with vegetables and meat. You must make sure the chef has adapted it for you with wheat-free soy sauce.

As a rule, Chinese chefs thicken with cornstarch. But many condiments and pickled items are imported from China, which makes it virtually impossible to know what's in them.

Before you give up on China, look for chrysanthemum soup, a light chicken soup afloat in chrysanthemum petals, or one of the egg drop, egg curd, or ginger broth varieties, which should be free of soy sauce. Forget the Szechuan favorite, hot and sour soup. It's always made with soy sauce, unless you have done your homework and have a willing chef to make it for you with gluten-free tamari.

Peking duck, with its deep mahogany lacquer of honey, is gorgeous when prepared properly. This dish can be made with barley molasses as well. Make sure you know the difference. Forgo the plum sauce unless you know what's in it. Pass up the hoisin sauce entirely. Tea-smoked duck is also very good and should not be prepared with anything but spiced salt, lemon or orange, rice, brown sugar, and black tea leaves. Remember what I said about the sauce. Any sauce.

Dim sum is Chinese for "dough." Stay away from these savory dumplings.

Read your fortune before passing the cookie to someone else. It should say, "Confucius say, have the dragon eye pudding for dessert." This Shanghai classic is usually made with rice flour. It wouldn't be as much fun if I told you what *longans,* or dragon's eyes, are.

Beth Hillson's General Tso's Chicken

Before you give up on Chinese cuisine, try this wonderful dish from Beth Hillson, the Gluten-Free Pantry's star chef and lover of all things Asian. It follows the Chinese principles of quick cooking over high heat and all it needs is hot jasmine rice to soak up the ginger garlic sauce. Who needs to go out when you can stay in and eat like an emperor?

Serves 4

8 boneless, skinless chicken thighs

MARINADE
1 egg, lightly beaten
1 tablespoon cornstarch

SAUCE
2 tablespoons wheat-free soy sauce
2 tablespoons rice vinegar
2 tablespoons water
1 large garlic clove, minced
1 teaspoon fresh ginger, minced
½ teaspoon red pepper flakes
Corn, peanut, or safflower oil for stir frying

1. Cut chicken into 1-inch pieces. Combine egg and cornstarch in a large bowl. Add the chicken and coat with mixture. Let stand 15 minutes at room temperature. Combine sauce ingredients and set aside.

2. Over a medium high flame, heat 3 tablespoons of oil in a wok or large frying pan. When oil begins to smoke, add chicken in small batches. Sauté until golden brown. Pour off all leftover oil.

3. Return chicken to wok or frying pan. Add sauce and stir mixture for 1 minute. Serve hot over rice.

German

German food isn't just hard to swallow on a gluten-free diet, it's the "*wurst.*" There's bierwurst, bratwurst, blutwurst, bockwurst, knackwurst, leberwust, mettwurst, weisswurst, zungenwurst, and just plain wurst—approximately 1,500 kinds of wursts, or sausages, all containing who knows what.

Then there's *bier.* A different kind for every man, woman, and stein in Germany.

If the bier and the wurst don't get you, the spaetzle and schnitzels will, weiner and holsteiner among them. There are dozens of *brotes* (breads), including pumpernickel, and there is sauerbraten, pfeffernusse, pfannkuchen, pastete, nudeln, nockerl, knödel, kuchen, kasekuchen, lebkuchen, baumkuchen, elisenlebkuchen, and gulasch. Never mind what all these words mean. To you, it's German for "you can't order it."

Not everything is verboten—you can have cabbage or potatoes, for example, as long as they're not swimming in cream sauce or encrusted with noodles.

Bottom line: All the really good German dishes are loaded with flour or bread crumbs or beer or something else that will make you feel empty right down to your liederhosen.

Have some strawberries *mit schlag,* which is with whipped cream. Or maybe just a nice slice of Muenster cheese and a glass of *wasser* while you're thinking about where else to go that won't make you cry.

Greek

Forget the kasseri cheese appetizer called *saganaki opa.* It's delicious. It's dramatic. It's flamed at the table. And it's full of bread crumbs.

Order *hummus,* a garlicky purée of chickpeas and sesame seeds (tahini) mixed with olive oil; *tzatziki,* whipped yogurt with cucumbers, lemon juice, and garlic; *taramasalata,* whipped Greek caviar with olive oil and lemon juice, or *babacunuch,* a dip of roasted eggplant with garlic, oil, lemon, and tahini. These are traditionally served with pita triangles, but in your case, they are just as delicious with chilled cucumber slices. Cucumber is the mainstay of traditional Greek peasant salad, so you shouldn't have a problem asking for a side order. If you prefer bread with your dip, toast some triangles of gluten-free bread or corn tortillas, or take along your favorite crackers.

Go crazy with briny Greek olives and feta, the salty and reasonably low-fat national cheese. Dolma are grape leaves stuffed with rice, and they are usually gluten-free. Ask first.

Stay away from *avgolemono*, which is a thick Hellenic lemon and egg soup with rice and chicken both, unless you can be positive it has been thickened with egg yolks only. Avgolemono is also served as a sauce for other Greek dishes, including the more substantial entrée of grape leaves stuffed with beef and lamb and rice, so it is important to establish its ingredients before cooking.

Pastitsio and moussaka are the Greek variations of lasagna. Both are held together with béchamel sauce, which is thickened with flour, and *pastitsio* usually contains pasta called orzo. Never confuse orzo (pasta) with ouzo (a very strong drink).

While *spanakopita* (spinach pie) should be an obvious no-no, some Greek restaurants make a variation that is a bubbly casserole of rice, spinach, and feta cheese minus the filo dough. As with every cuisine, all thick sauces are suspect and must be explained before you order any Greek stew or braised dish.

Plaki means anything on a platter or planked and usually refers to baked or grilled fish. Grilled fish à la Greque usually involves no more than olive oil, garlic, and lemon and is as heart healthy as it is gluten-free. *Gyro* is marinated, spiced meat, sliced very thinly. I, personally, do not trust it.

Skordelia is another name for mashed potatoes so garlicky and good, you'll probably cry with happiness for having had the sense to order them. Make sure the chef didn't take a shortcut and used nontraditional thickeners.

I don't miss Greek desserts because I've never really liked the overly sweet baklava and other syrupy filo dough pastries or the equally sweet *galakto-bouriko*, a baked custard with the same potential for toothache.

I always ask about the raisin rice pudding or homemade yogurt with honey and walnuts. Once assured that these are gluten-free, order these more traditional and less waistline-thickening endings to a Greek meal. Once in a while, you'll find a Greek restaurant that serves a traditional almond paste cookie made with no flour. When you do, buy a bag to take home and get the address and phone number of the bakery.

Indian

Warning: Once you fall in love with India, you may never come back. To experience the subtlety of exotic spices, mild with fiery hot, sweet with tart, and the gluten-free perfection of fragrant basmati rice is to appreciate why for centuries Europeans risked life and limb to travel to this magical country. Cardamom, coriander, cumin, ginger, turmeric, cayenne, and cinnamon are the grace notes of Indian cuisine, and, as often as not, the cuisine of this predominantly Hindu culture features vegetarian, dairy, as well as gluten-free dishes.

The basic principle of Indian cooking relies on searingly hot quenched by soothing and cool. Most dishes are usually served all at once, so the diner can decide how much of each temperature is appropriate. Desserts are deliberately mild and fragrant after a meal of such stunning contrasts. While it is true that many Indian chefs grind their own seasonings to make curry, their magical potion, there are too few of them to consider. If you can tolerate curry (many celiacs are sensitive to commercial curry powder), welcome to the land of vindaloo, tandoori, papadum, masala dosa, dal, raita, and mango chutney.

In traditional Indian kitchens, curry is based on something called ghee, which is really clarified butter, melted and skimmed of its foam several times. Ghee butter is the foundation for all the variations, none of which should contain flour. I say *should*, and I will say it until it is firmly in your mind, because in an age of shortcuts, your health depends on asking each time.

Curries range from mild to hair-curling. Never ask for very hot unless you know what that particular chef's definition of this is. You can always ask for something a little hotter next time. If you are sweating from the top of your head to the soles of your feet, it's already too late.

The vindaloo style of cooking tends to be the spiciest, while tandoori refers to the clay oven or tandoor used to prepare less fiery dishes, such as chicken marinated in lemon, yogurt, garlic, and ginger.

Basmati is often the rice of choice in Indian cooking, and it is sweeter and more fragrant than the standard grain.

Raitas are the yogurt sauces that cool the hot dishes. They are usually made with cucumbers and watercress, but can be made of bananas or bananas and coconut, or eggplant and potatoes. They are always soothing and put out the fire nicely.

Biryani is an eggplant and saffron rice casserole based on ghee, and dal is a thick purée of moong (yellow split peas) or *urhad dal* (lentils) that is a staple food in India and one of the highest concentrations of protein you can get. Lamb and goat are familiar items on Indian menus, but vegetable dishes feature prominently as well, because so much of India's population is vegetarian for religious reasons.

Watch out for *uppama*. It contains farina.

Always ask what chutney contains before trying it. Some exotic versions of this condiment contain pickled fruits and vegetables that have spent time in vinegar, which does not contain gluten, but some celiacs report being sensitive to.

Khagina is an Indian omelet; *akuri*, scrambled eggs; *aki*, a poaching liquid; and *pakoras*, spicy vegetable fritters, usually held together with lentil flour. I said "usually." Never order a pakora without first making sure it's safe. Ditto for *dosa*, a rolled lentil flour pancake filled with potatoes and spices.

Puri, chapati, nan, kulcha, roti, and *paratha* are all breads made of excluded flours. The crispy fried spiced wafers called papadum, however, are not. They are traditionally made from lentil flour. At the risk of beating you over the head, ask.

Desserts in India are really exotic. Stay away from the usual suspects and experiment with *rasmalai*, a sweetened cottage cheese dumpling served with thickened milk, or *gulab jamun*, cardamom-and-saffron spiced balls of milk curd in sugar syrup served hot.

There's always Darjeeling tea or the spicy minted variety called *masala*, but you really can't call yourself adventurous until you've tasted *masala lassi*, a traditional spiked buttermilk drink, or *mango lassi*, a wonderful yogurt drink with mango.

Sara Pluta's Pakoras
with Sweet and Spicy Chutney

Light and full of healthy fiber, chickpea is often the flour of choice for Indian delica-
cies as evidenced by these savory fritters from star chef and food writer Sara J. Pluta,
reprinted here with permission from *Living Without* magazine. The secret to these
golden fritters is good, healthy oil and the best spices you can buy. A visit to an Indian grocery is an exotic adventure, but you will find cumin, turmeric, cayenne, and
fresh cilantro in most American markets as well. Served with sweet and spicy chutney or cool, cucumber raita, these make a dazzling first course for a traditional Indian dinner of *sambhar* (a curry of red lentils and rice) or lamb *biryani* or can be
served with cocktails for an exotic change of pace.

Serves 4 to 5

- ⅔ cup chickpea flour
- ¼ teaspoon baking soda
- 5 tablespoons cold water
- ¼ teaspoon ground cumin
- ¼ teaspoon cayenne
- 1 teaspoon salt
- ¼ teaspoon turmeric
- ½ cup cooked potato, diced small
- ½ cup onion, finely chopped
- 2 tablespoons fresh cilantro, chopped
- 2 cups canola oil

1. Mix together the flour, baking soda, and water until smooth. Add
cumin, cayenne, salt, and turmeric.

2. Mix well. Add potato, onion, and cilantro.

3. Heat oil in wok or other deep saucepan until very hot, 350 degrees.

4. Add a tablespoon of batter at a time to the hot oil. Fry until golden,
about five to seven minutes. Remove with slotted spoon. Drain on paper towels and serve hot with chutney.

Sweet and Spicy Chutney

This chutney is the perfect foil for pakoras, but is equally at home as an accompaniment to grilled meats, chicken, and fish and Indian traditional casseroles. Look for tamarind concentrate in Indian grocery stores or in the specialty foods section of a large market.

Makes 1½ cups

1 cup raisins, currants, prunes, or other dried fruit such as apricots, pears, or pineapple
1 tablespoon tamarind concentrate
6 to 8 tablespoons water
½ teaspoon ground ginger
¼ teaspoon cayenne
¼ teaspoon salt
1 tablespoon lemon juice

1. Combine all ingredients in a blender and process until smooth.
2. Put mixture in a medium saucepan and bring to a boil and simmer covered for 10 minutes.
3. Serve as an accompaniment to pakoras, or over basmati rice.

Cucumber Raita

This cool combination of yogurt, mint, and cucumbers is a staple on Indian tables. It is served alongside meat or vegetable dishes to tame the heat of spicy food.

Makes 2½ cups

2 cups plain yogurt (soy or goat yogurt may be substituted)
½ teaspoon ground cumin
Pinch of cayenne or black pepper
½ teaspoon salt
2 tablespoons onion, minced
2 cucumbers, seeded and diced
3 tablespoons mint leaves, minced

Mix all ingredients together and chill until ready to use.

Italian

If you can't see past the pizza and the pasta with tomato sauce on a typical Italian menu, you will undoubtedly go home disappointed and hungry.

Always ask for risotto. Even if it's not listed on the menu, you may find a willing chef who is grateful for the opportunity to honor such a request. More than a meal, this classic rice dish is virtually a ritual in northern Italian kitchens, and it is even more ubiquitous than pasta in Turin, Milan, and Venice, and from the Alps all the way to the Adriatic, where the best short-grained arborio and carnaroli rice are found. When it is prepared properly, it is rich, creamy, cheesy, savory, satisfying, and everything you miss about pasta.

Try polenta. This wonderful cornmeal dish can be served soft and mixed with cheese and any number of savory sauces, or it can be cooked and sliced, then grilled and served as an accompaniment to roasted meats and other dishes.

My idea of the perfect Italian meal is to start with a light Parma ham and melon or an antipasto plate of tuna, salami, provolone, mozzarella, artichoke hearts, prosciutto, calamari, mushrooms (make sure they are not stuffed with bread crumbs), hearts of palm, olives, and anchovies.

Follow this with a small "pasta" portion of risotto with wild mushrooms or spring vegetables and a salad of tomatoes, fresh mozzarella, and basil with some good olive oil, a grind of pepper, and a splash of balsamic vinegar. It doesn't get better than *osso buco* (veal shanks) on a bed of soft polenta for your main course (as long as the shanks have not been floured first or the brown sauce thickened with flour), unless, of course, you have ordered a veal chop accompanied by grilled polenta with sun-dried tomatoes and mushroom or grilled *tonno* (tuna) marinated in olive oil, rosemary, basil, and garlic and served with *broccoli di rape* and rice.

If nothing but pasta will do, bring your own and ask that it be served with shrimp, mussels, clams, and scallops, an eggplant sauce, or a spicy *puttanesca* sauce, or placed under an order of garlicky shrimp scampi. (Don't forget to ask the chef to put on a fresh pot of boiling water for you.) Any safe sauce on the menu is yours for the asking with the price of a box of your favorite brand of gluten-free pasta and an affirmative response from the chef. Most Italian vegetables are done simply in olive oil and garlic, which makes them naturally gluten-free.

Desserts are as tough in Italian restaurants as they are everywhere else, but you never know when you are going to run into *croccante*, crunchy Italian pralines served with espresso or crushed over gelato, Bolognese rice cake (take care there are no bread crumbs lurking on its bottom), *monte bianco,* quite literally a mountain of chocolate and chestnut that has been snowcapped with whipped cream, or *zabaglione*, an airy concoction I have always believed to be made of Marsala wine and clouds, but which are really egg yolks and sugar beaten into a froth.

If you see coffee *granita* on the menu, you may not even care what is offered for dessert. This frozen Italian slush of sugar and very strong espresso, topped with whipped cream or milk is dessert enough for any serious sweet lover. Take care the whipped cream is only that.

If no such goodies appear, order your favorite gelato, a rich Italian ice cream that should be free of fillers (ask!), and always inquire how the cheese-cake is made (every once in a while you will find a light ricotta cheese cake made with no flour at all), and make sure you have your own biscotti.

Chickpea Socca

In Nice and Italian seacoast towns, on the border where national tastes blur, these *socca* or pancakes are the French version of fast food. Street vendors serve them with anchovies, black olive *tapenade*, hard-boiled eggs and *saucisson*; they are as ubiqui-tous as McDonald's, but so much better for the heart. Not too bad for the waistline, either. These versatile crepes can be used for chips, dips, as a substitute for bread for dipping into a pool of good olive oil, and come courtesy of chefs Bryan Sikora and Aimee Olexy of Django, Philadelphia. The thinner the batter, the crispier the *socca*, the thicker the batter, the softer the result. A heavy cast iron crepe pan makes all the difference.

Makes 20 Socca

 1 cup chickpea flour
 1 cup water
 ¼ cup olive oil
 1 tablespoon salt

1. Mix all four batter ingredients and pour into hot crepe pan, tilting to coat pan in an even layer.

2. Cook on one side until golden brown. (For thicker crepes, you may have to flip and cook on the other side.)

3. Remove from heat and set aside to crisp in a warm place (near pilot light or in a warm oven that has been turned off).

Japanese

If you love sushi or sashimi, you're in luck as long as you remember to bring your own wheat-free soy or tamari sauce or make sure it's provided at the restaurant. Do you remember the difference? Sushi is raw fish with rice. Sashimi is raw fish without rice. I like to order sashimi and a small bowl of brown rice when I eat Japanese. Take a little bit of the rice with a bite of the fish. It's not so filling that way, and brown rice offers more fiber than white. It's always good to bone up on the menu before you jump in. You never know what you might end up with otherwise. A basic course in sushi . . .

Akagai: Red clam
Amaebi: Sweet shrimp
Anago: Sea eel
Aoyagi: Skimmer clam
Ebi: Shrimp
Hamachi: Yellowtail
Hirame: Fluke
Hokkigai: Surf clam
Ika: Squid
Ikura: Salmon roe
Katsuo: Bonito

Maguro: Tuna
Mirygai: Giant clam
Saba: Mackerel
Sawakani: Baby octopus
Shake: Salmon
Tako: Octopus
Tamago: Egg omelet
Tobiko: Flying fish egg
Unagi: Clear water eel
Uni: Sea urchin

There are also lobster rolls, California rolls, avocado rolls, Alaska rolls, tuna rolls, crab sticks, and salmon rolls. These are rice, fish, and vegetable combinations that are often sauced. Ask first.

Tofu is soybean curd, a high-protein source that is featured prominently in Japanese cuisine and is absolutely tasteless until seasoned, fried, sautéed, or sauced. At that point it takes on the flavor of the food in which it is cooked. Always ask how tofu is prepared, as there is a strong probability that it has been soaked or stir-fried in soy sauce.

Mozuku is seaweed served with sweet vinegar, which invariably is rice vinegar and should be safe to order if soy sauce has not been added.

Avoid anything that is described as "tempura" unless you can be sure how the batter is made. Some Japanese chefs use rice flour for their fried dishes to give them a lighter taste, so it is entirely possible your favorite is one of them. Others keep rice flour on hand and may agree to do yours to order. Find out before you cross this dish off your list.

Beware of *soba*. These buckwheat noodles often contain a mixture of buckwheat and wheat flour. Never order *udon*, a wheat noodle. Look for rice sticks or rice noodles and ask that they be used in your soup.

Miso soup is soybean broth with tofu, and *wakame* and *sumashi* is clear chicken broth. Check for soy sauce before ordering these and always ask which type of *miso* is being used.

Gyoza is a fried meat dumpling that contains flour and soy sauce, but *edamame* is usually steamed soy beans with no soy sauce added.

Anything *teriyaki* is glazed, *yakatori,* glazed and skewered; and *sukiyaki* is a method of preparing vegetables, chicken, beef, or seafood in a souplike stew à la bouillabaisse. Order none of these. They're full of soy sauce.

There is surprisingly little gluten on a Japanese dessert menu. Green tea ice cream is refreshing and often homemade, with no fillers and stabilizers, and fried bananas with honey are quite good. *Yokan* is not for everyone, but for those who need to know, it's sweet bean jelly.

Mexican

Enchiladas, tortillas, carne asada, salsa, guacamole, *carumba*! Not to mention masa harina, huevos rancheros, nachos, tostadas, and good old rice and beans. This is the land of corn and plenty and mole sauce. Mexico is a gluten-free paradise.

A note of caution: If you are one of those rare birds who are sensitive to chili powder, don't even think of going Mexican. It's in everything. Sorry, *amigo*.

It is very important to find an authentic Mexican restaurant and not one of the ubiquitous burrito factories dotting the landscape. The reason for this is simple. The less formularized and processed, the safer it's going to be for you. Besides, places like these are American, not Mexican.

Real Mexican cuisine uses masa harina (a cornmeal soaked in lime), tomatillos (small green tomatoes), corn husks, which are traditionally used to serve tamales, guava paste, hominy (a cereal made from corn), and flat corn bread called tortillas, which are usually homemade and bear no resemblance to the tasteless versions found in fast-food restaurants and on supermarket shelves.

Homemade salsas bear little resemblance to those watery concoctions found in the grocery stores. Fresh ingredients and good nonprocessed cheddars and Jack cheeses are used in everything from nachos to quesadillas, Mexico's answer to pizza. These are usually made with the larger flour tortilla but can easily be made with its smaller and gluten-free cousin. Learn to spot the difference between these two tortillas from across the room. (Hint: Corn is yellow and smaller than flour, which is white and large.) In fact, almost any dish that is made with a flour tortilla can be made with a corn tortilla. Be careful, though, that the rest of the ingredients contain no gluten. Always ask if the chili contains any flour, as since some Mexican chefs start their chili from a *roux*.

A typical Mexican menu might include *gazpacho,* spicy chilled soup made of puréed tomatoes, peppers, cucumbers, and spices. Ask the waiter to leave off the croutons that sometimes accompany this dish. If you've forgotten and are served soup with croutons, don't pick them out. Ask for a fresh bowl.

Chile relleños can be made with bread crumbs or not. Make sure you know which you are ordering.

Most Mexican sauces—salsa verde, salsa rojo, salsa casera—do not contain flour. Guacamole sauce or dip is made from avocados, and mole is a spicy sauce that includes cocoa.

Beans *(frijoles)* are a mainstay of Mexican cuisine. *Frijoles refritos* (refried beans) are typically not made with any thickening, but traditionally they are fried in lard, so beware if you're counting fat grams, watching your cholesterol, or are a vegetarian.

As with all unfamiliar cuisines, avoid any chilis, stews, or dishes that appear to be enrobed in a thick sauce. They may contain flour. Cornstarch is often used as a thickener in many Mexican recipes as a substitute for wheat flour. Always ask before you rule something out.

Authentic chorizos, spiced Spanish sausages used frequently in Mexican cooking, usually contain tequila, wine vinegar, and hot chilis among other spices. Never eat a chorizo whose ingredients cannot be accounted for.

The traditional Mexican dessert custard is a caramel pudding called *flan,* which should be safe if made from scratch. Ask before you order it. Or have something simple and refreshing like a mango.

Rick Bayless's Quesadillas Asadas

There is no greater authority on Mexican cooking than Rick Bayless. Star chef and owner of Chicago's Frontera Grill and Topolobampo, he has made a career interpreting the depth and timeless flavors of old Mexico. These crusty griddle-baked *quesadillas* from his Julia Child Cookbook Award–winning *Rick Bayless's Mexican Kitchen* (Scribner) serve as a wonderful introduction to a country that is as near to heaven as a celiac can come.

Quesadillas are the grilled cheese sandwiches of Mexico. Though you can make them with ready-made tortillas, the difference is worth the trouble of making them yourself. With peppery roasted *poblano rajas*, these cheesy, chewy stuffed tortillas are a marvel of texture, spice, and heat. Simply lay a thin circle of dough onto the griddle, spread on the filling, fold it over and bake until crusty. Served as a casual main dish or as a late-night snack, and laced with a spoonful of tangy salsa you've got a party dish you'll want to repeat and perfect and improvise upon, maybe even invest in a tortilla press.

Makes 12 quesadillas, serving 4 to 6

FOR 2 CUPS ESSENTIAL ROASTED POBLANO RAJAS

- 1 pound (6 medium-large) fresh poblano chilis
- 1 tablespoon vegetable or olive oil
- 1 large white onion, sliced ¼-inch thick
- 3 garlic cloves, peeled and finely chopped
- 1 teaspoon dried oregano, preferably Mexican
  Salt, about ½ teaspoon

1. Roast the chilis directly over a gas flame or 4 inches below a very hot broiler until blackened on all sides, about 5 minutes for open flame, about 10 minutes for broiler. Cover with a kitchen towel and let stand 5 minutes. Peel, pull out the stem and seed pod, then rinse briefly to remove bits of skin and seeds. Slice into ¼-inch strips.

2. In a medium (8 to 9-inch) skillet, heat the oil on medium to medium-high flame, then add the onion and cook, stirring regularly, until nicely browned but still a little crunchy, about 5 minutes. Add the garlic and oregano, toss a minute longer, then stir in the chilies and heat through. Taste and season with salt.

Note: Rajas can be made 2 days ahead; cover and refrigerate.

FOR QUESADILLAS

   1 pound (2 cups) fresh masa for tortillas or 1¾ cups masa harina
        mixed with 1 cup plus 2 tablespoons hot water
2½ cups (about 10 ounces) shredded Mexican Chihuahua cheese,
        or other melting cheese such as brick cheddar or Monterey Jack

1. Cut two squares of medium-heavy plastic (a garbage bag works well) to cover the plates of your tortilla press. If necessary, knead a few drops more water into the masa to give it the consistency of a soft cookie dough, then roll it into 12 balls. Cover with plastic. Divide the cheese into 12 equal portions; cover with plastic.

2. Turn on the oven to the lowest setting. Heat a large griddle or heavy skillet over medium heat. Use the tortilla press to press out the dough one by one between the two sheets of plastic. Peel off the top sheet, then flip the uncovered side of the tortilla onto your hand (the top of the tortilla should align with your index finger, and fingers should be slightly spread to give support).

3. Carefully peel off the plastic, then, with a gentle, swift motion lay the tortilla on the hot griddle. Evenly sprinkle on a portion of the cheese, leaving a ½-inch border all around so cheese doesn't run out onto the griddle, then lay a portion of the rajas down the center. When the tortilla comes free from the griddle (it will take about 20 seconds), use a spatula to fold it in half, and gently press the edges together, more or less sealing them.

4. Move the quesadilla to the side to continue baking as you begin the next one. Continue making and folding quesadillas, letting them bake on the griddle until crispy/crunchy and nicely browned (the *masa* on the inside will still be a little soft), 2 to 3 minutes in all.

5. Keep finished quesadillas warm on a rack set on a baking pan in the oven. When all are made, line them up on a warm serving platter or wooden board or a basket lined with a napkin, and serve with salsa below.

ESSENTIAL CHOPPED TOMATO-SERRANO SALSA

12 ounces (2 medium-small round or 4 or 5 plum) ripe tomatoes
     Fresh serrano chilis to taste (roughly 3 to 5, or more if you like it spicy)
12 large sprigs of cilantro
 1 large garlic clove, peeled and very finely chopped
 1 small white onion
1½ teaspoons fresh lime juice
     Salt, about ¼ teaspoon

1. Core the tomatoes, then cut in half and squeeze out the seeds if you wish (this will give the sauce a less rustic appearance). Finely dice the flesh by slicing it into roughly ¼-inch thick pieces, then cutting each slice into small dice. Scoop into a bowl.

2. Cut the chilis in half lengthwise (wear gloves if your hands are sensitive) and scrape out the seeds if you wish (this will make the salsa a little less spicy). Chop the chilis as finely as you can, then add them to the tomatoes.

3. Carefully bunch up the cilantro sprigs, and, with a sharp knife, slice them ¹⁄₁₆-inch thick, stems and all, working from the leafy end toward the stems. Scoop into the tomato mixture along with the garlic.

4. Finely dice the onion with a knife, scoop it into a small strainer, then rinse it under cold water. Shake to remove excess water and add to the tomato mixture.

5. Taste and season with lime juice and salt, and let stand a few minutes for the flavors to meld.

Middle Eastern

Bulgur wheat is a big deal in the Middle East, as in *kibbie nayee,* the national dish of Lebanon. And tabbouleh. Forget falafel as well.

If you can get beyond the obvious no-no's, there is *emjudra,* a dish of lentils and rice cooked in onion broth. Many Middle Eastern restaurants serve *ej-jee,* a Lebanese omelet flavored with mint and onions. *Hummus tahini* is the Israeli and Egyptian version of mashed chickpeas and crushed sesame seeds, and while *baba ganoush* is spelled differently in Greek, it's still puréed eggplant with sesame dressing. This is a big favorite in Syria and Turkey as well.

Greek olives are called *zatoon* in the Middle East. *Laban* is said to be an authentic yogurt made from a thousand-year-old culture. I didn't think it tasted a day over five hundred years myself. As in Greek restaurants, cucumbers abound in Middle Eastern restaurants. Ask for your own plate and enjoy the dips.

Maza is the Armenian, Turkish, and Greek answer to antipasto. Mixed dishes are always good because you can discuss their contents when you order and ask that any unsafe dishes be left out and extras of the gluten-free dishes added. Some celiacs make a deal with their dinner partners, order two plates, and rearrange to suit. I am not a fan of this method. There is always the possibility of getting errant gluten mixed up with your portion.

Marinades are usually yogurt, garlic, and lemon in this part of the world, but do check first before you order the *kabobs.*

Pass up the pastry tray and have a piece of *halvah* or *halawah,* Lebanese sugar and sesame paste candy, a glass of rose water, or maybe a nice cup of *kawhwee,* the dark Turkish coffee that is usually served by the thimbleful, for good reason.

Russian

With my apologies to Russian friends, this is the land of bitter winters, little sun, and stick-to-the-ribs food that contains enough gluten to make all of Eastern Europe queasy.

Siberia seems to be the dumpling and noodle capital of the world with *pelmeni, verniki, haluski,* and *manti.* With breads and savories such as *kulebiaka, khachapuri, pirozhki,* and *pirogs,* Russian stroganoffs, Ukrainian crepes, *blini,* and all the thick cabbage and beet dishes of the Baltics, you may ask yourself what's left. Plentski.

Georgian rice and lamb pilafs are fragrant and filling and are made with nuts and candied orange peel. One in particular, from Azerbaijan, can be made with an egg, potato, pumpkin, or bread crust. Make sure you know which one is being used. Or better, ask that yours be prepared with egg, pumpkin or potato.

Borscht or *kologniy* is always good.

Say *nyet* to *tabbouleh.* This bulgur wheat is often prepared as a pilaf. Always make sure your pilaf is made only with rice.

Have a Russian omelet with sour cream and caviar. Or stuffed prunes. Lamb stew with chestnuts and pomegranates is a traditional Azerbaijani dish that should not contain wheat flour as a thickener, but as you know by now, you must ask.

Every country has its version of polenta, and Moldavian cornmeal mush is really very good.

Kasha and wild mushroom casserole is a hearty dish as long as you can be sure the buckwheat groats aren't mixed with unsafe grains.

Rice-stuffed grape leaves are Russian, as are stuffed apples, quinces, peppers, and pumpkins. Lamb is often used for stuffing as well. These dishes do not contain bread crumbs or any flour thickeners, but check with the kitchen anyway.

Mashkitchiri is literally mashed mung beans, vegetables, and rice.

Ask about the marinade before ordering kabobs and forget dessert. Have some halvah with a glass of tea.

Of course, there's always good Russian vodka. *Nasdrovia!*

Scandinavian

It's very cold in this part of the world, and there is quite a bit of fish, especially codfish. For this reason, you will find quite a lot of pickled and salted food. This means vinegar, so if you are still avoiding the stuff, you may want to pass on the smorgasbord, the traditional Scandinavian buffet table.

Moving beyond the stereotype, you should find Danish hot buttermilk soup, apple soup, cherry soup (*kirsebaersuppe*), and summer vegetable soup thickened with nothing but cornstarch. Swedish meatballs usually contain bread crumbs. You won't know until you ask. If you have to ask about beer soup, you should not be allowed to go out to dinner.

Gravlax is Swedish marinated salmon, and it's generally worth the high price. You will find reindeer, whale, and venison on menus in Scandinavian countries, and you may find these meats in Scandinavian American restaurants. If you do and can handle it—I draw the line at Rudolph—don't get so caught up in your ability to try new things that you forget to ask how they are prepared.

Danish ham is a real treat. Watch for mustard and bread crumbs in the coating and Madeira sauce in the glaze. Madeira is based on a brown stock that can, in turn, be based on a *roux,* or flour, paste.

As in all the restaurants in the world, watch out for sauces.

In the land of the midnight sun and lots of celiacs, Norwegian prune pudding is traditionally thickened with cornstarch, and Swedish rice porridge, a traditional Christmas dessert, should be gluten-free, as should Danish prune custard.

Akvavit is the traditional firewater of Scandinavia.

Ikea sells a mean gluten-free almond torte.

Spanish

While the Spanish have had an enormous influence on Mexican food, Spanish food takes its cues from the great cities of Barcelona, Valencia, Malaga, and Granada along the Mediterranean and from the dusky sweetness of North Africa just beyond.

All over Spain, bars and bistros called *tascas* serve the tapas, or small appetizer dishes that are the national snack. Their American cousins are cropping up in cities all over the United States, where it is the custom to drink sherry, share gossip, and order from extensive menus of foods served in very small portions.

Proceed carefully. It's easy to be overwhelmed by such small portions and the speed with which they arrive at the table. In the casual, often-rollicking spirit of these places, some gluten may slip by. Bypass the obvious and maybe not so obvious offenders—*empadillas* (turnovers), *emparedos* (small sandwiches), *croqetas* (croquettes), or any other puffs, pancakes, or balls.

Stick with simple dishes containing foods you can readily see—such as Spanish antipasto, garlic shrimp (*gambas al ajillo*), clams in tomato sauce (*almejas al diablo*), mussels marinated in red wine, capers, and pimiento (*mejillones a la vinagreta*), eels in garlic sauce (*angulas a la bilbaina*), or smelts. Order chorizo if you can ascertain how it was made. Some tapas restaurants serve miniature tortillas, which are not tortillas at all, but flat Spanish omelets served in wedges. Always ask about fillings before you order. Always ask about everything. If English is a problem in your local tasca, *pregunta* is Spanish for question. *Yo tengo preguntas*: I have questions.

If you are dining in a more traditional Spanish restaurant, there is always paella, the rich dish that is the centerpiece of Spanish cuisine. There is *paella a la Valenciana* with chicken and seafood, *paella marinera* with seafood only, *paella huertana de murcia* with vegetables, and *paella de codornices y setas,* featuring quail and mushrooms. *Fideua de mariscos,* a paella of noodles and shellfish, is best avoided.

Zarzuela de marisco is a spicy and spectacular shellfish stew served over rice.

Try one of the endless varieties of the hearty and filling Spanish tortillas or omelets. As everywhere, be wary of sauces and stews. Always ask the chef how either is thickened before ordering it.

Marzipan, the almond sugar candy, came to Spain by way of the Moors and is on many Spanish menus. In fact, so many Spanish candies are made with almonds, sugar, coconut, and eggs and no wheat or gluten that it is advisable to find a good Spanish-American market and stock up.

Skip the pastry cart. As always, ask before you order the *flan,* or explore the baked apples, bananas with honey and pine nuts, or pears in dark Spanish wine, prunes, and apricots. For once, you will not be sorry you ordered fruit.

Thai

The contrasts are sharp in this part of the world. Four-alarm curries, fiery chili pastes, searing peanut sauces, coconut milk, and lemon grass are the grace notes of this interesting food.

Spring rolls are often made with rice wrappers, which can be used for your own delicious purposes, for enfolding shrimp and green onions held together with fish sauce and lemon grass. Bean thread or rice sticks are used in place of wheat noodles, with tofu instead of chicken or beef. Pineapple and tapioca make fried rice distinctly Thai, and lemon grass soup can lull the diner into a false sense of security, a subtle prelude to the heat of any number of Thai curries.

Pad Thai is a classic dish made with rice noodles (*ban-pho*), egg, bean curd, bean sprouts, and green onion topped with ground peanuts. There are many variations on the rice noodle, as well as rice pancakes and spicy fritters of corn and potato.

The difficulty of dining safely on Thai cuisine is in the sauces. Clear fish sauce contains no wheat, but hoisin sauce does. Soy, tamari, and thick fish and peanut sauces are often used and can be a problem. If you love this food as I do, my best advice is to sit down with your local Thai chef and figure out together what you can eat and what you can't. If language is a problem, use your Thai dining card, page 500, in the appendix. Most Thai dishes are individually stir-fried, so it's not as if your diet is affecting the entire night's business. Naturally, you must be a good enough customer to make it worthwhile for the restaurant to clean the stir-fry pan and start over for you, and you should be considerate of peak times.

You will not be sorry you took the trouble. Fresh, homemade Thai rice noodles alone are worth the effort.

Pad Thai

Say hello to the national dish of Thailand. Crunchy, soul satisfying, spicy and sweet, this sauté of rice noodles with shrimp and bean sprouts couldn't be easier to make. Start with lettuce wraps or a simple salad spiked with lemon grass. The spicy version here is studded with peanuts compliments of Beth Hillson, star chef and founder of the Gluten-Free Pantry.

Serves 4

½ cup peanut oil
12 large shrimp, peeled and deveined
4 eggs, lightly beaten
2 cups softened rice noodles (soak noodles 1 hour in cool water, drain and measure)
1 teaspoon paprika

½ cup fish sauce
½ cup sugar
½ cup rice vinegar
½ cup ground unsalted peanuts
8 green onions, cut into 1-inch pieces
1 cup fresh bean sprouts, rinsed and drained, plus ¼ cup fresh bean
       sprouts, rinsed and drained for garnish
4 garlic cloves
6 to 8 dried red chili peppers or 1 teaspoon red pepper flakes
       Lemon wedges, for garnish

1. Heat oil in a large frying pan or wok over high heat until the oil begins to smoke. Add shrimp and sauté for 1 minute. Break eggs over the shrimp and allow to sit for 1 minute, then scramble mixture.

2. Add the rice noodles and paprika; stir briefly. Add fish sauce, sugar, rice vinegar, and peanuts. Sauté for 30 seconds. Combine bean sprouts, green onion, garlic and red peppers (or pepper flakes) to mixture. Toss to heat. Remove from heat, place in serving dish and garnish with bean sprouts and lemon wedges.

Learn More

There is nothing like a good cookbook to inspire experiment. Here are a few that will start you on the road to a well-rounded International library.

Indian Cooking by Madhur Jaffrey (Barron's)
Rick Bayless's Mexican Kitchen by Rick Bayless (Scribner)
The Essential Cuisines of Mexico by Diana Kennedy (Clarkson Potter)
Risotto from the Williams-Sonoma Series (Simon & Schuster)
Essentials of Classic Italian Cooking by Marcella Hazan (Knopf)
Quick & Easy Thai by Nancie McDermott (Chronicle Books)
Basic Asian by Cornelia Schinharl, Sebastian Dickhaut, and Kelsey Lane
    (Silverback Books)
The African Cookbook by Bea Sandler (Carol Publishing)
The Rice Bible by Christian Teubner (Viking)
The Food of Venice by Luigi Veronelli (Tuttle)

PART IV

Can We Talk?: Emotional, Social, and Family Issues

your cheating heart

You always hurt the one you love.

—THE MILLS BROTHERS

In the beginning, you will want to cheat. And many of you will, no matter how reasonable or convincing the arguments to the contrary.

Why would any celiac in his or her right mind want to do that?

It's not because we're dumb, or dense, or more self-destructive than the next person. It's because we want our old lives back. It's because we want to be normal (whatever *that* is). It's because food is the most primal instinct we have.

This is not a four-week ten-pounds-off kind of thing. This is not something we choose. The gluten-free diet is for life and therein lies the problem.

Compounding the problem is the fact that for more and more of you, the gluten-free diet is not the welcome relief it was to me—the end of suffering—but a sudden and terrible shock.

Not having severe symptoms or, in some cases, no symptoms at all, is great for your health, but not so hot for your resolve. It's much easier to stick to something when it's the antidote to suffering. Much easier to resist a slice of pizza when the penalty for eating it is thirty-seven trips to the bathroom. It's hard to demonize something that never really made you that sick in the first place.

Recently, my husband and I sold our house to a nice young couple who each wore the map of Ireland on their happy faces. At the closing, a tray of pastries was brought in for the occasion and I, of course, declined, saying, "No thanks, I'm a celiac." (I don't really expect everyone to know what that is, but it's my little contribution to making people aware of the word.) At that, the young and clearly pregnant wife smiled and said, "I'm a celiac, too. But I don't have symptoms and my doctor says I can have gluten."

"Who's your doctor?" I asked.

Well, you may have guessed. The person who told her she could have Danish pastry was none other than my doctor, too.

At that point, I came to my senses and decided it was probably not a good idea to lecture the person who is giving you a great deal of money for your house. I dropped the subject, signed the papers, accepted a nice bottle of champagne from our real estate broker, and tried not to be upset by the sight of a pregnant celiac munching a sticky bun.

I did tell my doctor though, first chance I got, who vented his frustration. "You have no idea how many people just don't hear what I'm telling them."

"Did you know she's pregnant?"

"Oh, God," he said, horrified at what could happen.

Mother and baby did just fine, but I haven't given up. Since my new house is a mere three blocks away from the old one, I will occasionally slip a gluten-free order form through my old mail slot with the really good items starred. Sometimes, my husband and I walk past the old house on our way to our favorite Italian restaurant, a serving of my gluten-free pasta tucked in a pocket. The stubborn look on her face when I show her my rice pasta and rave about how good it tastes is all I need to know about not getting through to this person.

Some of you will stash cookies in kitchen drawers, or eat a cheeseburger, roll and all. Friends will wonder why the front seat of your car is full of crumbs, why your briefcase smells of Krispy Kremes, why there are chocolate chips in your bed. In the middle of the night, you might shave the side of a lemon pound cake as I once did, telling yourself the thinner the slice, the safer the serving.

Denial is a powerful river that has to run its course.

Equally powerful is forgiveness. If you do have a lapse, accept that you are human and fallible and cut yourself a break. Instead of beating yourself up and engaging in what I call the "bad dog" syndrome, give yourself a hug, acknowledge how hard this gluten-free thing really is, and start over, resolving to get a better handle on what makes you want to go off your diet.

The urge to cheat may be intermittent, striking only when you fly through time zones or visit the zoo. It may hit you when you least expect it, passing a bakery or watching a child eat an ice-cream cone. I must confess, I have had two self-inflicted relapses since my own diagnosis (two in twenty years isn't bad). One can be traced to a vacation in Cape Cod and the irresistible corn and lobster bisque (I knew I should have asked if it was thickened with flour, but I didn't want to know the answer) and another to being home alone with a truffle cake sent for Christmas by a well-meaning but unenlightened business associate. I may be weak and disgustingly human, but even in desperation, I have my standards.

Was it worth it? Not really.

Would I do it again? Not in a million years, especially now with so many really good gluten-free foods readily available.

For one thing, I know just how haywire a system can go because of celiac disease. I've also learned that if denial is acknowledged and given its due, it will eventually, albeit begrudgingly, turn into acceptance.

But you're not there yet.

❥

It's okay to hate the people who try to stop you, even if those people are those nearest and dearest. It's normal for people who love you not to want to see you become ill again or to risk your future health. It's normal for friends and family to become quite unhinged when they witness what they know is a deliberate attempt to do yourself in with a bear claw. This, in turn, will upset you because, as everyone knows, a good defense is a good offense, and anyone who has ever watched the daytime talk shows also knows it is impossible to save another person from self-destruction.

If you cheat enough, friends might even try an intervention, and take turns telling you how much they love you and how sad it makes them to see you eating gluten. No matter how people choose to let you know you are doing something dangerous, you will meet their anger with your own. You will insult them and accuse them of trying to control you, and a fight will ensue. Everyone will remember the whole episode as dumb and stupid, but then so is cheating.

Even when your family and friends think your actions stem from ignorance, absentmindedness, or a temporary lapse in judgment, they will automatically assume you want to be saved, which, as you know in your cheating heart, is not always the case. Best to acquire some skills and take a good, hard look at what makes you tick.

Saving Yourself from Yourself

Anti-Cheating Strategy No. 1

No matter how much you might regret it later, tell your traveling companions about your diet.

The world can be a dangerous place for people like us, and it is very hard to resist seeing travel as a suspension of the rules. No one knows you, so who will know? You will. Before the urge to cheat hits, in the airport while you're waiting to board the plane, tell your companions you're a celiac. (You did order a gluten-free airline meal, didn't you?) Carry nibbles for your room or on the road; pack something sweet of your own for dessert. Offer your companions any bread or muffins that come with your meals. If you are traveling alone, break all the rules of etiquette (this is an emergency), and tell total strangers more than they want to know about your diet—the flight attendant, the person sitting next to you, the waiter at your hotel, the manager of room service. Who cares what they think? You'll never see them again.

When it comes to vacations, the danger is not restricted to staying in hotels, getting to and from a place, or even attempting to order new and odd-looking foods in foreign countries. Any holiday from routine and the responsibilities of work for more than a long weekend qualifies as a potential trouble spot, even if that means sitting on your own front porch with a pile of books or sleeping in your backyard hammock for a week.

Anti-Cheating Strategy No. 2

Pack your own gluten-free cookies, cakes, pies, and pizza, the gooier the better, eat too much of them, and come home as fat and guilty as everyone else.

Vacations are extremely tricky. We work hard, save our money, fly to Disney World, book a cruise, or rent a cottage in the woods. We drive, fly, hike, bike, sail, or swim off and forget all our worries and restrictions for a few weeks. We overspend, overeat, overplay, overindulge ourselves, our kids, our spouses, our friends; even the dog comes home with a T-shirt he'll never wear. We overdo it all, vainly trying to squeeze out two weeks of pleasure among fifty weeks of pain.

Restraint doesn't seem to have much of a say on vacation because the word *no* never seems to make it into the suitcase. I think this is because holidays are so hard to come by and are so tied up with feelings of deserving.

How often have you overheard one vacationer say to another about an ice-cream sundae, a mai-tai, or a Rolex, "Oh, go ahead, you deserve it"? How often have you said this yourself? My point exactly. Trouble is, what you deserve is not necessarily what is good for you. Tell yourself, while you may be on vacation, your CD is not.

Anti-Cheating Strategy No. 3

See how many gluten-free festive desserts you can invent. (Anniversary rice pudding, the "I Can't-Believe-I'm-Fifty" hot fudge sundae, bon voyage banana boat, retirement bombe, rehearsal dinner torte, and the divine wedding dacquoise just to get you started.)

Life's Big Moments are fraught with every emotional opportunity to cheat. Phrases like, "Hey, it's my birthday" and "It isn't every day you get married, turn forty, retire, celebrate a century in the armed forces, get divorced, have a baby, join a convent, get arrested, win the lottery, land a part in a movie" are dead giveaways that there is trouble ahead.

To make matters worse, it is virtually impossible to attend or be the guest of honor at any of these occasions without prolonged exposure to cake. Even worse, if you happen to be the bride or the groom and have let your in-laws talk you into a wedding cake you can't eat. I don't even want to think about the lifetime of concessions in store for the person who can't or won't made demands on his or her wedding day. (If this is the case, reread chapter 2 immediately!)

Anti-Cheating Strategy No. 4

Don't bother the bereaved or similarly preoccupied person with your problems. Just bring a nice gluten-free covered dish, keep your hands out of the bagel chips, and say something nice about the deceased.

This may sound odd, but funerals are dicey for cheating potential. I think it's because the enormity of death makes all of our petty concerns seem trivial and food is so central to the process of grieving. Custom dictates that each mourner contribute to the mountain of food, thus ensuring enough leftovers to help the family get through the first difficult days without having to worry about cooking.

How do you explain your gluten problem to a person who has just lost a loved one? You don't. You put something on your plate for appearances and before you know it . . . it's gone.

The only way to be sure this doesn't happen is to bring something you can eat.

Anti-Cheating Strategy No. 5

Tell the boss about your gluten intolerance and just happen to mention how important strict adherence to your regimen could be to the containment of health insurance costs for the company.

Job pressure is another big obstacle to self-control, especially the insidious variety found at the average downsized and outsourced corporation. Everyone is paranoid about everyone else. The boss says "Jump" and a chorus answers, "How high?" The boss says, "Let's go for burgers" and before you know it, you're tucking into a double cheeseburger on a sesame seed bun. You tell yourself you're doing it in the name of job security (only the healthy survive).

Tell yourself this: No one has ever been fired for refusing to eat bread. If you are, you probably have a landmark lawsuit, which will be waged on CNN.

Anti-Cheating Strategy No. 6

Figure out how many hours are lost to the company while your coworkers are out having pizza or huddled in front of the building puffing cigarettes. Contrast this with the cost of a refrigerator, a set of safety seal storage containers, and a toaster for your office.

Working late with nothing but a vending machine, a few takeout menus, and a hole as big as Cleveland in your stomach is not conducive to staying on the straight and narrow. Keep a box of cereal, crackers, and something that packs a big protein wallop, such as peanut butter or a box of gluten-free energy bars in your desk. Make sure you wash your utensils carefully, wipe jars, reseal packages, and close lids tightly. It won't be good for your career to be seen spraying Raid into your drawers or listing "desk extermination" among your business expenses.

If you're lucky enough to have a private office, I would strongly advise investing in a small refrigerator and keeping it stocked with bottled water, fruit, and your favorite gluten-free snacks. Otherwise, using the one in the employee lounge or cafeteria will do, as long as you label your food with as much guilt producing poignancy as possible. "Please don't steal this. It's the only food I can eat!" is always effective.

Physical vs. Emotional Hunger

Sometimes even the tiniest twinge of deprivation can push us over the line and trigger an eating episode with the usual emotional roller coaster—anger, happiness, sadness, boredom, thirst, water retention, success, failure, gloom, loneliness, envy, apathy, feelings of abandonment, something as life-shattering as the loss of a loved one, or as trivial as the loss of one's keys. Then there is feeling loved too little, too much, or not all. The discovery of a few unwanted pounds can do it and so can a particularly nasty bout of PMS, a fight with the boss, or a full-blown midlife crisis. Just about anything can weaken your resolve and leave you face down in a plate of chocolate-chip cookies.

It's impossible to control something you don't understand, so it's important to look carefully at what motivates the urge to cheat. Is it real hunger, which usually announces itself suddenly, loudly, and often painfully? Or is it emotional hunger, which creeps up on you and doesn't seem to have as much to do with food as it does with the need to fill the place that feels most empty?

Physical hunger is not a rational thing, but rather an irrational, animal need that lives in the dark and tangled pit of our stomachs and speaks to us in a low, rolling growl. True hunger does not respond well to do's and don'ts, shoulds and should nots, or diet restrictions of any kind, especially one that bans the glutenous belly fillers that satisfy it so quickly. Like Popeye, the hungry stomach "wants what I wants, when I wants it."

There's an old saying in diet circles: "It's not what you're eating, it's what's eating you." Unlike physical hunger, emotional hunger is not so easy to appease. The stomach rarely growls. There is no sudden pang, no sharp pain propelling you into the kitchen or to a forbidden buffet table. Something else, far more primal, moves us to this kind of eating. If in addition to simple appetite appeal the food we are considering carries with it feelings of love, warmth, happiness, fullness, satisfaction, comfort, and safety, if it stirs memories of any kind and it also contains gluten, it may be virtually impossible to resist.

Emotional hunger is insidious. It creeps up on you while you are watching television, in the middle of an argument, during a moment of sadness and loss. It takes advantage of you when you have too much work and too little time, when you have the flu, a broken foot, tennis elbow, a dented fender, or whenever you feel most sorry for yourself. It arrives with your divorce papers, the new car agreement, the mortgage application, the promotion, or the pink slip. It can explode in a sudden desire to eat everything in sight, and it can show up right after a filling meal because emotional hunger doesn't come from the stomach but from the heart or the head or the psyche. It comes from wherever we keep our pain.

Like anything that comes from deep within your emotional programming, this kind of hunger is a powerful force. One minute you are a normal person eating three gluten-free meals plus snacks a day, and the next you are chowing down an entire pizza with extra cheese or working your way through a box of glazed donuts. You are an emotional hostage, hating yourself more with every bite.

If you don't spend some time figuring out which emotions or situations trigger this dangerous behavior, you will never be free of it. Even if you have never indulged in this kind of naval gazing in the past, this is the time to start.

Unexamined emotional hunger is one of the reasons some people become obese, alcoholic, drug-addicted, fools in love, abused, and worse. It's why you have no idea why you would even consider doing serious harm to yourself with a spring roll.

Compounding the problem is our national preoccupation with healthy eating, moderate exercise, and normal body weight fed to us in media messages that bombard us with images that do not add up. Every day we turn on our televisions and see too many people eating far too much to be so thin, giving permission to the emotionally hungry celiac in our private hearts.

Anti-Cheating Strategy No. 7

Understand that the way to your cheating heart is through your stomach. Keep it reasonably full at all times, but not so full that you get fat and acquire other problems. Eat enough to keep your brain from sounding the eating alarm.

If you are truly hungry, the sight of any food, including off-limits food, will trigger an uncontrollable urge to consume. Sadly, there are many people in the world and right here in the United States who experience this kind of hunger every day. And every day, the rest of us get up and go to our refrigerators because we only think we're experiencing it.

Anti-Cheating Strategy No. 8

Forget:"You are what you eat." Remember: "You eat what you feel."

There are as many behavioral cues in one's life as there are breaths in each day, and it would be impossible to discuss the derivation of every impulse. The following chart may help you clarify your own personal list of emotional land mines. When a truck hits you, it's very important to get the license plate and a good description of the driver. It's just as critical to know what's driving your behavior and to understand the difference between what's felt and what's real. While these interpretations may not always apply to you, they should offer some serious food for thought.

Feeling	Reality
My life is empty.	My stomach is empty.
I can't have anything.	I can't have this corn muffin.
I want to crunch a pretzel.	I want to bite your head off.
I'm so angry, I could eat everything in the house.	I have trouble expressing my anger, so I eat bread instead.
I need pasta.	I need comforting.
I want to hurt you.	I am hurting me.
Others try to control me.	I see assistance as control.
I need to eat this pie.	I need attention.
You don't care if I eat this cookie.	I need to talk about why I want to eat this cookie.
If I get sick and die, then you'll love me.	If I get sick and die, no one will love me.
Why me?	Why not?

On closer inspection, you may find that the various feelings behind the urge to cheat express themselves in the need for different foods. If you watch and listen carefully, you may be able to match the food craving with the feelings. It's different for everyone, but the list below may strike a familiar chord. Make sure you have the gluten-free equivalents on hand for those cravings that ring true.

Pretzels, chips, bread sticks	=	Anger
Pasta, noodles	=	Sadness
Cocktail mix nibbles	=	Denial
Ice cream, anything frozen	=	Pain
Muffins, toast, cereal	=	Romantic love
Gravy, stuffing, sandwiches	=	Mother love
Anything with butter fat	=	Unrequited love
Bite-sized cookies, nuts, M&Ms, or other miniature foods	=	Anxiety

Anti-Cheating Strategy No. 9

Suffer.

I know a rather unusual therapist who holds the revolutionary view that the only trouble with most people is that they've never learned how to suffer. He says that, as a culture, we have dedicated ourselves to the notion that psychic pain is preventable. An entire self-help industry has sprung up around the misguided belief that if we try harder, we can deflect or postpone or even wipe out suffering altogether.

Building on that hypothesis, one could say that most self-destructive behavior is a subconscious unwillingness to acknowledge what is really going on, and that it is a repetitive and futile attempt to avoid the unfamiliar territory of our own feelings and be enlightened by the lessons of experiencing them deeply.

If you doubt this, all you have to do is watch someone dating the same type he or she just divorced to see what great and destructive lengths people will go to avoid learning something about themselves through their angst. Still unconvinced? Watch an angry ex-smoker light up after a fender bender in the parking lot.

A friend of mine is fond of saying about life "No one gets out of it alive." Isn't it easier to stop spending enormous amounts of energy on the struggle to remain unaffected by our suffering? Why not surrender to it, feel the pain and move past it, maybe even learn something in the process?

The next time you experience sadness or hopelessness or anger about your gluten-free lot in life (or anything, for that matter), and you feel like crying, slamming a wall, whining, or hollering your head off, find a private place and do it. Let your feelings happen, instead of keeping them under a tight lid. If you're unaccustomed to doing this, you will become extremely uncomfortable during the first few minutes of this exercise. Resist the impulse to push your feelings away. The whole process shouldn't take more than fifteen minutes. My guess is that when you find out what's really going on, you will forget about the unsafe food.

Anti-Cheating Strategy No. 10

Make a stack of photocopies of the "cheat sheet" on the next page, and fill it in every day for two weeks.

Patterns will emerge. Associations will be made. A particular time of day may reveal itself to be more dangerous than another, one activity more fraught with temptation than another. The results may surprise you.

Be specific and do whatever it takes to tell the truth. If you ate standing up, say so. The more specific you are, the more insight you will gain. You will begin to take control over those times you are most susceptible to going off your diet.

Anti-Cheating Strategy No. 11

Acknowledge your cheating with forgiveness. And start fresh.

Whenever you begin to lose touch with the emotions that drive your cheating behavior, make some fresh copies of your cheat sheet and start over, and don't fall into the oldest trap of all. You know how this goes: "I've already had half a pie, so why not be a total idiot and finish it off?" This, of course, is followed by: "I feel sick now because I'm bad, so why don't I eat something really bad and make it worthwhile getting sick over?" Blah. Blah. Blah. Blah. It doesn't matter whether you're talking about pounds, as in "I'm never going to be thin, so why don't I eat this?" or talking about gluten: "I'm already miserable; why not finish off the pizza?" It all comes down to being able to stop the downward cycle by acknowledging that you are human and forgive yourself and start over. When viewed this way, weakness itself can become a strength.

DAILY CHEAT SHEET Date _____

	Foods Eaten	Time Eaten	Where Eaten	With Whom	In Response to Physical Hunger? (Rate level from 1 to 10)	In Response to Emotional Hunger? (Rate level from 1 to 10)	Symptoms
Breakfast							
Midmorning Snack							
Lunch							
Afternoon Snack							
Dinner							
Miscellaneous Food Consumed (List of all picking, nibbling, noshing, vendor food. Remember, eating over the sink, cleaning plates, and finishing the kids' sandwiches count!)							

_____ I did not cheat at all today. _____ I cheated a little today. _____ Gluten disaster.

_____ I resolve to forgive myself the weaknesses of today and to start again tomorrow, committed to my health, determined to end my self-destructive behavior, and to be as resourceful in finding gluten-free foods I will enjoy as I am in finding the foods I sneak.

_____ Not perfect, but better than before. I will try harder tomorrow.

_____ Congratulations! Keep up the great gluten-free work.

Comments:

Dieting: The Double Whammy

Many people are malnourished when they are diagnosed with celiac disease. After diagnosis, the emphasis is on rebuilding health, strength, and muscle, which means resuming a normal body weight, which in turn means eating pretty much anything you want for a while.

At five feet eight inches and a whopping ninety pounds, hair cropped to about an inch all around to encourage new and healthier growth, my husband dubbed me "Q-Tip with Chocolate Shake." The good news is that we eventually *do* gain weight. And that, of course, is the bad news as well.

Some people do this gradually over a long period of time, slowing down at what is easily maintained, while others just keep on gaining. The experts say this is due to the fact that for many celiacs, the body is absorbing food properly for the first time, based on how little or how much damage the intestine has sustained during the active or even quiescent phase of the disease. In other words, we may have eaten a lot, but the food never really got absorbed. Add to that calories, grams of fat, level of activity, age, and whether the metabolism is still racing or has been turned down by the thermostat of time, and bingo, you've got yourself a weight problem.

I have my own theory on the subject, of course, and it's simple. What is unattainable is suddenly attractive. People who rarely ate bread, cookies, pasta, or pie now can't get enough of the gluten-free varieties, full of fat, white flour, and sugar. Suddenly, we are loading up on foods we never ate in the first place, just because we can't have their mainstream counterparts. No wonder the pounds pile on.

Like many young women in the 1970s, I associated carbohydrates with unwaiflike, unfashionable figures. I nibbled cottage cheese, fasted occasionally, ate hard-boiled eggs or bananas, and drank black coffee with everything, attributing my wafer-thinness to good genes and exceptional willpower. Now I never miss a meal and rarely pass up the opportunity to enjoy a new gluten-free something or other and, like everyone else in American over the age of consent, I find I must diet.

Dieting is never easy, but for people who know eating just enough gluten to develop symptoms is the quickest route to skin and bones, it can be an especially tempting reason to cheat, kind of like having your cake and eating it, too. Don't be shocked. I know you've thought of it.

Anti-Cheating Strategy No. 12

Find a really terrible photograph of yourself taken while you were sick. The next time you are tempted to eat pasta in order to lose weight, make note of your rib cage pushing through your shirt, your sunken eyes, your lackluster skin. Remember how sitting at your desk bruised the "buttons" of your spine, how sick you felt. Understand there is such a thing as being too thin.

The current demonizing of carbohydrates will no doubt give sway to something else equally insane. We have become a nation of test sticks fully conversant in all the colorful nuances of ketosis. While it's certainly easier to order a gluten-free meal nowadays—hamburger, no roll, no fries, salad with a little balsamic—I've got to believe that we're going to end up paying the piper for eating all that fatty, not to mention expensive, red meat, cheese, and overprocessed low-carb food. Complex carbohydrates are good for us as are most foods (except those containing gluten) in moderation, especially fruits and vegetables. I'm not a doctor or expert on nutrition, but I predict we will have a veritable explosion of heart disease and cancer from our misguided belief in what may only be clever marketing. My experiment with the lure of quick weight loss certainly did work, but the cost was total cholesterol that shot up to 259 from 150. Liquid diet shakes are not only unrealistic—the minute you eat real food, you regain the weight—they are particularly dangerous for celiacs. If you can find one of these highly sugared potions in a flavor that's gluten-free, you are doomed to consume only that flavor, reducing an already impossible diet down to its barest bones. This cannot be good for you.

Forget Jenny Craig or Nutri-System or L.A. Weight Loss, or any of the programs that require you to buy food at franchised centers. Food labeling laws do not apply to products that are sold privately. Not only will it be difficult for you to find something you can eat, you will have no idea how many calories, carbs, and grams of fat each meal contains for when you're ready to go it alone.

Many of these companies count on your regaining the weight. When your bottom line expands, so does theirs. Enough said?

Programs like Weight Watchers are a bit better. While it's true that you can't eat most of the packaged products pitched at these weekly meetings, the plan is not dependent on them. The language changes frequently to make the program sound new, but this old-fashioned support group approach teaches moderation and portion control through the use of daily points. Members learn very quickly how to effectively "eat their points." It's quite possible to fashion a healthy gluten-free diet using this method. Not to mention the weekly public weighing to keep you honest.

Anti-Cheating Strategy No. 13

A yo-yo is a toy, not a word to describe your eating habits.

Losing and gaining, then losing and gaining is terrible for your body, not to mention that many people lose their gallbladders because of yo-yo dieting. And hasn't your body been through enough lately?

Remember this: The faster you lose the weight, the faster it comes back. The more you starve yourself, the more efficiently your body stores calories as fat against the day it finds itself starving once again. Basically, your body knows what you're going to do to it and behaves like a squirrel in the Antarctic. Failure is a breeding ground for cheating and you don't want to go there.

Besides, you're already on a diet for life. Who needs another one?

If you have recovered so well that you now have a weight problem, my advice is to lay off the gluten-free desserts for a while, ditto for the muffins and the high-fat cookies. Eat enough high-quality, lean protein and fiber and lots of fruits and vegetables in small meals spread throughout the day, so you never end up standing at the sink and eating everything in the refrigerator. Cut down on calories, watch the fat and sugar, and start a moderate exercise program. Before you embark on any exercise plan, though, see your family doctor or your gastroenterologist.

I would strongly advise newly diagnosed celiacs not to go it alone when starting a gluten-free diet and/or a reducing diet, but to seek professional nutritional counseling in the person of a registered dietician to help you make changes you can live with long term. A professional will help you design your diet with an eye toward health and balance, as well as recovery and achieving an ideal weight.

The same goes for those of you who need to put some more meat on your bones. Forget those high-calorie shakes, quick fixes, and power powders with labels that read like the Oxford Unabridged. Even if you find a shake that's gluten-free, they're full of chemicals and things best left in the lab. It may be boring, but eating well-balanced meals with enough of the nutrients you need and taking vitamin mineral supplements is going to get the job done in the long run. Again, seek professional help to ensure you're doing the right thing.

The only way to stop the yo-yo is to cut the string.

Thank You for Not Smoking, Drinking, or Eating Red Meat, Fats, Sugar, Carbs, Caffeine, and Chocolate

Any form of self-imposed deprivation, act of willpower, or abrupt change in lifelong patterns can put a severe strain on your carefully maintained equilibrium and trigger a gluten-cheating episode. It really doesn't matter what you give up or why—cigarettes, diet sodas, alcohol, animal protein, or lollipops. One big no-no in your life is enough. Two can put you over the top.

During the first two weeks of any voluntary substance avoidance, it is quite common to experience the urge to shift addictions, or if that is too strong a word, pleasures. Experts report that recovering drug addicts begin drinking, reformed drinkers suddenly crave chocolate bars, eschewers of meat yearn for sugar, and so it goes. Here's how to make sure you don't move from cigarette puffs to puff pastry.

Anti-Cheating Strategy No. 14

Get rid of every no-no in the house.

Forget what your grandmother taught you about wasting food. Be merciless. Serve only gluten-free meals. Send the family out for breakfast, lunch, and dinner, if necessary. So what if you blow your budget, you're worth it.

Anti-Cheating Strategy No. 15

Never try to tough it out alone.

Tell everyone around you what you are giving up and why, and ask for their support and understanding before you start. Join a support group or start an informal one of your own. Find a like-minded friend and do it on the buddy system. Confess that you might want to cheat on your gluten-free diet and ask to be saved ahead of time.

Anti-Cheating Strategy No. 16

Take up needlepoint. Or weaving. Or painting. Or juggling.

This may sound silly, but you can't cheat if your hands are busy with something you really enjoy. It is impossible to eat gluten while doing these things. I don't count years when I speak of my own success staying off cigarettes, nor do I tell horror stories of eating English muffins while caught in the throes of gluten withdrawal. I count needlepoint pillows and chair covers and beach bags and eyeglass cases.

Whether you have told yourself there is no flour in a certain dish you simply had to have, just nibbled the edges of a cookie, or walked into an Italian restaurant in broad daylight and brazenly ordered a heaping bowl of linguine and clam sauce, there is one final strategy that may help . . .

Anti-Cheating Strategy No. 16

Remember that success is getting up one more time than you fall down.

You're only cheating yourself.

fear of frying, gluten accidents, and other tough situations

If anything can go wrong, it will.

—MURPHY'S LAW

With all the wonderful gluten-free foods available, awareness of CD growing daily, and your considerable skill and creativity in making sure you have enough to eat, negotiating life without wheat should be a piece of cake. It should be, but even the most resourceful, self-assertive, and organized celiac finds herself painted into a nutritional corner from time to time, buffeted by life, love, business, family tradition, sibling rivalry, spiritual belief, and organized eating. Life passages like going to college, falling in love, and getting married are especially difficult for someone who needs to know not only where his or her next meal is coming from but also exactly what's in it. It's all about equilibrium, perspective, emotional honesty (with oneself), knowing where the pitfalls are, and always, a healthy sense of humor.

Fear of Frying

With apologies to Erica Jong, fear of frying, or *gustaphobia*, as I like to call it, is the abnormal fear of eating in other people's homes and/or restaurants. Many celiacs, especially those who were severely sick before diagnosis, develop this problem. In its advanced phase, people are known to become reclusive and unable to engage in the most innocent breakfast, lunch, or supper without getting the sweats and sneaking into friends' pantries to read labels. Paranoia becomes a way of life. It's human nature to get a little nervous about gluten in the weeks and months following diagnosis, but when it goes on and becomes a way of life, it can be disabling, not to mention socially isolating.

I have received many letters about this condition, so many in fact that I was inspired to give it a name. One person in particular, who turned out to be a friend of mutual friends, wouldn't accept their dinner invitation unless I came too, and she could watch me eat. Watching another celiac eat and not keel over is a good strategy for getting over gustaphobia.

Another way to vanquish this crippling condition is to invite a veteran celiac to join you for dinner or lunch at his or her favorite restaurant. This way, you can watch how ordering a good and safe gluten-free meal is done. If your buddy is on friendly terms with the chef, by all means, ask if you can go see where your food is prepared. Practice asking the questions that will ensure your meal is free of gluten and go over the menu together so you can learn how to spot dishes that are safe and cooking techniques that require bread crumbs, thickeners, roux, or other flour-based sauces. This can be a wonderful confidence booster.

Shopping with a partner helps a lot, too. Reading labels and asking questions together is a good way to discuss the irrational fears that crop up, i.e., the label is lying, what if some gluten got in by accident?, the product is cross-contaminated, the staff doesn't care. It's good to "shadow" this person for a while, so you can see how it's done. I imagine a service pairing new celiacs with veterans, kind of like the Big Brother/Big Sister organization. If you find yourself declining dinner invitations and avoiding social engagements, pondering the cost of a personal food taster or wondering if the breeze can spread hot dog bun particulate matter from your neighbor's barbecue, call your local support group and ask for the name of someone who lives nearby. Down the road, you can show your gratitude by doing the same for another newly diagnosed person.

I would also recommend a vacation from Internet bulletin boards. For every person who posts an item about something being gluten-free, or asks a perfectly reasonable question, there are ten vitriolic responses about why it couldn't possibly be or why the questioner is a complete idiot, celiac saboteur, or spy for the gluten industry. It's enough to drive a thinking person crazy. You don't need to worry about things like whether or not "turtle breath" is GF, as one poster put it, or if opening one's mouth while walking down the bread aisle is dangerous. Celiacs can be just as wacky as anybody else.

Do share your fears about eating with friends and loved ones and give people an opportunity to allay them. Ask pals for their recipes, and for a peek at the labels on the products they use. Watch as they prepare your food. Tell them that if you seem to be picking at your dinner it's not personal, that you're just getting the hang of eating again. Even better, volunteer to help with the meal, so you can correct any inadvertent contamination. Remember, we're all afraid of something. I have a friend who's terrified of mosquitoes and when she's around we never dine outside. Another chum, who was once in a fire, hates candles. Trust close friends (family should go without saying) with your fear and allow yourself to be loved enough to be understood. Toughing it out, in this case, is not going to help.

Trust is contagious and one confidence usually inspires another. Tell the truth about yourself and you may learn that after cooking all that salmon for your best friend's heart, she's really afraid of fish bones.

The best medicine for fear of frying: do the frying yourself. Make lunch, brunch, or dinner or pack a picnic and show them all how gluten-free is done. But don't forget Helen who needs to cut back on her sodium and Peter with the cholesterol problem. Remember to include something for lactose intolerant Louise, and don't make it too fattening for Freddie who's always ten pounds away from a different life. Take care of other people and they will take care of you.

The Rubber Chicken Dinner

Even the most well-ordered celiac life holds a few business and association lunches or dinners, especially in election years, during which you find yourself at a table with total strangers trying to figure out how to cheerfully watch them eat. The hospitality industry calls these affairs "captive feeding," and for good reason. Very little control can be exerted on what comes out of a kitchen that may be serving two or three banquet rooms at once. What does come out is often inedible, whether it's gluten-free or not.

As speaker after speaker drones on about the company's profits, the charity's good deeds, the association's honorees, or the candidate's promises, by all means keep busy. Rinse your eggs Benedict in your mimosa. Move everything around on your plate like a person with obsessive-compulsive disorder, and camouflage the mess with your napkin and a sprig of parsley. But don't march into the factory-sized kitchen and expect them to make you something special, unless you have a high tolerance for frustration, enjoy cardboard food, or miss the gang in anger management class.

I attended one of these dinners in Clearwater, Florida, given by a hospice to honor their volunteers, among them my mother. Reluctant to mention my peculiar plumbing in front of her friends and colleagues, I asked one of the servers to wrap up my untouched steak "for the dog" who, I explained, was on a high-protein diet. I was so busy trying to hide that I wasn't eating, I hadn't noticed that no one else had touched his or her food either. The minute we got outside, my mother dumped my little tinfoil swan into the nearest trash can and gave me a wicked grin. "You don't want poor Barnaby to get sick, do you?"

Sometimes we get so absorbed in our little battles with gluten that we forget that nobody likes the food at these things. Those who do eat, often go home slightly queasy and wondering why they bothered. Nick Pritzker of the Hyatt Hotel family once told my husband, "Never eat in a hotel or sleep in a restaurant." This is good advice.

Invitations to banquets often arrive with dinner choices. By all means, check the plain chicken breast or the steamed vegetables, but don't expect to enjoy them and you won't be disappointed. If you want to avoid coveting the rock-hard roll on your bread plate, and telling yourself the cookie dough ice cream is safe, arrive full. Or promise yourself a nice meal afterward. (When I attended these things for business, I always treated myself to tea in the afternoon, complete with gluten-free scones, cookies, or something equally wicked.)

Look at it this way, it's only a meal, one of three squares each day. Next week alone, you'll get 21 opportunities to make up for it. If you're like me and prefer several smaller meals spread out over the course of a day, you'll get 35 chances.

Sooner or later, someone will ask you why you're not eating. Do not tell the truth. The truth will lead you down a path you don't want to go, especially if the table is full of gossipy industry colleagues. Even if it isn't, the truth will inevitably prompt some kindhearted person to flag down a waiter or scurry into the kitchen trying to help you. You do not want this.

Have some fun instead. If you don't know anyone at your table (or you do and don't care what they think of you, or they're in cahoots with you), please feel free to choose from the following responses:

"I have a bet with my (husband, sister, best friend, boss, etc.) that I can lose the most weight in one week, which ends tomorrow. I want to win."

"I'm giving up dinner (or breakfast or lunch) because I need an extra hour in my day." (Feel free to invent an interesting list of activities you now have time for: fencing, polo, tap dancing, building a home biosphere, etc.)

"My hypothalamus is on the fritz."

"Have you seen the kitchen?"

Smile sweetly and tell them you're on the color diet and that today is blue.

If you really want to start trouble, say something that seems to make sense, but really doesn't. Say you're "politically opposed to mass feeding," then go to the restroom when the fight breaks out.

"How could anyone swallow after that speech?" is always nice, provided the speaker or the speaker's spouse is not sitting at your table.

If you're in the mood for mischief and think you can carry it off, you have my permission to use something I invented during a monotonous radio advertising award ceremony during which microphone-shaped ravioli were served. When the person next to me asked why I wasn't eating, I lowered my voice down to a conspiratorial whisper and leaned close. "I didn't want to ruin the meal by bringing it up, but I guess you missed that *60 Minutes* story on ravioli (feel free to substitute appropriate entrée). It's a miracle we're all still alive."

More often than not, the less said, the better. Sometimes it's enough to answer a question with a shrug, a charming smile, and a simple, "I'm not hungry right now." Who can argue with that?

What's important here is this: having a gluten-free meal, or any meal, for that matter, is not an inalienable right and in situations like this, you're not going to get one until after it's over.

Go home, kick off your shoes, and heat up a nice, gluten-free pizza.

A Gluten Accident

Oops. Sounds like a toxic spill, doesn't it? Well, it is, in a way. And it's a whole lot more serious than missing a meal. Or is it?

Doctors disagree. Most say if it's an isolated incident, it won't affect the course of your condition at all. But if you've just been diagnosed and not completely healed, or exquisitely sensitive, getting an inadvertent crouton or crumb or dose of cereal filler you hadn't counted on may cause a nasty reaction. The lucky ones report cramping, feeling nauseous, or getting dizzy the minute they've eaten something containing gluten. I say lucky because if you know you're going to feel lousy when you cheat, well, you're less likely to. Others, like me, need a repeat of the offending substance before problems like bloating, itching, mouth ulcers, and brain fog kick in, while other celiacs say they don't react at all, at least on the surface.

By now I hope it's been drummed into you that whether you have a hair trigger or get delayed symptoms, or suffer not at all, frequent ingestion of gluten will cause serious damage over time. This is especially important information for the celiac who wasn't all that sick in the first place. If the insult is repeated often enough, you will compromise your health whether you're consciously aware of it or not.

But an accident is just that and they happen to all of us. Many years ago, before I had the hang of the diet and knew better, I decided it would be healthy for me to add brewer's yeast to my morning tonic. I know what you're thinking. Jax! We all make honest mistakes in the beginning. There's no shame in it.

At first I felt fine, then I noticed, to put it as gracefully as possible, that bathroom visits were increasing while the rest of me was decreasing at the alarming rate of five pounds in four days. It wasn't long before I realized the morning drink was the culprit. I tell you this not to be indelicate but to illustrate how symptoms of gluten ingestion are different for everyone.

I should have, but did not run to my doctor. Nor did I worry about lymphoma. I did not demand a full body scan, or beat myself up or poll other celiacs for the doom and gloom report. I did not panic. I applied logic to the situation. If something was in my gastrointestinal tract that shouldn't be there, I figured the idea was to get it out as fast as possible before it had a chance to do any more damage to my nicely healing villi. My solution was to drink gallons of water and take a ton of fiber, which is exactly what my doctor would have said was fine to do had I asked him. He also would have said to do nothing and wait for nature to take its course. Being proactive seemed to help, or at least I imagined that it did, and now if I think I've gotten something I shouldn't have, this is what I do.

As it happens, I am not alone in my willingness to apply common sense and creativity to a situation like this. In a recent posting on an Internet celiac list, celiacs reported do-it-yourself remedies to this common situation. Many share my belief that a good dose of psyllium husks or some other fiber will do the trick. Some celiacs believe in charcoal; that it "sucks the gluten right out of the intestines." Other strategies include Pepto-Bismol, L-glutamine, papaya, pineapple, and other digestive enzymes, bananas, avoidance of rich foods for a few days, a glass of wine for cramping, plenty of water, extra B_{12}, acidophilus, ginger, heavy foods to move gluten out of the system faster, light foods to rest the stomach, soothing teas like chamomile or mint, and extra calcium, magnesium, and zinc.

Before you rush out to buy one of these supplements or products or undertake a change in diet, understand there is absolutely nothing medically sound or sanctioned in the aforementioned. Nor is there proof that these strategies work better than doing absolutely nothing and simply waiting for the gluten to leave your system naturally. You will never read about them in a medical journal or a serious article on celiac disease. Whatever you feel best doing is the right thing to do as long as it doesn't make the situation worse— i.e., if you have diarrhea, don't take laxatives.

Understand that a gluten accident isn't just about getting sick for a brief period of time, it's about being afraid that it won't go away. I believe the urge to doctor ourselves, albeit with unproven remedies, is really about regaining control. That's just human nature.

The best medicine for a gluten accident is letting your doctor do periodic blood screening, especially in the months and years following diagnosis. If you are getting gluten, whether unwittingly or not, it will show up on the test. This way, you can rest easy knowing that a rare accident may cause a reaction, and most likely won't cause irreparable damage.

A Drink with the Boys and/or Girls

I haven't smoked for so long, I really can't remember when I quit. But even back in the dark days, when the idea of smoking was considered sophisticated, even attractive, I knew I ought to cut it out. After a few days of going cold turkey, I accepted an invitation for cocktails from a friend who owned a very popular bar.

I was never one for hard liquor, but I do enjoy a nice glass of wine. I knew how obnoxious an ex-smoker can be, so I sipped a nice merlot and tried not to mention the smoke swirling around me. By the second glass, I was attempting to swallow smoke rings floating by, and by the third, I was mooching cigarettes from everybody around me.

I quickly learned that alcohol is a substance that weakens resolve and is not a friend to someone trying to kick a lifelong habit. Eating gluten certainly qualifies as a lifelong habit. I dared not drink another drop of wine until I was well over cigarettes, and I avoided it again when I was diagnosed as a celiac.

In many ways it's easier now for a nonsmoker than it is for a celiac to go out for a social drink. Many bars and restaurants outlaw cigarettes, but there's no rule about the bowls of pretzel nuggets, nuts, pigs in blankets, nachos, and those little pizza things set out for happy-hour nibbling. This is not to say you have to become a hermit, but if you find yourself in a place where one drink turns into two, you could be headed for serious trouble, especially in the weeks and months just after diagnosis when you're still feeling sorry for yourself. Even more so, if you weren't that sick to begin with.

My best advice is to stay out of situations involving drinking until you've got your diet well under control. This way, if you do get a little buzz going, you're not going to fall apart and eat something you shouldn't. Your eating habits will be second nature by then.

If passing up an invitation or two isn't in the cards, nor is drinking fizzy water for the duration, follow this variation on an ironclad rule: Friends don't let friends eat gluten.

Give someone you trust strict instructions, in writing so it's official, making it clear that if you get a little *sloshy* and are tempted to eat a pretzel or an egg roll or some other unsafe bar food, this person has your permission to stop you. If you must, carry a snack-size bag of gluten-free pretzels for when the munchies hit, and don't forget to ask the bartender for a clean bowl. Ditto for nuts, fruit mix, corn kernels, or whatever is nice and salty and makes you feel part of the crowd.

Socializing often taps into our deepest feelings about identity and pleasure. In the weeks and months following a change as drastic as going gluten-free, it's smart to make a list of those occasions or situations that might leave you feeling weak or sorry for yourself and prepare a strategy ahead of time.

Perfect the drop-in, the fine art of arriving late, and leave early. This isn't really as tough as it sounds. Show up at the very edge of rudeness, talk to everyone you can, especially the person who organized the evening, then leave. Everyone will swear you were there the whole time. I used to use this tactic to successfully avoid the rubber chicken lunch altogether. I'd show up for the cocktail time, talk to absolutely everyone I could, especially clients who would report back to my boss that they saw me, then skedaddle the minute the banquet doors opened.

Volunteer to make the arrangements for the after-work cocktail party and supply your own snacks. And forget the mixed drinks. You really don't want to have to climb over the bar to read the mix label. Stick with tonic and something or a glass of wine and don't overdo it, at least until you've got your diet and feelings of deprivation under control.

Communion

I got into trouble in the last edition of this book by saying that from time to time I take the host and feed it to the birds after church. Some people wrote to say this was wrong and one irate nun called my behavior "a desecration." I meant no offense. Inspired by a childhood fascination for St. Francis and his love of all God's creatures, I sincerely believed and still do that I am honoring the mystery of the mass by allowing "the body and blood" to make its way back into the universe.

But I haven't always given the host back to nature. The wafer from my father's memorial mass is still in a little box with his missile and letters of con-
dolence. My mother's, too. I can't imagine how saving such a memento could
be wrong. I've never felt, as many Catholics do, that my participation at mass
is diminished in any way by my not being able to eat the wafer. If I'm in a
church that offers a chalice, I try to get up there quickly before crumbs accu-
mulate and take a sip of wine and decline the bread. If God doesn't know I've
got a problem with gluten, who does?

This is a troubling issue for many, though, fraught with tradition and
church rules that cannot be broken, as one poor Catholic child found out recently in a much-publicized refusal to allow the little first-time celebrant a
gluten-free host. Once, while attending mass at the shrine of St. John Newman in Philadelphia, I went up to the rail, received the wafer in my hand, lowered my head, and walked away. My plan was to give it to my husband who
knelt to my left, or to one of my parents who sat to my right. But as I walked
away from the altar, a deep voice boomed at my back. "Consume the host!"
The voice reverberated in the quiet chapel. I froze in my tracks and popped
the wafer straight into my mouth. My shocked family stared.

"I thought it was the voice was God," I whispered, amazed that anyone
would shout at me to do such a thing across a quiet church. We were in God's
house, not to mention in the presence of a saint, who is given credit for more
than one miracle. I figured anything could happen.

The priest in question was an old-fashioned hard-liner straight from Ireland, where the idea that a sip of wine, as Monsignor Thomas Hartman wrote
in Long Island *Newsday*, can count as the body *and* blood of Christ. For young
children taking Holy Communion for the first time, he says most priests will
consecrate some grape juice as a substitute for the wine and the wafer. Most
likely, the poor man thought I was some kind of perverted host abuser. Of
course, you know from reading the preceding "gluten accident" what I did
when I got home.

The point is, you may find yourself in conflict with church authority as
you find your own way of participating in this important sacrament. You will
also come up against the bias of what other members of your church say is appropriate. To this I can only say I remember vividly the children on my street
saying I wasn't Catholic because my parents sent me to public school. In my
opinion, people like this, including small-minded priests, don't matter. What
does matter is your belief and your relationship with it.

The best way to handle the situation is to sit down with your priest or
minister and decide what to do together. By all means, tell him or her how

important it is for you to participate as much as you can. If you are comfortable taking wine and skipping the bread, do so. But ask the priest if you can take the first sip to avoid crumbs in the chalice. If you would prefer a more traditional host, ask if you can supply a gluten-free wafer for consecration.

One Presbyterian community with several members who are either celiac or wheat-allergic solved the problem by ordering gluten-free bread from a knowledgeable local baker, who prepares it for communion. This way no one feels left out. If your congregation is large, post a note on the church bulletin board and you may find yourself with more company than you imagine.

Anglican St. Thomas Church and the Cathedral of St. John the Divine in New York serve gluten-free communion wafers. United Methodist, Christian Reform, Lutheran, Episcopal, and many other protestant denominations will accommodate the special diets of its parishioners. Ask and you shall receive.

The American Catholic Church (as opposed to the Roman Catholic Church) offers its members a gluten-free host made by Ener-G Foods and is sold 50 to a box (www.ener-g.com).

If you and your doctor decide that the new low-gluten host sanctioned by the Roman Catholic Church is for you, by all means talk to your priest and make arrangements. While this wafer is considered safe by some American celiac experts, remember it is made with a very small amount of wheat starch allowable in Europe and in keeping with canon law. This low-gluten host is still controversial among many Catholic celiacs who wonder aloud with more than a little anger at how the church came to the conclusion that only wheat bread qualifies as communion, but allows an alcoholic a sip of grape juice instead of wine.

If you decide this is the way for you to go, contact the Missouri Benedictine Sisters at (800) 223-2772 or altarbreads@benedictinesisters.org.

If not, there are priests to be found who will bend the rules and consecrate the gluten-free host quietly and out of public view, as one unidentified priest did for a New Jersey youngster whose First Communion was recently and quite publicly invalidated by the Diocese of Trenton. The priest will then place it in a small container (these are found in stores where Catholic religious articles are sold) and put it in the chalice for your consumption at mass.

If you choose not to partake, don't let anybody make you feel guilty. Heaven knows, this is a matter between you and The Boss.

Going to College

Finding, then getting into, the school that's right for you is stressful enough, and that's nothing compared to staying in. For many of us, college is where we learn to do our own laundry, balance a checkbook, live on a budget, and pay the credit card bill for the first time in our lives. With no one around to enforce homework, keeping up our grades is suddenly in competition with falling in love, drinking beer, attending fraternity and sorority parties, organizing pranks, going out for burgers, pulling all-nighters, organizing and participating in political rallies, developing social awareness and other activities crucial to the undergraduate experience. We learn quickly the value of establishing priorities and developing organizational skills.

For many of us, college is also the first time we are totally responsible for our meals. It's easy to sleep through breakfast and fall prey to the late-night junk food, binge eating, and constant grazing on high-calorie, high-fat foods. Easy to pile on the dreaded "freshman fifteen."

This first taste of freedom is heady, like the longest day of the year when even the sun doesn't play by the rules. We are still experimenting with who we are in college. We try on alternative futures like new clothes. It is exciting to discover our interests, our skills, our passions. Plans change as quickly as the weather. We are young enough to believe we can get away with eating pizza. It's a wonder we graduate at all. Doing it gluten-free is nothing short of a miracle.

The best argument for staying on the diet is this. Gluten not only affects our bodies, it affects our minds. Your brain is the organ you need to have in peak shape if you want to go the distance. You don't need brain fog when you're cramming for finals. You don't need fuzzy thinking when you are singled out by that professor you've got a crush on to explain Einstein's Theory of Relativity. You don't need it when you're reading your work at your first poetry slam. And you certainly don't need to discover a few years later that you did yourself irreparable harm.

And speaking of brains, the more you know about your diet, the better off you'll be away from home. If you can't explain exactly what you need, how can you expect someone to serve it to you?

It's hard, you say. Of course it is. But when you take into account that gluten-laden beer is the lion's share of that freshman weight gain, the picture brightens. Avoiding it not only keeps you healthy, it keeps you slim and gorgeous while everyone else is looking pudgy. Myself, I have always hated the taste of beer. I discovered letting it go flat and pouring it over my ironed-flat hair gave it an incredible shine.

As for other alcoholic beverages—we all know drinking under the age of twenty-one is against the law. There, I've said it. Okay.

Most college parties are BYOB along with a big bowl (garbage can, in some cases) of something potent and unspecified. Bringing your own bottle of wine or other gluten-free potable will not only ensure that you don't get any gluten, it just may keep you from swallowing something even more dangerous and waking up in the rosebushes.

In many ways, living in an off-campus apartment is easier for celiac students. Apartments have freezers and microwaves and toasters, and most university towns and cities have good health food stores for stocking up on gluten-free foods and snack items. Much easier to control what you eat in an apartment than in a dorm where dinner is in the cafeteria. Advertise for a like-challenged roommate. With 2.2 million of us out there, nobody's ever the only celiac.

But if your heart's set on experiencing the communal way of life, it's best to negotiate your needs and the meal plan before you move in. If you make it clear that your food is for a medically diagnosed condition, and not a "preference," you may be allowed to have a small freezer or a microwave or a toaster not usually sanctioned for dorm rooms. If you ask, you may be given a corner of the cafeteria freezer for your GF foods, and if so, you've got a great introduction to the commissary manager for when you explain your diet and ask for special treatment.

Celiac disease is covered under Section 504 of the American with Disabilities Act and you can force the college to comply with your needs. There's nothing less conducive to bending the rules than a university administrator made to feel a student is going to sue. I say if you can avoid invoking, or talk your parents out of invoking, this powerful disability label, by all means, do. A sitdown with the housing director, food service manager, and director of student disabilities ought to do the trick.

I would contact a celiac support group near the campus. They're going to know much more about where to get food than anybody at school. Ask for a list of celiac-friendly food stores and restaurants. Ask for a written explanation to give the school cafeteria chef or manager. Who knows? There may even be a pizza place in the area that will top your gluten-free version or make you one from scratch.

Whatever you do, don't try to hide the fact that you're a celiac. Another important conversation to have is with your roommate. Call as soon as you get his or her name. Will he or she respect your special food and not raid your supply? Let him know it's okay to eat in front of you. Tell her it's like being a vegan or a macro without the gluten. If you feel the situation will be trouble, ask to be reassigned.

College life is spontaneous, always carry something in your backpack in case. Go to home.bellsouth.net/p/PWP-glutenfreeforever and get some tips from an actual gluten-free college student. But keep in mind that CD affects different people in different ways. Another fun Web site is www.celiac chicks.com, which proves you can be totally cool *and* gluten-free.

Dating

Dating and its cousin, Falling in Love, are food-intensive situations, full of insecurities, emotional baggage, appetite issues, candlelight, and lots of cheese and wine. Short of dating other celiacs (www.meetup/celiac.com), how does a well-adjusted, gluten-challenged person go about experiencing love and all its derangements?

Well, for starters, never lie about being a celiac, even on the first date. Yes, I know. Any condition with the word *disease* in it makes you sound damaged, ill, or, worse, contagious. No matter. It's who you are. Of course there will be a cad or caddess or two who will make gluten jokes and dump you because you're not quite perfect. Consider yourself lucky or chalk it up to natural selection (what would they do in a real emergency?). Move on.

Lies always come back and bite you. How would you feel if someone you really liked didn't trust you enough to share his peanut allergy? Or if you found out months later, he or she was a little phobic in tight places, an orphan, afraid of the dark, or liked to eat foods in alphabetical order? Our differences are what make us unique, special, lovable, ourselves. Repeat that ten times before your next date.

Casual dates are the easiest—meeting for coffee, seeing a movie, going cycling, visiting a museum, rock climbing, walking in the park—but sooner or later, all dates end up with food. This is not because the participants are hungry, it is because dinner is a good excuse to look our best and stare at each other over plates of food, preferably in the flattering light of candles. If you're doing the inviting, pick a place that's best for you, one you've already checked out (see chapter 8, "How to Get a Chef to Eat out of Your Hand"). If you're the one being asked, use the opportunity to say you need to be gluten-free and ask if the restaurant is accommodating. Your date's response is a great way to measure his or her level of generosity and concern for the needs of others.

As the relationship develops, add more details to the gluten-free story. If you were sick, don't give all the gory details on the first date. And whatever you do, save the conversation about what happens to you if you eat gluten for when you know him or her better. Nothing like gastrointestinal talk to take the bloom off the rose.

My husband's mother was more than a little strange. When I look back, I see that my clever boy added a little something about her with each successive date. By the time we met, there was nothing she could do to shock me (and she did plenty) or to change how I felt about her son. Being a celiac is like that. A little at a time as the friendship develops.

Over time, a special diet can show you a person's heart in a way nothing else can.

Consider George of *Foods By George* and his girlfriend, Ceil. When Ceil got sick with CD and ended up in the hospital, she was inconsolable after hearing she could never have pasta again. George was so distraught at the idea of his darling being miserable, he promised he'd invent a pasta she could eat. He did just that and it turned out to be a pasta, then a pizza, then a ravioli we *all* could eat. Ceil got better, they got married, and we all ate happily ever after.

If dating turns Serious or possibly even to Love, there is usually a period where the throat closes up and nobody eats. At least that's what a poll of friends and past experience tells me. You both eat nothing at all and live on long, soulful looks or you eat everything in sight and not get fat, enjoying briefly the white-hot metabolism of lovers. If you do break up, I guarantee it won't be about gluten. If it *is* about gluten, consider yourself better off without this person.

If the only logical step after Dating and Falling in Love is Setting the Date, there are many wonderful gluten-free bakers who'd be happy to pipe rosettes onto a gluten-free extravaganza for the wedding. And yes, the reception can and should be gluten-free. Don't alter a standard menu to your needs, contact one of the chefs, caterers, and cooking schools listed in chapter 9 and create a gluten-free reception no one will ever forget. If you can't get a glorious gluten-free meal on your own wedding day, when can you?

The Holidays

Drum roll here. This is the Big One.

Family holidays are the most stressful situations for any celiac. It doesn't matter whether it's Thanksgiving or Christmas or Hannukah or Passover, Kwaanza or *Seinfeld's* famously fictional holiday, Festivus. Nor does it matter whether you have just been diagnosed or have been gluten-free forever.

Centering on food, but often having very little to do with it, family feasts are loaded with baggage.

The list of uninvited guests is long. There is sibling rivalry, oedipal struggle, withholding of love, dispensing of love, mother love, father love, competition, overfeeding, avoidance issues, you-love-him-best issues, love-me, love-my-stuffing, your sister's pregnant and you're not even married yet, and the ever-popular, if you're special then I must not be, and its kissing cousin, if you're damaged then we must all be, to name but a few. Of course, none of these things are on the table where you can see them. All anybody can see is turkey, stuffing, plum pudding, rugelach, matzoh, and gluten as far as the eye can see.

Time and time again, I hear the horror stories. One sister promises a gluten-free stuffing (see page 416 for recipe), then denies she ever promised it.

Another family lays on the guilt—how could you ask for special treatment when I'm so busy cooking for so many?

One celiac is asked to bring her own food to her brother's house. Another is asked to arrive after everyone has eaten.

Some families simply stonewall the problem, serving the meal with no alternatives, as if nothing has changed.

Friends who are unkind to us soon find themselves on the outs. So how come we don't hold our families to that same standard? Blood gets away with more than water is the plain truth. No matter how dysfunctional the behavior, no matter how rude and insensitive, these are the only people you've got. We can pick our friends, but not our relatives.

I don't buy it. If you've explained your diet, provided information, offered to make a dish or two, and shown where gluten-free products can be purchased, you have every right to expect something special. Look deep into your heart here and consider your own response to the problems of others and answer honestly. Are you willing to change your routine for others? Or are you so concerned with gluten that you've forgotten Uncle Bob's lactose intolerance or Auntie Kay's aversion to cigarette smoke? Are you as flexible as you want others to be?

Do you work with your family about what you can eat or do you set traps? Do you eat what they make, then tell them you got sick later? Be honest. Have you set them up to fail? Have you shared with your family how important it is for you to feel included, how isolated you feel when you come to these occasions? And I don't mean saying something snide after they've let you down, but before, in an open and nonadversarial way.

Have you phoned the one who's cooking to make arrangements well before the holiday? And have you offered to pay the extra expense for gluten-free products? Has your family experienced a really good gluten-free meal at your house? (If you don't make your own food in your own house, what reason does your family have to do so?) If you've answered yes to all these questions and you can honestly say you've been as truthful about your feelings and expectations as you can and you are still made to feel unwelcome, then you must bring the situation to a head.

It is perfectly appropriate to turn down family invitations until the people who claim to love you put their actions where their mouths are. In fact, it's preferable. I don't mean telling the folks you're busy or you're going elsewhere. If you don't show up, you owe it to yourself and to them to say why.

Confrontation is not easy for most people and most of us will do anything, including filling up a cooler with gluten-free foods and dragging it to a family party, to avoid it.

One way to start is to ask, simply, "What's this really about?"

Rarely is the problem about food. You may find out that it's about the time your little sister's friend wasn't welcomed sufficiently at your house. Or it's about a mother who holds her position in the family by keeping her children at odds with one another. (This is what Franz Joseph did to hang on to the Austro-Hungarian empire for so long.) It could be about family tradition being more important than the family itself. Or it could be about jealousy or how miserable one sibling feels when the other is given attention. Sometimes admitting that one family member isn't perfect puts the entire family's worth in question; this is especially true of a problem that's genetic. The word *denial* rears its ugly head.

In one family I know, an older sister's refusal to give her brain-injured brother special treatment stems from her little-girl grief at seeing her father's joy at having a son and believing she had been replaced in his affection. Of course, it doesn't make sense blaming a baby brother for a parent's failure to ease that transition, but sibling rivalry rarely makes sense. One celiac I know, a beautiful and accomplished surgeon, was treated badly by her siblings because it was the only area where they felt superior. Cruelty to people you love comes from a dark and tangled place.

It would be nice to think that diffusing family conflict is simply a matter of emotional honesty, that having a heart-to-heart about the real issues underlying the offense would do the trick. But some wounds have been buried under kneejerk behavior for so long, that it would take an army of Dr. Phils to bring them to the surface.

Sometimes, the best way to be heard is to stop speaking. Make it plain, without starting World War III, that you will not be accepting any more invitations until such time as the family starts acting like one where you are concerned.

Offer to have the dinner at your house next year so you can show everyone what a holiday meal everyone can eat looks like. (Don't bluster about this, either, be prepared to do it even if you have to learn how to cook or have it catered or Big Sis or Cousin Sal has been doing the particular holiday for years.) If your family is the kind that needs a knock on the head, leave mid-meal. If you're away from home, go to a hotel, if necessary. If you can't afford that, go up to your room and pack a bag.

Whatever you do, don't sit in the corner while everyone else chows down on foods you miss. Don't pick and snipe at the person after the fact. Don't lie and say it's okay when it isn't. Don't indulge in equally selfish behavior. And never let gluten jokes, or other passive aggressive behavior, such as "Oh, I forgot crackers for you," go unremarked. No one forgets another's happiness on an important holiday, unless they mean to.

In some families, tough love is the only love that matters.

Enablers, Worry Warts, and Other Oddballs

It's the grandmother who can't stand to see her little darling go without. It's the friend who never could lose that twenty pounds. It's the wife who practically tastes her husband's food before he eats it, who learns everything there is to know about celiac disease for him. It's the mother who's so afraid you'll get sick again she won't feed you anything. In my own family, no matter how carefully I explained the gluten-free diet to my parents, they'd ask questions like, "Are you sure you can have those strawberries?" At every meal, they'd point to some innocuous dessert and say, "There's sugar in that, you know." Their concern, while endearing, sprang from their fear of screwing up, and became a kind of paralysis, which I finally broke through by leaving information for them to read and sending baking mixes, pasta, and other gluten-free products to them for my visits.

What affects us often sends a shudder through those closest to us. What happens to romance when eating cake at midnight is no longer allowed? Will you still be friends if you can't go to the mall and eat sticky buns while you shop? Any change as important and defining as this one shakes the foundation upon which a relationship rests. The gluten-free diet doesn't just alter life for the celiac, it changes the rules for everyone in her world.

Your significant other may not be able to say, "I miss our midnight raids on the cookie jar." It may be easier to tease you into having "a little bite." Keep some ice cream in the freezer, along with a few slices of fattening gluten-free cake, and reassure your sweetie that some things never change—it's still the two of you in your pajamas against the world in the middle of the night.

Ditto for your slightly diet-challenged best friend. She may push you to eat a slice of pizza or something equally bad because your diet has made her feel alone with her weakness.

The worst way to deal with this is to become holier than thou. Let her know that while your gluten-free diet is non-negotiable, you're still able to enjoy something wicked, just as long as that something is made with safe ingredients.

When a child is involved, he or she can end up being the flash point for issues between adults. The most common conflict is the daughter-in-law deemed hypervigilant by a doting and disapproving grandmother. Very often the real problem has nothing to do with the child at all, but rather the potent issues of grown children forming lives and rules of their own. Nevertheless, otherwise sane adults can turn a child into an emotional football.

The best way to nip this potentially dangerous situation in the bud is a family conference that makes it clear the child is to be gluten-free no matter whose opinions are to the contrary. Having said that, young parents need to be open to hearing how dismissive and dictatorial they may sound to grandparents who managed to raise them without dire consequences. Love is the key here. And respect.

Overly nurturing people are another breed entirely. You have a gluten accident and they ask, "How could I have let this happen to you?" They think it's their fault somehow for not being vigilant enough. While this kind of concern is seductive, especially when you're sick, it's also controlling. Just as the bully is often insecure, so the nurturer often has control issues. It's important to know the difference between genuine care and something not quite right.

I hate to make generalizations, but men who are diagnosed with CD often let their wives or mothers or even daughters take responsibility for their diets. In my experience, women seem to be hardwired to do this; in fact I have found myself counting grams of fat for a husband who couldn't care less.

If you don't believe this, go to a health spa and see how many women offer the odd male guest one of the measly four shrimps on their plates.

All well and good, but the trouble is, the celiac never becomes adept at the diet and whether consciously or not, blames all lapses and setbacks on the other person. What you end up with is the alpha male who doesn't have a clue about what to eat and thinks it's beneath him to worry about it, or the sickly perpetual victim who is guaranteed attention by his abdication of responsibility. Either way it's not healthy.

We've all seen the wife out for dinner with her husband telling the waiter what her spouse can and can't eat. The husband sits passively by, until she nixes something he really wants, and he calls her a nag. This is called buttering both sides of your bread. You can't relinquish control and keep it at the same time.

There's an old joke told by a Catskill's comic. Husband and wife are eating dinner in a fancy restaurant. When the waiter asks the man if he has enjoyed the meal, the man shrugs and says, "I don't know. Ask her."

Many of us allow ourselves to be taken over by a caring partner because it taps into a bigger need—to be loved, to be understood, to be the sick one and get all the negative attention that implies. There's nothing wrong with it, just know that for every enabler and over-giver, there is someone on the other end allowing it to happen. It takes two to tango.

Change one detail about a relationship and the whole relationship goes tilt. We've seen it all before, one partner quits cigarettes and the other smokes at the computer they share. One goes on the wagon and the other one sweetly asks, "Pour me a drink, will you?" A friend of mine whose career depended upon her thinness on camera came home furious and humiliated after her boss took her out to dinner to tell her she was getting a little too plump for the anchor chair. (Interesting choice of venue, wouldn't you say?) She took to her bed and her husband, whose own career wasn't as stellar, coaxed her out of it with a big pot of spaghetti.

Going gluten-free requires great sensitivity to the needs of others. Just as you have been shocked into a sudden change, so you must understand how your transformation affects people close to you. No matter what I hear to the contrary, I refuse to believe any grandparent, husband, wife, friend, lover, or colleague ever deliberately sets out to sabotage, enable, smother, pacify, confuse, undermine, deliberately misunderstand, or turn on you because they want to see you suffer. They do it because they feel threatened or excluded or dispensable or unloved. Most people inflict pain in order to keep from feeling it. (I'm not talking about people who are dead mean, inherently evil, mentally ill, or anyone who is a serious sociopath. I'm talking about people you love and who love you.)

Cook up a big pot of something comforting, pour yourselves a glass of wine and talk about it. Really talk about it. Make it clear that you appreciate the help, but at the end of the day the gluten-free diet is yours and yours alone. If you mess up, it's your fault, and if you don't, it's to your credit.

As long as you both realize it's not about food, you'll be fine.

sex and the celiac

I'll have what she's having

With apologies to Nobel Laureate Gabriel Garcia Marquez, I present to you a true story I like to call *Love in the Time of Semolina*, a cautionary tale about romance and gluten.

Once upon a time, a certain young poet of my acquaintance, a handsome and frail twenty-five-year-old celiac I'll call Byron, fell for a robustly beautiful Italian girl (let's call her Teresa) with doe eyes, glossy black hair, and skin the color of the Umbrian earth.

CD had hit him hard, and by the time the doctors solved the mystery of his rapidly failing health, Byron had lost a lot of weight and was quite ill. There was much work to do if his badly scarred intestine was to return to normal. His focus, up to that point, had been on finishing graduate school, regaining his strength, and learning how to live gluten-free, scrupulously avoiding even the slightest whiff of anything that could keep him sick. In fact, until he met Teresa, Byron rarely ate out, preferring to heat up his own food or defrost one of the meals his mother prepared and wrapped for him every Sunday.

In Teresa's big southern Italian family, pasta wasn't merely a food, it was a form of worship. Pasta with olive oil and garlic, *livornese* with olives and capers, *puttanesca* with fresh tomatoes and hot peppers, *bolognese* with ground pork, veal and beef—all were made with nothing but the finest semolina flour. When told that Byron could not partake of their boisterous family meals, Teresa's family shook their heads sadly. "Ah, *celiachia*," said Noni, remembering how many children were affected by this odd complaint when she was a girl in Naples.

Byron was drawn to Teresa's beauty, but also to her vibrant good health; just being around her made him feel better. As for Teresa, with her big Mediterranean heart, she wanted nothing more than to make her beloved well and strong again. She turned her kitchen into a gluten-free paradise, hand-stirring risotto and polenta and cooking big pots of gluten-free lasagna and brown rice pasta. She even made gnocchi from scratch the way her mother had taught her, cutting out the dumplings with a whiskey glass.

When the couple sat down to dinner, she to the real thing, he to his gluten-free version, Byron blessed the day he'd found such a beautiful and generous soul.

"You are the most wonderful woman in the world," he'd say, kissing the tips of her fingers, knowing how lucky he was.

To put it as delicately as possible, it wasn't long before the young pair got past the hand-holding stage. But alas, whenever things became amorous, Byron's stomach churned and he had to rush to the bathroom with the kind of problem that can really take the bloom off a budding romance.

Too embarrassed to reveal his sensitive plumbing to Teresa, he would make a hasty retreat, leaving her to wonder, as many young girls would in her situation, what she'd done to drive him away.

Byron couldn't imagine what he was reacting to. He was scrupulous about his diet. He carried his lunch to school and avoided the cafeteria as he has been warned to do. He ate before going to parties and checked the ingredients of all the vitamins, cold remedies, and prescriptions in his medicine cabinet.

The only time he truly enjoyed eating was with Teresa, who never mixed her food with his, was careful to cook his pasta in a fresh pot of water, and even bought a second toaster oven for her tiny apartment, so her crumbs wouldn't mingle with his. No one else cared for him like that, except, of course, his mother.

Byron's mother, who almost lost her mind with worry as she watched her son fade away before her own eyes, then nearly burst with joy to discover he was a celiac and not dying after all, had her suspicions. Could a girl who was raised on that much pasta exude the stuff straight through her pores? She hated to be an overbearing mother and meddle in such personal matters, but her son's health was at stake.

She remembered her own courtship, how fascinated she and Byron's father were with every freckle, every finger and toe, every hair on the other's head, how they wanted to eat each other up, not unlike toddlers who put every object of desire into their mouths. She wished he was still with her to talk to him man to man, but he had died young, and she always suspected his death was related to undiagnosed celiac disease, something she was trying to keep their beloved Byron from doing.

"Does Teresa brush and floss her teeth before kissing you?" she asked her embarrassed son.

"Ma!"

"Well, does she?

Byron glared, but his mother could not be dissuaded.

"It could be it's her lipstick you're sensitive to, or her face cream, or body lotion or talcum powder," she said, plunging on despite how awkward this was for both of them. "Whatever it is, you need to talk to her about it. And you need to tell her the truth."

Despite his profound discomfort at having his mother talk to him this way, Byron promised he would.

"There's something I have to tell you," Byron told Teresa the next night.

Her heart dropped, but she listened patiently as Byron stammered and stumbled through his explanation of what happened to him after they kissed for a while.

"I thought it was me," she said, relief swimming in her beautiful eyes.

"Oh God, no," he said, "I love you."

Out went her old cosmetics. In came a new supply of gluten-free, hypo-allergenic lotions, creams, cosmetics, and pretty lipsticks that did not change Byron's desire to kiss her. With a lifetime supply of plain dental floss, and his and her electric toothbrushes, the young couple found an unlikely and surprisingly sexy source of togetherness. Teresa washes carefully after touching unsafe foods and they have been known to shower together to avoid wasting water and time.

As far as I know, there were no more incidents and in the spring, Byron proposed, presenting Teresa with a modest diamond solitaire she wears with pride. As soon as they finish their degrees, they will have a big fat gluten-free wedding and a honeymoon in Teresa's ancestral village where much brushing and flossing and kissing will go on.

The moral is this: not everything you put in your mouth is food. When you're a celiac, the concept of being lovesick takes on a whole new meaning.

"Not that there's anything wrong with that," as Jerry Seinfeld is so fond of saying.

As long as you play it safe, there's no reason you can't play.

How to Safely Love Your Gluten-Free Lover

When bees do it, it's cross-pollination. When allergic humans do it, it's cross-contamination. Not a romantic phrase, but nevertheless apt. We know how much can happen to a food before it hits your plate—french fries having a bath in oil used for onion rings, an errant crouton, a flour-dusted raisin, a knife that's just cut another sandwich, a grill or a cutting board that didn't get wiped down. But what about food that was never *on* a plate? A kiss stolen over a plate of pasta and, before you know it, you're ingesting something you hadn't bargained for.

Where does lipstick color go when it fades?

It goes straight into your stomach. Unless, of course, it goes into his.

To compound the problem, many celiacs are sensitive to other substances besides gluten. Peanut and wheat germ oil–based cosmetics, skin creams, aluminum in deodorants, talc made from wheat starch, fragrance and chemical-laden air fresheners, toxic cleaning products, and formaldehyde in carpeting all contribute to problems. For the truly sensitive, just breathing something toxic is enough to cause itchy throats, wheezing, and yes, kissing the fingers that have just licked the cake batter out of the mixing bowl can really put a pall on any romantic plans.

We've all heard the stories: a woman with shellfish allergy goes into anaphylactic shock after kissing her boyfriend. Child with peanut allergy plays spin the bottle and keels over. Or as my poor friend Byron so well knows, a little kissy-face and wham, an hour in the bathroom.

The only way to avoid a nasty and potentially embarrassing situation is to do what my young friend so bravely did. Have a frank conversation with your partner about the following hygiene matters and intimate behavior, then have some good, clean fun. So . . .

- Brush, floss, and rinse your mouth after eating foods your partner is sensitive to; not only will your breath be sweeter, your mouth will be healthier, thus even more kissable.
- Make sure all your shared vitamins and supplements are gluten-free.
- Use hypo-allergenic and fragrance-free soap, cosmetics, shampoo, and styling aids and personal products.
- Wash any body part that has been powdered, creamed, conditioned, shampooed, gelled, made up, dusted, fluffed, slicked, or has touched any gluten-containing substance that can get into the wrong place.

Not that I am a prude, but this is, after all, *The Gluten-Free Bible,* not *The Joy of Celiac Sex,* so I won't go into all the ways one can unwittingly share food or list all the means by which otherwise inedible products can get into your stomach. Besides, if I have to tell you, this chapter isn't for you anyway.

Kahlil Gibran once said, "Let there be spaces in your togetherness." I would add to that, let there be no cereal in your spaces.

It's embarrassing, but what is the alternative? We have had to learn how to talk about safe sex. We can handle this.

Inevitably, all this fooling around leads somewhere. With good planning and a little luck, baby makes three. Well, maybe not.

Fertility Problems and CD

Sometimes, no matter how hard you try, no matter that you have taken your temperature, figured out when you're ovulating, or even stood on your head for half the night to help the whole thing take, good news still eludes you.

The experts say infertility is one of most commonly overlooked problems in undiagnosed celiacs. A U.K. study at the Derbyshire Royal Infirmary found that late onset of menstruation and early menopause in female celiacs not following a gluten-free diet may contribute to infertility by shortening the reproductive period in a woman's life. And researchers report that men with CD may have reversible infertility due to impotence, hypogonadism (decreased functional activity of the testes), abnormal sperm motility, or androgen resistance that resolves or improves when gluten is withdrawn.

Doctors in Finland studied female hospital patients of reproductive age complaining of primary or secondary infertility or those who had experienced two or more miscarriages and discovered subclinical celiac disease and iron deficiency anemia in a small percentage of this group. No CD was found in the control group, yet women suffering from infertility problems were found to have CD at a rate ten times higher than the prevalence of CD in the normal population. The study concludes that silent celiac disease should always be considered in women with unexplained infertility.

Another study at Orebro Medical Centre Hospital in Sweden goes so far as to say that even treated CD, in either of the parents, can have a negative effect on pregnancy.

Dr. Peter H. R. Green, director of the Celiac Disease Center at New York's Columbia-Presbyterian Medical Center, agrees. In a recent article in *The Lancet,* he states that undiagnosed celiac disease is indeed associated with delayed periods, cessation of periods (amenorrhea), premature menopause, recurrent miscarriages, and fewer children. The article goes on to say that CD may be associated with babies of low birth weight, increased infant mortality, and a shorter duration of breast-feeding. Dr. Green adds that infertility in men can be associated with CD and that male celiacs tend to have children with a shorter gestation and lower birth weight than those without the disease.

Indeed, many unscientific surveys point to the same conclusion. Scratch below the surface of the celiac community and you will hear sad stories of miscarriages and infertility, especially among older celiacs and those with long-standing undiagnosed disease. Post a question on this subject on the Internet and you will be deluged by tales of difficult pregnancies, miscarriages, and fetal defects. You will hear from one woman after another desperately trying to get pregnant and finding out, years too late, that undiagnosed celiac disease was the culprit.

Most experts agree that more research needs to be done, especially among American celiacs. Screening needs to be widespread and routinely given to women in their reproductive years in order to avoid these tragic circumstances.

A new physician survey fielded at Thomas Jefferson University Hospital in Philadelphia attempts to accomplish just that. The researchers hope to highlight discrepancies between clinical investigation and practice in an effort to more precisely identify and treat individuals with celiac disease and make screening part of the routine workup of infertility. In other words, they want to get your internist, your gynecologist, and your obstetrician up to speed on something that could be so easily prevented.

All this is well and good. But your biological clock is ticking now. A few pieces of common sense from the experts:

- If there is a history of miscarriage or difficult pregnancy in your family tree, follow your diet to the letter.
- Make sure your iron, zinc, folate, and other important vitamin and mineral levels are checked before you conceive.
- If you smoke, quit.
- If you drink, don't.
- Discuss your plans with your gastroenterologist and, if necessary, redo blood tests to make sure you are not getting any gluten.
- If you've just been diagnosed, wait until your gut is healed and you know you're absorbing normally to try to get pregnant.

Remember that most of the problems reported in these studies are among *undiagnosed* celiacs or those not compliant with the diet. Write this down and put it in the drawer with your home pregnancy kit.

The Pregnant Celiac

So let's say congratulations are in order.

In an article in the Celiac Disease Foundation Newsletter, Michelle Melin-Rogovin, program director for the University of Chicago Celiac Disease Program, says the most frequently asked question by recently pregnant celiacs is whether or not they should stay on the gluten-free diet during pregnancy.

Go figure.

She reports that many new mothers-to-be believe the diet will deprive their developing fetus of the nutrients it needs and hurt the growing baby. Nothing could be further from the truth, she says. In a study of 25 patients and 60 pregnancies, researchers found that 21 percent of women who were not on the gluten-free diet experienced pregnancy loss, and 16 percent of women experienced fetal growth restrictions.

Citing a large Danish study with 211 infants and 127 mothers with celiac disease, Melin-Rogovin tells us researchers found that the mean birth weight of children born to mothers on a gluten-containing diet was significantly lower than babies born to mothers without celiac disease. Interestingly, this same study determined that women on the gluten-free diet gave birth to children weighing more than those born to mothers without celiac disease.

In another study that looked at the effect of the gluten-free diet on pregnancy and lactation, she tells us investigators learned that women with celiac disease who were not on the gluten-free diet experienced pregnancy loss at a rate of 17.8 percent, compared to 2.4 percent of women with celiac disease who were on the gluten-free diet.

The news is not so good for the undiagnosed celiac. In a study published in *Gut*, Italian researchers at the University of Naples Federico II found that up to 50 percent of women with untreated celiac disease experienced miscarriage or an unfavorable outcome of pregnancy, but that after six to twelve months on the gluten-free diet, unfavorable outcomes of pregnancy occured at the same rate as that in the general population. They conclude that celiac disease is more common than most of the diseases for which pregnant women are routinely screened, and that unfavorable events, like miscarriage, low birth weight, and neural tube defects, may be prevented by a gluten-free diet.

The article further states that although spontaneous abortion has no specific cause, celiac disease may be suspected from the finding of persistent iron deficiency and abnormal weight loss during a first, but more often, a second pregnancy. Women with undiagnosed celiac disease seem to have an 8.9-fold relative risk of multiple spontaneous abortions and low birth weight babies compared with treated patients.

The study concludes that a gluten-free diet resulted in a 9.18-fold reduction in the miscarriage rate and a reduction in the prevalence of low birth rate babies from 29.4 percent to zero. Of 112 pregnancies in women with untreated celiac disease, 20 ended in miscarriages compared with two of 22 in patients on a gluten-free diet. Similarly, six babies were stillborn in an undiagnosed group compared with none in a group on a gluten-free diet.

There is much discussion about whether or not neural tube defects, i.e., spina bifida, anencephaly, and other serious fetal abnormalities like Down syndrome, congenital heart defects, and mental retardation as a consequence of anemia is linked to undiagnosed celiac.

In a letter to the editors of *Gut*, emphasizing the need for health care professionals to recognize and treat the manifestations of CD in women of reproductive age, Dr. K. K. Hozyasz of the National Research Institute of Mother and Child in Warsaw, suggests, that "coeliac disease should be considered as a cause of birth defects associated with folic acid deficiency, for example, spina bifida, orofacial clefts, heart defects, in the offspring of women of short stature." He goes on to say that "a low plasma level of folic acid is a common finding in newly diagnosed patients and there are good theoretical reasons for hypothesizing that coeliac disease could also be a maternal risk factor for birth defects."

Researchers at the University of Naples put a finer point on the issue. While not denying the fact that undiagnosed and untreated celiac disease may be a severe cause of discomfort, i.e., anemia, associated diseases and unfavorable outcome of pregnancy in clinically evident patients, there is sufficient proof that after one year on the gluten-free diet the majority of these women enjoy a successful pregnancy. On the other hand, those cases identified only by screening, which are the majority, do not have major clinical complaints, and hence it is expected that they may not ever manifest overt disease or severe complications in reproductive performance.

Is there a better reason to take your supplements, check your levels of folic acid and not cheat on the diet? I don't think so.

There's More to Eating for Two Than Avoiding Gluten

In a recent CSA *Lifeline* article, dietician Gloria Scarparo advises pregnant celiacs to supplement the gluten-free diet with a daily dose of 1,200 mg of calcium combined with low-fat dairy products. Since iron deficiency is relatively

---

Busybody Alert

· ·

If you are reading this book, most likely you know you're a celiac. I cannot emphasize enough the need for you to do whatever it takes to get your newly married sister, brother, cousins, aunt, or uncle to read this chapter. As you know by now, if there's one celiac in the family tree, there's bound to be more. Make a scene if you have to, but get anyone in your family who is experiencing fertility problems or has family plans in the making to a gastroenterologist (see page 362 for a listing of celiac-friendly doctors) to be screened for CD. If you can spare someone you love unnecessary heartache, think what a wonderful godmother or godfather you'll make.

---

common in pregnant women, she suggests at least 30 mg of iron daily. Good sources of iron are spinach, liver, peanuts, and dried fruit. Eaten with foods that are high in vitamin C, such as bell peppers, broccoli, citrus fruit, kiwis, and strawberries, iron is absorbed more efficiently.

Folate or folic acid is one of the most vital vitamins for the unborn child in the first trimester and Scarparo suggests that the pregnant celiac should get at least 400 micrograms daily. Folate works to prevent serious birth defects and is crucial for the embryo during its growth phases. In its natural state, folic acid is found in hazelnuts, walnuts, almonds, cabbage, beets, asparagus, spinach, gluten-free grains and cereals, citrus fruits, bananas, melons, and kiwis.

Gluten isn't the only troublesome food for pregnant celiacs. The American Pregnancy Association recommends the following guidelines of foods to avoid during pregnancy (yes, there's more than gluten to worry about):

Raw meat. This includes sushi, undercooked seafood (forget about that seared ahi tuna for a while) or uncooked beef or poultry as it puts the celiac mother-to-be at a higher risk of toxoplasmosis and salmonella.

Deli meat. Deli products pose their own problems for the gluten-free, but for the pregnant *and* gluten-free they're a no-no. These products have been known to be contaminated with Listeria, which has the ability to cross the placenta and may infect the baby, or cause blood poisoning that may be life threatening.

Liver. There is some concern about the amounts of vitamin A in liver. Large amounts of vitamin A have the potential to pose a risk to an unborn baby. The safest approach is to avoid eating liver.

Fish contaminated with mercury. Fish containing high levels of mercury should be avoided. These include shark, swordfish, king mackerel, fresh tuna, sea bass, and tile fish. Canned tuna is considered safe, but no more than six ounces of albacore tuna a week should be eaten. Mercury consumed during pregnancy has been linked to developmental delays and brain damage.

Fish exposed to industrial pollutants. Avoid fish from contaminated lakes and rivers that may be exposed to high levels of polychlorinated bipheryls (PCBs). These fish include bluefish, striped bass, salmon, pike, trout, and walleye. Contact the local health department or Environmental Protection Agency to find out which fish are safe to eat in your area.

Raw shellfish. The majority of seafood-borne illness is caused by undercooked shellfish, which includes oysters, clams, and mussels. Cooking helps prevent some types of infection, but it does not prevent the algae-related infections associated with red tides. Raw shellfish pose concern for everybody and they should be avoided altogether.

Raw eggs. Raw eggs or any foods that contain raw eggs should be avoided during pregnancy because of the potential exposure to salmonella. Caesar dressings, mayonnaise, homemade ice cream or custards, hollandaise sauces, and unpasturized eggnog should be avoided.

Soft cheeses. Imported soft cheeses may contain bacteria called Listeria. Cheeses to avoid are Brie, Camembert, Roquefort, feta, gorgonzola, and Mexican style *queso blanco* and *queso fresco*. Soft non-imported cheeses made with pasteurized milk are safe to eat, as they do not contain gluten.

Unpasteurized milk. Again, this may contain Listeria, which crosses the placenta and may lead to infections or blood poisoning.

Pâté. Another possible source for the bacteria Listeria.

Caffeine. Although most studies show that caffeine intake in moderation is okay, there are others that say caffeine may be related to miscarriages. Avoid caffeine during the first trimester to reduce the likelihood of that happening and afterward limit caffeine to fewer than 300 mg per day. Caffeine is a diuretic, which can result in water and calcium loss, so make sure you are drinking plenty of water, juice, or milk rather than caffeinated beverages.

Alcohol. There is NO amount of alcohol that is known to be safe during pregnancy and during breast-feeding. Prenatal exposure to alcohol can interfere with the healthy development of the baby and depending on the amount, timing and pattern of use, alcohol consumption during pregnancy can lead to fetal alcohol syndrome.

Unwashed vegetables. While vegetables are safe to eat, it's essential to scrub them thoroughly in order to avoid exposure to toxoplasmosis which may contaminate the soil in which they are grown.

Herbal remedies. Certain herbal remedies like goldenseal and mugwort may be associated with uterine contractions and should be avoided. Take nothing without checking with your doctor first.

Cigarettes. The news gets worse about cigarettes. Don't even breathe near one.

A recent *New York Times* article aptly named the paranoia of pregnancy "The Nine Months of Living Anxiously." Yes, it's normal to worry about everything you put in your mouth during this time. The author did a Google search on the key words, "pregnant women should avoid" and got almost 7,000 responses. Everything from tanning salons to hair dye (play it safe and use vegetable dyes while pregnant), to time spent in a hot tub or sauna, kitty litter and phthalates (chemicals found in many industrial and cosmetic products, including hand creams, nail polish, perfume, and hair spray).

The FDA just added farm-raised salmon to the list of banned foods because it contains higher levels of PCBs and dioxins than what is considered safe by the Environmental Protection Agency.

According to a study reported in the *American Journal of Clinical Nutrition,* high-glycemic foods like white bread, highly processed grains, and potatoes may increase a woman's chances of having a baby with spina bifida or some other neural tube defect, and the strongest link was seen among obese participants. Women in the group who ate the most high-glycemic foods had four times the risk of delivering a baby with spina bifida. We can only wonder how much more they could have learned if all the women in the study had been screened for celiac disease.

H_2O is another issue. Mothers-to-be in Washington, D.C., have been advised not to drink tap water in certain neighborhoods. To be brutally honest, government water standards are often lower than our own. Filtered or bottled water is never a bad idea for anybody. For pregnant celiacs, it's common sense.

All this and gluten, too. What with all of these no-no's, it's amazing how easy it is to pack on the pounds.

She's Not Heavy, She's My Mother

In case you were wondering where all the extra weight goes and why it's so hard to see your feet, some fascinating facts from the American Pregnancy Association:

Baby = 7 pounds   Maternal breast tissue = 2 pounds
Placenta = 1 to 2 pounds   Maternal blood flow = 2 pounds
Amnoitic fluid = 2 pounds   Fluids in maternal tissue = 4 pounds
Uterine enlargement = 2 pounds   Maternal fat stores = 7 pounds

That's almost 30 pounds without even accounting for pickles. Or the gluten-free ice cream.

To Breast-Feed or Not

There are those weird breast pumps and embarrassing leaks back at the office and there's the problem of what to do when baby is hungry in public (tuck yourself in a corner somewhere and wrap a shawl around both of you). Some friends won't invite you out (what kind of friends are they?), and some husbands feel just plain left out of all that bonding. You can't leave the little tyke with anybody for very long because you're dinner for the next year or so. Still, the good reasons far outweigh the inconveniences, not the least of which, according to ProMom.org, is a breast-feeding mom will lose the baby fat much faster than a formula girl.

Besides, there is nothing like looking at your chubby, healthy baby and knowing you did that all by yourself.

The American Academy of Pediatrics says the average length of time for breast-feeding is twelve months or longer, depending on the mutual desire of the parties. This is another good reason to be at least a year out from your CD diagnosis. Undiagnosed CD often cuts short a woman's period of lactation. The longer you are on the gluten-free diet, the more likely you will have enough milk for the whole time.

Here, from ProMom.org, are some more good reasons to consider breast-feeding.

1. Breast milk is the perfect infant food. It can never be tampered with. There are no nutrients missing, nor are there ingredients that will be proven to give rats a headache or worse ten years from now. Its safety can never be questioned, nor can it ever be recalled.
2. According to the American Dietetic Association, breast-feeding encourages bonding and stimulates the release of the hormone oxytocin, which is responsible for stimulating contractions, milk ejection, and maternal behavior.
3. Breast-feeding helps decrease insulin requirements in diabetic mothers.
4. Breast milk is always the right temperature. No bottles to heat up. No accidental burns.
5. Breast-feeding makes for less smelly diaper changes. It's true. In side-by-side tests of breast-fed vs. formula, the natural baby won by a nose.
6. Breast-feeding satisfies baby's emotional need to be held, cuddled, and cradled. Some hospitals have programs where volunteers hold sick babies whose families cannot come every day.
7. Not breast-feeding may increase a mother's risk of breast cancer.
8. Breast milk lowers risk of baby developing asthma.
9. Breast-fed babies get fewer cavities.
10. Breast milk, because of its protective antibodies, is believed to confer immunity to disease and aids in the development of a healthy immune system. Breast-feeding may delay or reduce the risk of developing celiac disease.

Oh, yes. Breast milk is 100 percent gluten-free.

Before you know it, you will say hello to your feet again. And to the creature you can't stop marveling at, whose tiny toes and fingers fit in your mouth.

Isn't that how we got started on this subject?

When your new little person gets to the teething stage, there's a lovely gluten-free rusk in the next chapter, while you're waiting to find out if he or she takes after Mama or Papa in the gluten department.

There are no gluten-free names. May I be so bold as to suggest Jax if it's a girl? Or even if it's not.

Learn More

For more information, referrals, and support:

American College of Obstetricians
and Gynecologists
409 12th Street
P.O. Box 96920
Washington, DC 20090
www.acog.org

American Dietetic Association
120 South Riverside Plaza
Suite 2000
Chicago, IL 60606
(800) 877-1600
www.eatright.org

American Pregnancy Association
1425 Greenway Drive, Suite 440
Irving, TX 75038
(800) 672-2296
www.americanpregnancy.org

Centers for Disease Control and
Prevention
National Center for Environmental
Health
*Folic Acid Now: Before You Know
You're Pregnant* (publication
#99-0204, order # 099-6069)
www.cdc.gov

Food and Drug Administration
Center for Food Safety and Applied
Nutrition
www.vm.cfsan.fda.gov

International Council on Infertility
Information Dissemination, Inc.
P.O. Box 6836
Arlington, VA 22206
(703) 379-9178

La Leche League
1400 North Meacham Road
Schaumburg, IL 60173
(847) 519-7730
www.lalecheleague.org

National Foundation for Celiac
Awareness
224 South Maple Way
Ambler, Pennsylvania
(267) 625-5505
www.celiacfoundation.org

National Institutes For Health
9000 Rockville Pike
Bethesda, MD 20892
www.nih.gov

National Maternal and Child Health
Clearing House
2070 Chain Bridge Road, Suite 450
Vienna, VA 22182
(703) 356-1964
www.circsol.com/mhc

Nursing Mothers Council
P.O. Box 1463
Palo Alto, CA 94303
(650) 599-3669

U.S. Department of Agriculture
(USDA)
Food and Nutrition Information
Center

National Agricultural Library
1031 Baltimore Avenue, Room 304
Beltsville, MD 20705
(301) 504-5719
www.nal.usda.gov/fnic

Promotion of Mother's Milk, Inc.
www.promom.org

Vegetarian Resource Group
P.O. Box 1463
Baltimore, MD 21203
(410) 366-8343
www.vrg.org/index.htm.

mama's little baby
can't eat shortnin' bread

Pat-a-cake, Pat-a-cake, baker's man,
Bake me a cake as fast as you can;
Pat it and prick it, mark it with a B,
Put it in the oven for baby and me.

—*Traditional nursery rhyme*

My friend Louise believes bananas are the root of all evil in the world. As a child, she couldn't digest them properly and got a terrible rash. Her well-meaning parents made matters worse.

Instead of telling little Lou that her particular plumbing wasn't banana-friendly and that she'd best avoid anything even remotely banana-flavored, they warned that even the merest whiff could kill her. Whenever a Chiquita Banana commercial shimmied across the family's tiny black and white TV screen, they leapt to their feet and pointed to the shameless hussy who would spell doom for their darling girl. "I'm Chiquita Banana, and I'm here to say," Louise's parents would sing, wagging their fingers and rolling their eyes at the dancing character in the Carmen Miranda hat, "a banana will kill you in the most horrible way."

To this day, the poor dear quakes at the sight of a fruit bowl. She has never enjoyed a hot fudge sundae, knowing the makings of a banana split lurk nearby. Nor has she ever experienced the pleasure of a thick chocolate shake or a fruit smoothie on a hot day for fear of a banana-tainted blender. She considers the idea of a Caribbean vacation with all those plantains and banana trees tantamount to a trip to Dante's inner circle of Hell. Her first husband once took her to a fancy New Orleans restaurant that specialized in Bananas Foster. Let's just say her second never made *that* mistake.

Granted, poor Louise is an extreme example, one that would be best served by twenty or thirty years in the company of a good therapist. But her case is also one that illustrates how the presentation of a dietary restriction, especially one as important and rigid as the gluten-free diet, can have a lasting effect on how a child views the world as an adult. It begs the fundamental question for parents of children who must learn to avoid gluten. How do you teach the importance of avoiding certain foods and substances without creating a phobia that can ruin your child's life? Is she afraid of it? Or is she simply mindful of what might happen if vigilance is not observed?

Children are like tofu. They tend to absorb whatever flavor they are exposed to. Are you a panicked parent or an optimistic one? Are you a worrier or do you take a laissez-faire position? Do you blame or do you take responsibility? Would you say you are controlling or easygoing?

If possible, try to respect the offending food and its place in the lives of others without demonizing it. Easier said than done when you're trying to keep your little darling from getting some accidental gluten. There really are no bad foods, only tummies that have trouble digesting them. Just as there are no bad animals and flowers and trees, only skin and eyes and noses and respiratory systems that are sensitive to them. Food isn't the illness, the illness is.

Like blue eyes, red hair, brown skin, long fingers, flat feet, freckles, the proclivity to play the piano or tell stories, our special characteristics make us unique. The child who grows up seeing his sensitivity to gluten or dairy or peanuts or any other food as something foisted upon him by a hostile world is more likely to grow up feeling victimized by his dietary restrictions, rather than be individualized by it. The lucky ones who are taught to see themselves through the prism of that which makes them special are more likely to take responsibility for their diets and grow up celebrating, not being ashamed of, this part of themselves.

While this may seem a little too philosophical for a youngster to absorb, consider the alternative: what if you were raised thinking pasta could kill you and you discovered you had accidentally eaten a noodle? Perspective is important here. One accident does not death by pasta make. This is your fear, not your child's. There's a fine line between teaching a healthy respect for the repercussions without creating a person who's afraid to eat.

Much as we wish we could, we can't guarantee our children safe passage in a dangerous world. No one can do that. But we can raise people who are not afraid of it, children who honor themselves by honoring their special needs and expecting others to do the same.

Take a good look at a child who picks the brightest crayons and boldly colors outside the lines. You'll see a parent willing to do the same.

❧

Let's kick things off with a few words from a medical expert who has guided hundreds of little celiacs and their parents through diagnosis and the adjustment to a gluten-free diet. Michelle Pietzak is a pediatric gastroenterologist at Children's Hospital of Los Angeles, assistant professor of pediatrics at the University of Southern California, and the West Coast director of the Center for Celiac Research.

What if My Baby Is a Celiac?

Michelle M. Pietzak, M.D.

If you are reading this book, you are already well ahead of the game. You are lucky to have heard of celiac disease, and luckier still to have the wit, wisdom, and insight of Jax Peters Lowell, novelist, author of *Against the Grain,* and twenty-year veteran of life on the gluten-free diet, before you. Given that the majority of American physicians still know very little about the condition that is quite common in Europe, the fact that you are here with *The Gluten-Free Bible* in your hands is a modern-day miracle.

How is it possible for the United States, a world leader in health care and research, to be so far behind its European colleagues in diagnosing CD? The answer lies in part with infant feeding practices and the misconception that this condition is rare and exclusively a childhood disease. But let's start at the beginning. How does CD affect children? Is treatment different for them? And, if CD is so common, why do I feel that I'm the only parent in America who spends two hours on every trip to the grocery store reading confusing labels?

Until recently, celiac disease has been strictly defined as an illness of early childhood that causes its victims to have diarrhea when they eat gluten-containing grains. Physicians were taught to look for children with potbellies and stick-thin arms and legs. Many believed, and some still do, that CD can be outgrown. We now know that children with CD do not always present with diarrhea and, in fact, may be chronically constipated. Many children do not look malnourished at all, and may even be overweight. No child ever outgrows celiac disease.

For parents who bring their children to my practice, I define celiac disease as an autoimmune condition that occurs in certain individuals who eat gluten. Autoimmune means that the body attacks its normal tissues, in the same manner as if an invader were present. The body is misguided in its defense system, and targets healthy, normal tissues, as it would an infection. The tissue primarily affected in CD is the gastrointestinal tract, but we now know that virtually any organ system in the body can be affected by celiac disease. So, while CD has been classically defined as *enteropathy* or a disease of the gut, I prefer to look at it the way we view a disease like lupus or type I diabetes: an autoimmune condition with a dietary trigger that can affect many different systems. If we broaden our definition thusly, many more cases of CD would be diagnosed. For example, people with dermatitis herpetiformis, the skin manifestation of CD, or neurologic manifestations of the disease, like seizures or depression, and those with no overt GI symptoms would be discovered promptly and treated appropriately.

The definition of celiac disease is evolving, but we have a firm grasp on certain facts. As in many diseases, both genetic and environmental factors must be present in the same person in order to make a diagnosis of CD. We know that two HLA genes, DQ2 and DQ8, must be present for the individual to develop celiac disease. The job of the HLA is to allow white blood cells to recognize "self" from "non-self." In the celiac, the "non-self" is the environmental trigger, gluten. Both genes must be present in order for an individual to develop celiac disease. If they are not, a child can eat all the gluten he or she wants, and will not develop the disease. Conversely, if no gluten is eaten, despite the presence of these genes, celiac disease will not be triggered. While this sounds simple, the immunology is quite complex, and we are just beginning to understand it. It is also quite probable that there are other genes and perhaps other environmental triggers, such as infections, which may play a role.

The good news, and it is great news, is that removing the trigger cures the disease. If a team of scientists could isolate and remove the environmental trigger for Crohn's disease or ulcerative colitis as easily as in CD or dispense with the need for insulin in type 1 diabetes, they would win a Nobel Prize. There are no cures for these conditions, only immune suppressive medications to treat symptoms, which are not without their side effects. This is why I always tell worried parents of celiacs how lucky they are their child's suffering is so easily remedied. When I am asked, "When will there be a cure?" (as I often am), my answer is always the same. "There is a cure, it's the gluten-free diet." No other autoimmune disease can make this claim. The gluten-free diet is challenging, but compared to a lifetime of medication, it's a piece of cake.

How do symptoms of childhood celiac disease differ from those in adults? As I have said, the classic (but actually rare) childhood presentation is that of a malnourished child with a loss of fat stores and muscle due to chronic diarrhea. However, this classic form was described before the advent of modern-day infant feeding practices. Because of food allergies, the American Academy of Pediatrics has promoted the delayed introduction of solids in the diet and encourages breast-feeding. These two factors may delay, or even prevent completely, the occurrence of CD. This is why "classic CD" is rare in the United States and this description is a misnomer.

Children with CD may be irritable, depressed, and have increased separation anxiety from their parents. Children soon learn that when they eat, they hurt, and may present with anorexia. Many little ones will vomit, or have what appears to be reflux, once they begin to ingest gluten-containing foods. If they vomit enough, they may not have diarrhea, because they expel the toxic gluten from above, and not below. Other pediatric GI symptoms include constipation, abdominal pain, and lactose intolerance, which can also be seen in adults.

What confuses physicians is that celiac disease can present outside the GI tract. These children never make it to a gastroenterologist, and often the condition is missed until GI symptoms develop. In the musculoskeletal system, a child may have isolated short stature, joint pain, dental enamel defects, osteopenia, or frank osteoporosis for unexplained reasons. A particular rash called dermatitis herpetiformis is the skin manifestation of celiac disease that can appear in adolescence. Iron-deficiency anemia with associated fatigue is very common in untreated CD and is due to malabsorption. The central nervous system may also be affected and we know that mania, depression, seizures, and various behavior problems occur in the celiac child with greater frequency than in other children. Many of these symptoms improve on a gluten-free diet.

We also know those children with type 1 diabetes, thyroid disease, and autoimmune arthritis and liver diseases are at higher risk for celiac disease. Unfortunately, many of these conditions can have GI symptoms of their own, which may confuse the picture. Three syndromes, which are usually diagnosed in childhood—Down syndrome or Trisomy 21, Turner syndrome (the absence of one X chromosome), and Williams syndrome—also have higher rates of celiac disease. Despite studies investigating these chromosomal defects, connections to CD are unclear.

Why subject a child to early testing? There are three reasons: cancer, nutrition, and the risk of developing other autoimmune conditions. Patients with untreated celiac disease have a higher risk of other GI cancers, as well as twice the mortality of their non-celiac brethren. One rare cancer in particular, enteropathy associated T-cell lymphoma, is very difficult to detect and treat and can be fatal. But despite the fact that the risk of this cancer is higher in untreated celiacs, the risk of nutritional complications is much greater. These include diseases that result from malabsorption of vitamins and minerals: osteoporosis (vitamin D), night blindness (vitamin A), neuropathy, ataxia, and other neurologic complaints (vitamins E and B_{12}), bleeding problems (vitamin K), and anemia (iron, B_{12}, and folic acid).

We also know that the duration of gluten exposure can determine a celiac child's risk for developing another autoimmune condition. Children diagnosed before the age of 2 have a 5 percent lifelong risk of developing such a condition. The same child who is diagnosed between 2 and 10 years has a 17 percent risk. And if the diagnosis comes after the age of 10, the risk jumps to 24 percent, which may explain why so many newly diagnosed adult celiacs already have another co-morbid condition like type 1 diabetes, Sjögren's syndrome, thyroid disease, or rheumatoid arthritis.

I believe all children whose first-degree relatives (mother, father, brother, sister, son, daughter) and second-degree relatives (grandmother, grandfather, aunt, uncle, niece, nephew, cousin, grandchild) are biopsy-proven celiacs should be screened with serum or blood antibody tests. Also, children with unexplained diarrhea, short stature, poor weight gain, anemia, joint pain, and osteopenia should be tested. Vague symptoms of other systems where there is a strong family history of autoimmune diseases or GI cancers should also be considered for testing. In my opinion, any child with another underlying autoimmune condition should be tested, as many of these diseases have associated GI symptoms, which mask the presentation of CD. However, treatment with immune-suppressant drugs may make antibody testing falsely negative, and may even partially treat the celiac disease. Likewise, a gluten-free diet that has been strictly adhered to for weeks or months may make serology falsely negative. This is why we like to test children who are currently ingesting gluten. Genetic testing, especially of young siblings or those who are already gluten-free, may be valuable. If a child is DQ2 or DQ8 negative, it is very unlikely that he or she will ever develop celiac disease.

Positive blood antibodies do need to be followed up with a small bowel biopsy, still considered the "gold standard," to confirm diagnosis. Why subject a small child to this invasive endoscopic procedure? Serology can be falsely positive in other conditions such as food allergy, GI infections, cystic fibrosis, and other autoimmune diseases and a biopsy can differentiate between these different conditions. Also, gluten removal and resolution of symptoms can occur with wheat allergy or gluten intolerance, and patients with these conditions do not have the increased risk, and therefore do not require increased surveillance for nutritional deficiencies, GI cancers, and other autoimmune conditions. Lastly, celiacs must be on a gluten-free diet for life. A child has another seventy or eighty years of eating ahead, and a parent better be sure there is good reason to be vigilant about gluten. A gluten challenge, which requires putting gluten back into the diet and repeating the biopsy after the gut has healed, is no longer recommended, unless the original diagnosis was in question.

In the research community we often hear the phrase, "the celiac iceberg." The analogy is apt as there is only about one-eighth of an iceberg's total mass peeking out of the water, while seven-eighths is submerged. Those children with classic symptoms who are getting diagnosed are only the tip of this iceberg. A prevalence study conducted by the Center for

Celiac Research at the University of Maryland found that 1 in 132 healthy
individuals has celiac disease. In children with symptoms, it was as high
as 1 in 40. Based on the 2000 U.S. census, and assuming the entire population is healthy, which we know it is not, this translates to approximately
2.1 million people with CD. Based on support group data, it is estimated
that, at the time of the study, about 15,000 celiacs had been diagnosed.
This means only 0.7 percent of celiacs have been diagnosed, leaving the
other 99.3 percent shuttling from doctor to doctor, with complaints that
continue to go unrecognized and untreated.

In Los Angeles where I practice, the average time for an adult to get a
correct diagnosis after first seeking medical care is twelve years. Twelve
years. I submit to you that this is more than just an iceberg; it is a national
tragedy. If a child is to grow to be a healthy adult, there is no time to waste.

For every one of you who hold this book today, knowing that your
child has CD or wondering if he or she will, there are another 140
"mama's little babies who can't eat shortnin' bread" and do not know it.
Be glad, be creative, read on, and weep for joy. You are in the capable
hands of a writer who knows what it is to live gluten-free and has never
forgotten we are all children at heart.

Language Matters

A good way to begin is to be mindful of what you say. "Don't eat that, it's bad,"
gets the job done, but it's much healthier to teach a child to say, "No thank
you, pizza doesn't agree with me." Or, "I'd like to have a brownie, but I can't."

Let's say your child is allergic to cat dander, as many are. Is it the cat's fault,
or is it the child's fault for forgetting to avoid petting it? When your baby comes
home from school with a tummy ache, does she admit, "I ate some cereal by
mistake?" Or does she place the blame elsewhere, saying, "They gave me cereal"?

The tummy ache may hurt just the same, but owning the mistake is what
prevents the next one. It's never too early for a child to learn to take responsibility for her behavior.

It's hard to recognize a child's needs as separate from our need to protect
them. But sometimes we unconsciously instill fear in order to assuage our own.
What parent has never said, "That cookie could kill you." This, too, will create the
desired effect. But it's manipulative and emotionally dishonest. Better to say, "I
worry that you'll be tempted to eat some gluten and get sick again." Or "It scares
me to think of you at a pizza party, even with your own pizza." Or "I'm afraid
your teacher will give you the wrong snack." Sentences that express concern for
another person, even a little one, should start with *I'm afraid . . . , I worry . . . ,*
or, *It scares me.* The only way to teach emotional honesty is by example.

Be honest with your fears and your child will see that it's okay to be honest with his.

It may not seem like a big deal, but don't let anyone refer to your child as sick or as a "patient." While it's true that CD is a disease, symptoms may no longer present. Children believe what adults say about them. If you don't believe this, reread *The Secret Garden*.

Of course you're afraid that your child will get some gluten and get sick, but it won't help to draw the curtain of your own fear around him. Worry that goes beyond reasonable concern creates another kind of illness. The idea is to raise a person who is not wounded by her problems, but challenged by them. Consider the case of the Olympic swimmer who won a gold medal in spite of a lifelong battle with asthma or the chef who allowed celiac disease to lead her to create the world's first gluten-free bagel. Who knows, a future entrepreneur could be inventing the gluten-removal meter in your kitchen this very minute.

No parent ever sets out to shape a banana-phobic Louise, but understanding our own fears can go a long way in not perpetuating them in our grain-challenged children.

Words count as much as deeds.

Why Doesn't Ritchie Get Itchy?

It's hard enough to be different, even when you're a grown-up. I hate being the one to have to interrogate the chef on absolutely every ingredient before I order and sometimes I just want to go along with the crowd, even though I know it could make me sick. Peer group pressure is a powerful thing at any age. But having special requirements at an age when conformity equals social acceptance and anything different is suspect and routinely ridiculed is tough for a child. I recall the exquisite torture and nerdiness of having to wear Hush Puppies when all the other kids wore Keds.

Despite your best efforts, no one can guarantee that your baby won't be treated badly by the other kids from time to time, but there are lots of ways a parent can keep a child from always feeling like the odd one out. One surefire way to help a child on a gluten-free diet forget he can't have mac 'n' cheese and ice-cream cones like everybody else is empathy. Explain that while Ritchie may not get itchy from pizza or Izzie may not get dizzy from pie, one can't drink milk and the other can't have a puppy. Janey may be able to eat a grilled cheese sandwich, but she can't play outside when the pollen count is high. Here are a few ideas to get you started:

- Make an imaginary pet for the friend who is allergic to cat or dog dander. Give it a name, buy it a collar, and walk it together.
- Invent a passive indoor sport for your child's asthmatic or environmentally sensitive friend to play when the air is unhealthy.
- Devise an allergy buddy system.
- One day treat everyone to dairy-free ice-cream sodas after school, another gluten-free cookies, nut-free brownies, and so on.
- Volunteer to make the gluten-free pizza crusts for the next party, instead of just supplying your child's. Network with the mother or father
  of the lactose- or peanut- or soy- or casein- or sulphite-allergic child,
  so every child gets his or her turn. This way you can help make sure
  your child is invited to parties and not be ostracized by overscheduled
  parents who have no time to supply gluten-free food.
- Start an allergy club and create a membership directory with Polaroid
  pictures. Sometimes the best allergy medicine is as simple as being
  aware that others suffer, too.
- Give all the kids drugstore masks on a windy day with heavy pollen.
  Create a theme—Zorro or *E.R.*
- Sing them this little ditty, with apologies to Anonymous . . .

> *Monday's child is gluten-free,*
> *Tuesday's child gets hives from tea,*
> *Wednesday's child can't bear cat hair,*
> *Thursday's child must gasp for air,*
> *Friday's child will wheeze and sneeze,*
> *Saturday's child is eggless, please.*
> *But the child born on the Sabbath day,*
> *Fair and wise, loves to say,*
> *"Thank you, God, that I'm this way."*

Teaching a child to see their friends' frailties, as well as their own, can go a
long way in countering the natural self-absorption that comes with any health
problem or lifelong diet. What better antidote to isolation than including and
celebrating everyone's differences? Honoring the restrictions of others does
something else, too. It teaches generosity and good manners, one of the most
valuable lessons any parent can give a child.

Pack Your Bags, We're Going on a Guilt Trip

My cousin, who is now a forty-five year-old man, was diagnosed with diabetes at the age of two. Until he was old enough to do it himself, his father gave him insulin injections because his mother couldn't bear to pierce her boy's perfect baby flesh. No one ever discussed the disease in the child's presence. My aunt compensated by never saying *no* to her son. My uncle's response was to watch life unfold through the gauze of a martini. All through high school, my cousin held his parents hostage, threatening to go off his diet whenever they attempted to set curfews, insist that he do homework, or try to enforce the rules most teenagers lived by. After being accepted at a college as far away from home as he could manage, my cousin insisted that his parents buy him a car they couldn't afford. When they refused to do so, he stopped taking insulin and almost died. The day he was released from the hospital, there was a brand-new Thunderbird convertible parked in the driveway.

How can you discipline a poor, insulin-dependent child or, for that matter, a poor cookie-starved toddler? You can and you must. If you don't, the monster you create is entirely your own doing. Here are the facts:

Fact #1: Genetics aside, your child's food intolerance is not your fault and all attempts at compensation will result in manipulation, no matter how sweet-natured the child is now.

Fact #2: No matter what you are going through as a result of your child's gluten-free diet, there is one incontrovertible reality. The problem belongs to your child and he or she will handle it the way his or her nature dictates.

Little People / Big Feelings

You may be so grateful that your child is well again (or that he or she doesn't have a life-threatening illness) that in your relief you may overlook the feelings of sadness and loss your child may be experiencing in the wake of diagnosis. A toddler does not have the verbal skills or insight to be able to articulate this, thus these feelings can take many forms—tantrums and other antisocial or aggressive behavior, anger, loss of appetite, moodiness, decline in school performance, feigned illnesses, picking fights, tears, refusal to eat or to play with other children, the sudden acquisition of an imaginary friend, or just plain bad behavior. The reaction may even manifest itself as colds, fevers, headaches, lack of energy, low-level malaise, and the one thing you fear most, cheating on the diet.

The problem is denial, and it's the first leg of the same miserable journey we must all travel before arriving at acceptance. It's why the man who has just had a heart attack sneaks cheese and cigarettes, while the rest of the family rants about his suicidal behavior. It's why an otherwise sensible woman like myself, knowing she will suffer serious gastrointestinal consequences, once tucked a piece of cake into her purse.

There is a period of mourning for children, too, and in our haste to see them get well, we forget that all they want is for things to be the way they were before. If a child is to honor himself by taking responsibility for his diet, he has to know it's okay to honor the sadness, anger, and loss of control that comes with it. It's important to create an environment in which the child feels safe enough to talk about these feelings with no judgment about how they are being expressed. If a child senses judgment, he or she will quickly get the message that only the feelings that don't scare Mommy and Daddy are okay and learn to suppress the others.

Try not to look at the behavior, but attempt to see what's behind it. Remember that difficult children are usually those who are having a difficult time. This rule applies to adults, too, who are just big kids with better vocabularies.

In the age of kiddie antidepressants, rampant ADD, and other convenient diagnoses for problems every growing human must face, parents are afraid and justifiably so, of having their children labeled "difficult" and unnecessarily stigmatized. Because of this, parents are sometimes reluctant to discuss behavioral problems with teachers, child-care professionals, and others until it becomes so obvious that the behavior becomes the issue, not the reasons motivating it. It takes a great deal of effort and sensitivity, but creating a chain of understanding and support for your child (the earlier the better after diagnosis), is not only possible, it's preferable to trying to "normalize" what doesn't feel normal to your child.

Watching a child's tantrum is like watching a summer storm. First comes the boom of thunder, then the crackle and hiss of lightning, then the rain, always the rain, cleansing and necessary. Try to remember that bad rhymes with sad.

Labels Have a Way of Sticking

Here's another banana story, this one true as well. As a child in England, my friend James was horribly allergic to cow's milk and wheat. He was a celiac, of course, but no one knew it yet. His arms and legs were skinny and emaciated, his belly distended, and he was pale and listless. In those days, it was believed a diet of rice and bananas was all a child like James could digest, and at home he was served an endless supply of this bland food. When he was barely a year old, the family attended a church picnic, where everyone in the village brought a covered dish and children and adults played lawn games and ate their fill. Fearful their ill child would get the wrong food from a well-meaning neighbor (these were the days when mothers fed and comforted the child closest to them without regard for maternity or potential lawsuits), but not wanting to keep the sad little boy home, James's father fashioned a sign, complete with pictures of little monkeys and bunches of bananas and hung it around the baby's neck. To James's everlasting embarrassment, the yellowed photograph of him wearing this sign survives in the family album to this day. A thin child in a diaper and a dopey sun hat sits on a plaid blanket on a patch of grass, solemnly staring into the camera. There is a sign around his neck bearing the words, "Please don't feed me, I've got my own bananas."

I've seen messages from parents posted on the Internet that advise other parents to label their children like UPS packages. I couldn't disagree more. There's no need for a celiac child, no matter how little, to be turned into a living Post-it note. By all means, send a toddler off to nursery school with a follow-up note reminding the teacher of his or her special needs, but only after you've made an appointment and explained the problem in person and offered to participate in the solution.

Ditto for the dietician who manages the school cafeteria, as well as the operator of the day-care center. Better still, supply the special foods yourself and ask that they be served to your child when other children are being fed. Without a great deal of fanfare, one parent solved the problem by supplying a laminated photo of her child with an explanation of his diet on the back. He knows to always ask for the tray with his picture on it and the cafeteria staff knows they aren't giving a gluten-free lunch to the wrong child. This is a great idea because the explanation only appears in the lunchroom where it counts and is not pinned to the poor child's sweater all day. How you present something like this is important. The goal is raise a child who believes the rest of the world wants his food, not the other way around.

A meeting with the school nurse is a good idea as well, so you'll know if your child is suffering any celiac-related symptoms during the day. And speaking of symptoms, the person who monitors the bathroom passes ought to be alerted ahead of time to save your child embarrassment should frequent bathroom emergencies still be a problem. A private signal between teacher and celiac can save a world of embarrassment for your child.

Short of food, ask that no undue attention be given to your youngster. Present the request firmly and in adult terms. A good example is, "You know how it feels when you're trying to lose a few pounds and the waiter carrying the plate of cottage cheese and the lemon wedge shouts, 'Who gets the diet plate?' Well, that's how my child feels, too."

The challenge is to convey the seriousness of the problem without exaggeration, which may cause your child to be stigmatized or treated like an invalid. Make it clear that celiac disease and the gluten-free diet limits only eating, not participating in normal school sports and other activities. This is a litigious world, and people may overreact to potential liability by shutting your child out of games, trips, and other healthy recreation.

You may be tempted to rush into every lunch, dinner, sleepover, school trip, picnic, party, and snack situation like a gluten attack dog, sniffing out every offending crumb before allowing your darling to participate in anything even remotely food related. It will certainly save your child any accidental exposure to the offending grains, but shining the spotlight of "special problem" can also cause great social angst. No little person needs that kind of embarrassment. Remember how you felt when your mother made you wear ankle socks with your first pair of heels?

Time and time again, children tell me how hard it is to be the focus of that kind of attention. You don't hear people saying, "Don't give Henry a glass of wine, he's an alcoholic." The same holds true for children. No need to explain to the other kids, unless they ask, or unless your child wants to tell them himself.

They Always Loved You Best

My father was as healthy as a horse. His brother George was allergic to everything. George got the cream. Dad got the milk. George got the nutrient-rich broth. Dad got the pallid remains of the chicken that made it. Little Georgie was shipped off to an aunt's seaside cottage for his summer vacation, while Jackie stayed in the hot city and got to play on "tar beach." Daddy grew up to be an athlete who wouldn't think twice about going back into the game with a broken bone. While Uncle George, even as a grown man, was afraid of getting a cold. Can anyone tell me why they hated each other? Or who was responsible for it?

Sibling rivalry. There's nothing you can do to banish this fact of family life. And you shouldn't try. It's the natural sorting out of things or, as Anna Quindlen so eloquently put it in her *Philadelphia Inquirer Magazine* essay on the subject of siblings, "They are, therefore I am not. We define ourselves in terms of our differences from those who share our life. As though our house-holds were theaters, as they are, we enter on cue and take the seat that is not filled. The clown, the thinker, the quiet one [. . . the celiac]. The role is cast. Sometimes our parents do the casting: Mrs. Portnoy turned her son into a prince, so his sister became a peasant."

When one child is the focus of so much special attention, it's easy for the others to feel slighted. A few ideas for keeping siblings from brooding:

• **Set up a kitchen cabinet or a separate shelf just for the gluten-free sibling.** Put it within easy reach; stock it with all the foods he or she needs and likes. This helps a child be less dependent on others, keeps his food out of harm's way, and sets boundaries for the rest of the family. Encourage sharing and don't make gluten-free goodies so sacrosanct that they become an argument one child always wins. Set up something equally special for the non-gluten-free kids, too. Remember, it's not fair to be able to eat your food *and* everybody else's.

• **Allow your gluten-free child to opt out of family events that are too difficult.** A sibling's ice-cream and cake party can be torture for a child who is forced to go or to eat something different from the others. But never cancel the event itself, or make another child feel guilty for enjoying it. The idea is teaching your little celiac to say so when it's not comfortable for him, rather than blame others for eating something in front of him he can't have. You don't want to raise a martyr, or a child who never had a birthday cake because his brother or sister couldn't eat it.

• **Find ways to give the others equal attention**. If you send your celiac to one of the gluten-free summer camps around the country, be especially sensitive to arranging an equally wonderful treat for the non-celiac child. Of course, this can seriously tap the little bit of energy you have after working all day, cooking, running errands, playing chauffeur, and having five minutes for yourself. Years from now you'll be glad you made the extra effort.

There is no finer reward for all your hard work than to see brother taking care of sister, sister tucking little brother under her wing, reading labels for him, explaining why he can't eat what others are enjoying. Watching them become friends as they grow, each one separate and unique, not resenting, but respecting and loving one another's differences as much as their similarities—this is the gift of emotionally intuitive parenting.

Which brings me back to my grandmother. She meant no harm, but by coddling one son and assuming the healthy one could fend for himself, it was she who set their lifelong animosity in motion. If she'd only cooked two chickens, one for the broth and one for the meat. If only she had stood up to her sister and refused to send one brother to the beach without the other. If only . . .

Childish, you say. Yes, indeed. There really is no other explanation for why my really smart and otherwise well-balanced father would buy a beach house to which he would never invite his brother, or why, for the rest of his life, he refused to be in the same room with a chicken.

Growing Up . . . and Out

Many children with celiac disease do not grow at the same rate as other children. Some shoot up as soon as the offending gluten is removed, others don't seem to be affected and remain at the bottom of the growth charts. While there is a great deal of controversy about prescribing growth hormones for these children and much disagreement about the dangers and long-term effects of such a regimen, it's never too early to teach that stature is never measured in feet or inches. Anyone can be tall *inside*.

Seeing to it that your gluten-free youngster gets the right foods and doesn't feel left out of social activities is hard enough. But how do you make sure that in preventing a relapse of one disease, you're not contributing to another? The statistics are alarming. Childhood obesity is on the rise. More and more children and adolescents are overweight, which not only puts them at risk for heart disease, arthritis, and other chronic disease as adults, but is causing problems like diabetes, hypertension, high cholesterol, sleep apnea, conditions that until now have rarely been seen in children. Part of the blame lies in high-fat and sugary snacks (high-fructose syrup, palm kernel oil, and other bad fats do just as much damage in gluten-free goodies as they do in the glutenous variety), but a lack of activity is equally responsible. Schools rarely provide a real workout at recess or in gym class and when the kids do get home, going out to play or ride their bikes often loses out to more sedentary pursuits like TV and computer games. Given this and the fact that many gluten-free products are packed with sugar and fat, a parent must be careful not to turn a sickly and too-thin child into an unhealthy and overweight one.

Ask any child, on the social discrimination scale fat trumps celiac for getting made fun of every time. It's never too early to start pudge-proofing your celiac. Stock the fridge with healthy snacks like fresh fruit, orange slices, or celery sticks stuffed with low-fat peanut butter. Gluten-free pretzels are a better low-fat choice than cookies and cakes, as are gluten-free energy bars, dried fruits, and whole-grain (brown rice) breads and rolls and muffins made with a minimum of fat and sugar. Try to keep sodas to a minimum and bear in mind that many fruit juices are little more than flavored water and sugar. Make up bags of nuts and raisins or gluten-free granola for snacking. Keep a big bowl of fresh salad in the fridge. Ditto for crisped raw veggies.

Cook healthy. Use half-and-half instead of cream and switch from whole milk to 1% or low-fat soy milk. Use olive oil for cooking, low-fat vegetable spreads, cream cheese, nut butters, and whole fruit spreads rather than butter, margarine, and high-fat mayonnaise. Avoid processed foods and buy leaner cuts of meat for the whole family, preferably those raised without hormones or antibiotics. If your child really hates vegetables, as so many do, be creative by making soups and offering snack-time veggies with dips.

Expose little ones to new foods frequently. This keeps them from developing a fear of unknown foods later on. And do buy children's cookbooks. Children are more apt to eat what they create.

Taste is an acquired habit. If you do these things gradually, you will help your child develop the taste for cleaner, more wholesome foods.

While you're at it (you're already scouring labels for gluten, anyway), look for hydrogenated or partially hydrogenated oil on food labels, which often indicates the presence of unhealthy trans fats. In the future, the FDA will make it mandatory to label these dangerous artery-clogging fats, but for now you must be a sleuth. Look for trans fats in baked goods (including gluten-free baked goods), chips, butter and margarine, even low-fat pudding and microwave popcorn. Also check for non-organic cottonseed oil, which may contain high levels of toxic pesticides.

By any other name, sugar is still sugar. Sugar sources include cane sugar, fructose, fruit juices, barley malt (a double whammy here—gluten *and* sugar), corn sweeteners, honey, maltose, and dextrose. All of it puts on the pounds, messes with insulin levels, and sets off a lifelong taste for more sugar. It's always a good idea to buy organic produce, but not everything warrants the extra expense. The term "certified organic" refers to the method of farming used, not the level of the pesticide in the final product. Visit the Environmental Working Group's Web site at www.ewg.org to find out what produce is better bought organic and what's safe to buy conventionally grown. (Hint: Organic bananas aren't really worth the cost, the peel keeps the fruit from any contact with pesticides.)

Celiacs are often more sensitive to food additives than other children. I've never outgrown my allergy to the Tartrazine Yellow dye found in food, as well as in some medications. The Center for Science in the Public Interest suggests avoiding sodium nitrite, saccharin, caffeine, Olestra, and artificial coloring, among others (www.cspinet.org).

Buy your picky eater a special dish with many compartments and let her experiment or "graze" among healthy offerings. Let your child be your helper (if you can stand the mess) and offer a taste of new foods as you go.

To teach portion control, a friend of mine serves bite-sized food on toothpicks, like Cher did in the movie *Mermaids*. Of course, you need to make sure your child is old enough to handle toothpicks safely.

Use non-food rewards. Instead of a high-fat treat for a good report card or chores done, offer stickers or a gadget for the bike or skateboard (exercise!). Celebrate special occasions with a trip to the movies or a day at the museum, or in the park, or children's theater instead of making a sugary, high-fat feast.

Make it a family rule never to eat in front of the TV, as well as not eating on the run. Good table manners include chewing slowly, no gobbling. Sit down together as often as schedules allow.

Sign your child up for after-school exercise and other physical activities. In addition to team sports, look into the neighborhood Y and churches and synagogues that provide safe, supervised places for playing ball, gymnastics, jump rope, and other physical games. Organize a neighborhood clean sweep or leaf-bagging day. Set a timer to go off after a half hour or hour of TV watching or playing games on the computer.

Just as some adult celiacs develop weight problems after diagnosis, due to increased absorption of food and the addition of gluten-free breads and cakes and cookies, etc., to our diets (all of a sudden we want what we can't have), so do children. Balance is the best lesson we can teach our children and the best place to learn it is at home, at an age when our eating habits are still forming.

Aunts, Uncles, Grandparents, and Other Saboteurs

I shall never forget the distraught parent who asked me what she should do about the mother-in-law who deliberately fed her celiac granddaughter gluten every chance she got. "You're too picky," she said when asked why she would do such a dangerous thing.

"She doesn't believe me, basically," the young mother told me. "She thinks I'm a hypochondriac and doesn't want her granddaughter growing up without foods other children eat. Not only was the child confused and sick, the conflict with his parents was causing the marriage to founder as well.

It just didn't make sense. Why would a grandparent deliberately set out to hurt a child she claimed to love? Careful listening unearthed some clues. The older woman frequently referred to her son and the fact that he has shown no such disease as a youngster. She often made reference to her daughter-in-law's family, their allergies and fussy ways. Was it possible that in denying the baby's condition, she was denying the possibility that she may have had a role in it?

On a wild hunch, I suggested that mother and daughter sit down and together write Grandma a letter. In it, they would assure the older woman that it was okay to be allergic to gluten; that it wasn't any different than being unable to eat sesame seeds like Grandpa and having to avoid salt as she had to or having asthma or arthritic knees. This was a letter full of love and understanding and it ended with forgiveness. "It's okay if you gave me celiac disease," the child wrote with her mother's help, "because you gave me freckles, too, and beautiful red hair like yours and a funny smile. If it weren't for you I wouldn't have my mommy and daddy and grandpa, too."

I received a letter from the mother some weeks later. The mother-in-law had phoned in tears. "I'm so sorry," she sobbed. "I feel so guilty, I didn't realize what I was doing."

We get all our good qualities from our families, as well as our weaknesses. We can't control what we pass along, but sometimes we compensate by refusing to see. Sometimes all it takes is love and being told it's all right.

Another young couple decided to raise their little boy on the macrobiotic diet. Little Aaron, who is also a celiac, has never tasted cow's milk. Not only that, he's never eaten meat or cheese, or has he had any white sugar in his three years of life. His favorite snacks are homemade brown rice treats and gluten-free cookies sweetened with fruit juice. He is the rare toddler who is partial to greens and tofu. His father is allergic to sugar and milk and his mother is so sensitive to dairy that she breaks out in terrible patches of eczema if she eats even the smallest spoonful of cottage cheese.

When it was discovered that Aaron was a celiac, his parents assumed he'd most likely inherit their problems, too, and started him off on a dairy- and sugar-free vegetarian diet. It was a good decision. The absence of sugar has given the tot a serenity not seen in children Aaron's age. As he happily swigs from a bottle of calcium-fortified soy milk and nibbles his scrambled tofu, we have to concede his sweet disposition may indeed give some credence to the argument that carnivorous eating begets carnivorous behavior.

But alas, no family, not even a nutritionally balanced macrobiotic one, is an island. Whenever this threesome travels through the Maine woods to Grandma and Grampy's house, trouble follows. The grandparents support their grandson's gluten-free diet, but think it's ridiculous and dangerous to raise a vegetarian baby and offer ice cream, candy, and chocolate milk every chance they get. Worse, they do it behind his parents' backs. This not only makes the child sick, fussy, difficult, sleepy, and confused, it makes his father and mother extremely angry.

"They eat like animals," says the young mother.

"They're killing themselves," growls Dad, "and they're trying to take us down with them."

"What do they eat?" I ask.

"Steak and mashed potatoes and bacon and eggs," the couple replies, their disgust plain.

"They think they're doing us a big favor by offering us a bowl of over-cooked vegetables." The husband shrugs.

I put the question delicately. "Have you ever served them meat at your house?"

"Of course not," they answer, horrified.

"Well, I don't drink," I counter. "Does that make it all right not to offer a glass of wine to my guests?"

They frown, not wanting to, but getting my point.

"Maybe you should," I suggest. "If you showed some respect for their food, they might not feel so threatened and do the same for you. Besides, would it kill you to cook a free-range chicken or fry an organic egg?"

Most families mean well. But when they feel judged, as these folks did, they dig in their heels and become saboteurs. Not because they're evil or they want to see their grand-babies sick, but because their way of life is being threatened. All they see is what they're doing wrong. They're made to feel unhealthy, outdated, politically incorrect, irrelevant, and old-fashioned. Instead of telling their children they're being self-righteous, rigid, and rude, they go underground. Validating themselves becomes more important than considering their children. This is called passive-aggressive behavior, and no matter that Ghandi glorified it when he kicked the British out of India, it's destructive and unnecessary.

Sometimes the solution is as easy as knowing that it's not about winning. It's about the other person's point of view, about simply being kind.

My friends now serve Grandma and Grampy chicken and apple pie (they just don't mention that it's the hormone-free, organic variety) and I hear the grandparents are becoming quite adept at making gluten-free tofu sandwiches for family picnics. The last time I looked, they were keeping a sharp eye on anyone who might inadvertently give little Aaron white sugar.

There will always be people who will pooh-pooh the importance of your child's diet. These are the same ones who pass the cheese plate to Uncle Louie who just had bypass surgery. Sometimes they do it because giving special treatment to other people is an emotional impossibility (if you're special, I must not be). And sometimes it's because they're just too selfish or lazy to bother. Scratch a little beneath the surface and you may find out there's a real fear of failing, so nothing is done at all. How you deal with family members really depends on how important they are to you and your family's well-being.

In most cases, an old-fashioned family meeting will do the trick. Gather your clan around you, and explain the seriousness of the problem. Offer comments from your child's doctor and pass out copies of articles on pediatric celiac. Then ask for their support in seeing to it that their nephew, cousin, grandchild gets no rude surprises while in their company. Do it as soon as your child is diagnosed, so the conversation does not coexist with an emotionally loaded holiday like Thanksgiving, Christmas, or Passover. Do give copies of the gluten-free diet to all parties. A family letter is good, too. One family I know made copies of their child's finger painting and sent it out as a holiday card with a little explanation tucked inside. Finally, a use for those "Dear friends and family . . ." we all get at the holidays.

Do send relatives a supply of gluten-free foods for visits. (Yes, it's expensive and worth every penny to see the smile on your baby's face when he's served his favorite foods at Grandma's house. It also gives them an easy way to re-order without you.) In fact, buy them a copy of this book to refer to about where to order from, as many have done with delicious success. In other words, help your family help you.

What if, despite your best efforts, the family does not take your child's diet seriously? You have no choice. You must make it brutally clear that they will not be welcome in your home, nor will you visit theirs, if they insist on ignoring the ground rules. It's surprising how tough you can be when your child's health hangs in the balance, tougher even than when it's you. Be firm and see how quickly family members get the message.

Playdates and Other Danger Zones

Hard as it is to believe, there are parents who will not invite your child to a party because making something special is too much work. Worse, there are parents who will break a playdate when they get wind of special requirements.

Sadly, an increasingly stressful and insensitive world has made this kind of bad behavior commonplace.

Adults in positions of power can be also cruel to children as a way of fighting with parents who make their jobs difficult. I would not advise threatening the dietician, camp counselor, teacher, or principal with lawsuits and other punishments as a way to getting them to take your child's requirements seriously. More likely than not, the opposite effect is achieved. Better to use some honey. Make it easier for the school dietician by offering to design gluten-free menus once a week or once a month. Give out the CSA/USA booklet, *Your Student Has Celiac Disease*. Post your phone number and e-mail address on the back for consultation. Offer to supply foods that can be kept in the school freezer. And don't forget nonedible supplies like crayons and finger paints and play dough little ones are forever putting in their mouths. Check out what brands the school uses and supply substitutes, if necessary.

In social situations, the key is letting other parents know that accidental ingestion of gluten could have serious consequences for your child without making people afraid to host him. Volunteer to supply pizza shells or cupcakes for birthday parties, picnics, and outings. When your child is invited somewhere, send a friendly e-mail thanking the parent for the invitation and take the opportunity to explain your child's diet. This is the time to offer to make something and be available for questions when menus are being planned. Never ask another parent to do something you are not willing to do for her child.

Conversely, when your youngster has a friend over for a playdate, always ask about his special requirements, if any. Always serve your child's special foods and make it really special. It's hard enough to have to say "no thank you" in someone else's house, you shouldn't have to do the same in yours. Yes, I know special foods are expensive, but your child's social standing and sense of well-being is worth it. Serve gluten-free pizza, sandwiches, make up a special cookie mix, and let all the kids get in on the act. The idea is to raise a child who believes everyone wants to eat her special food not the other way around.

Halloween

In the contract between parent and child, telling the truth is the Holy Grail of relationships. However, in the name of love and concern, a parent can always find a little wiggle room, especially if the benefits far outweigh the fib. There is no better time to invoke your right to tell a little white lie than on Halloween, where a well-meant treat can turn into a nasty trick for your gluten-challenged vampire, fairy princess, or denizen of Harry Potterdom.

Put yourself in Spider Man's tights. You're standing there in your mask and cape, looking just like the real thing, when the door opens and you shout "Trick or treat!" with the other kids. You offer your bag and in go all sorts of goodies, only to be confiscated when you get home. Or worse, you're left standing on the doorstep in your tutu while everybody gets candy and you get a lousy banana or a lollipop.

What's a parent to do?

Wave your own magic wand and play a trick on your child.

Before the big night, make up a big batch of your child's favorite gluten-free treats. Pay a sneak visit to the neighbors and give them each a sealed bag clearly marked with your child's name. When your child rings the doorbell, they've got a safe treat to put in your baby's goodie bag.

And remember your little munchkin will be in costume and may not be recognized by the neighbors. So don't forget a name tag. Cross your fingers behind your back and tell him pirates did this when they were raiding ships to avoid confusion. You get the picture. When he or she is thirty-three, you can tell your darling celiac the truth about how you put on sunglasses and a wig and crept around to the neighbors with a bag of gluten-free tootsie rolls.

I'm not kidding, there is such a thing. A few years ago, the folks at Miss Roben's circulated a gluten and dairy-free recipe for what they called Mock Tootsie Rolls, from a clever, but long-forgotten source.

Mock Tootsie Rolls

1 cup clover honey
1 teaspoon GF vanilla or ¼ teaspoon vanilla extract
2 cups cocoa powder
1½ cups milk substitute
1 cup confectioners' sugar

1. Microwave honey for 25 to 30 seconds on high. Do not allow honey to overheat and boil.

2. In a large bowl, combine honey and all other ingredients and continue to blend until mixture forms a soft, smooth ball. This will take a *long* time and while it may seem that more liquid is needed, resist the urge to add it.

3. Roll the blended taffy into log shapes and wrap in paper to resemble the real McCoy.

This is where the fun starts. You can call the Tootsie Roll people, tell them what you're doing and ask to buy some of their papers. But don't get mad if they refuse. Think of the lawsuits. Some nut makes a strychnine-laced version and passes it off as theirs.

You can also wash and reuse the original wrappers for your little switcheroo. (Now there's an excuse to avoid the Town Watch committee: "I'd love to, but I'm washing Tootsie Roll wrappers. . . .")

If you're going to be doing this often, you can go to a candy maker's supply house and buy a bunch of wax paper wrappers (maybe to share with your support group). Or, you can just get some candy paper and decorate it yourself. Call them *Ma's Famous Taffy Rolls* or *Tootsie Wootsies*.

Of course, you can invent a new tradition, the annual appearance of the gluten-free fairy perhaps. Ask an uncle or family friend to arrive in costume and transform all unsafe treats into gluten-free ones. Naturally, this requires that you supply said safe treats before the big switch, and it's wise to pick a fairy who's good at sleight of hand, is a bit theatrical, and doesn't mind wearing something silly.

If you do have a Halloween party to avoid the dangers of going door to door, make sure all the treats are gluten- and lactose-free, depending on your child's particular restriction. One well-known chef asked what kind of party her kids wanted and they said a cocktail party. Everybody dressed like grown-ups and, even better, acted like them (big lessons here about how we sound to our children). They sipped juice "cocktails" from martini glasses while grown-ups dressed as waiters tended bar and served the children canapés from trays. Eloise couldn't have done it better.

A party for pets is good, too, if you can stand the ruckus and all that hair. Another great idea is a Hollywood movie premiere party. Roll a red carpet down the front walk and let all the kids dress up as their favorite star or movie character. Rent a kleig light to sweep the sky. Let each parent wear a chauffeur's cap and drive each guest to your house (some will actually rent a limousine for the night). Interview each child as he or she arrives and film the event for posterity. Keep the fun going inside with prizes for best costume, best imitation, best performance, etc. Go to a trophy shop and buy some Oscar look-a-likes for the prizes.

There's always the haunted house tour, but these places may give your child some unsafe goodies, so why not transform your own house into a spooky one? Change all the light bulbs to eerie red or purple. Hang a "body" from the shower nozzle. Put a monster in a closet. Make a tape of something being dragged, like a chain, a bureau door slamming, a squeaky screen door, spooky voices, etc., and play it as background. Serve "eyeball" soup, wolf's bane, witch's brew (a little dry ice will make a punchbowl smoke). Go to a magic shop and get fake blood, cobwebs, fright wigs, a disembodied hand to put in the dishwasher or in the bathroom sink.

Obviously, the haunted house party is for older children, and not for toddlers who are prone to nightmares. Bigger kids will love it though, and the gorier the better.

Granted, this is a lot of trouble to go to, but Halloween is a big deal these days. You don't want your little monster to miss out just because of gluten. Besides, you're not just giving him something safe to eat for trick or treat. You're teaching a lesson in resourcefulness, magic, and love. Enough to last a lifetime.

A Word about Perfection

It's exhausting raising any child, much less one with a severe diet restriction. Here's the truth. Mother and fatherhood (let's face it, mothers, even working ones, still do most of the work) is too huge a job to do well all the time. Nobody has boundless energy; nobody can handle every situation, every time. Nevertheless, the myth of perfection haunts you. You drank a cup of coffee or a glass of wine during pregnancy. You forgot to play Chopin piano concertos or read Shakespeare's sonnets to her *in utero*. You let a phone call interrupt your child's dissertation on *The Stinky Cheese Man*, thus cutting short a career on the stage. Other parents seem to do all the right things, so how come you're so busy you can't even find your shoes?

I'm not suggesting that you should lower your standards. Of course, you are always going to protect your child from gluten in any form, work hard to keep day-care workers, teachers, dieticians, and other parents informed and on your child's side. Of course, you'll always try to be the best parent you can be.

But if you expect to raise a well-adjusted adult, one who sees the pursuit of perfection as the destructive folly it is, someone who sees rules not as ironclad but as flexible, bendable boundaries, you have to see things that way yourself.

It's okay . . .

to make eggs for dinner when you're too tired to cook anything else.

to stay in your pajamas until lunch time.

to cancel a playdate because you're too tired to get her there.

to blow off homework until after a walk in the park.

to let him stay up late because you got home from work late and wanted to play.

to fib about the time to get her to go to sleep early.

to create a diversion while you talk on the phone.

to make up a faster ending to a bedtime story because you want to go to bed, too.

When I was a child, my mother and I walked in freshly fallen snow the moment it stopped falling. Even if was two o'clock in the morning, she'd wake me up, bundle me into my snowsuit and take me into a world that was ours alone. This is one of the most vivid memories I have of her—muffled sound, crystalline white, softly swirling flakes, just the two of us wrapped in cotton batting, gleeful in our mittened abridgement of the rules.

When I was a parent myself, I asked my mother how she never lost her sense of play.

"Didn't you know?" She smiled.

"Know what?" I asked.

"That you taught me as much as I taught you."

Home Plate

Some foods make you fat.
Some foods make you thin.
Some foods taste so good,
They just make you want to grin.

By all means, teach your celiac to cook. The more participation, the more fun, the better your chances are of getting your little one to eat. Janet Rinehart of the Houston CSA chapter offers the following advice from the *Houston Chronicle*. First and foremost, make sure the recipe you choose is appropriate for the age level of your child. Read the recipe all the way through and make sure you have all the ingredients and equipment on hand, then lay it all out on the counter. Calculate how much time the job will take, including cooling time. Ask yourself if it will be finished for supper. Wash your hands. If you stop in the middle and pet the dog, wash your hands again. Ditto for touching raw meat, chicken, eggs, etc. Have towels at the ready—one for wiping up spills, the other for hand washing. Make sure everything is child height. Step stools come in handy here.

If the recipe calls for an herb, teach your child to learn its smell. Ditto for cheese. Decide if you like mild, medium, or sharp. Be patient. Of course, it's easier to do it yourself, but perfection isn't the point here. Explain as you go. Be part of the team. Whatever you do, don't yell. Even if the potholder catches on fire and the dog runs off with a chicken leg, laugh, fix, and laugh some more. Remember the only way to learn is by making mistakes. Wisdom, indeed.

And while we're on the subject of kids and food, let's face it. There isn't much a kid likes to begin with. Anything green, red, yellow, blue, beige, or gray, squishy fishy, spicy, smelly, dicey, ricey, cheesy, gooey, remotely unusual or not an Oreo cookie is greeted with suspicion and considered "yucky."

When you consider that the level of dining experience of the average grade-schooler is usually limited to cookies and milk, macaroni and cheese, peanut butter and jelly sandwiches, and the occasional Happy Meal, you begin to see the special difficulties of satisfying the gluten-intolerant palate.

In fact, it would not be an exaggeration to say that the smaller the child, the bigger the problem. The reason for this is simple. Adults can and do experiment. Children can't and won't for at least another fifteen or twenty years.

There's quite a bit you can do to ensure that your little one not only eats well but eats just like the other kids. If you do it well, one day you may even find your offspring has traded one of your creations for a set of stickers or the latest video game. On the following pages are a few tried-and-true, kid-tested recipes to start you off.

A Twice-Baked Teething Biscuit

I am told when my mother wasn't looking, my grandmother rubbed whiskey on my gums to ease the pain of a tooth cutting through. This gluten-free rusk is the perfect solution for a teething baby's justifiable bad mood. It was developed by Joe Garrera, master baker and recipe consultant to more than one of our favorite gluten-free bakeries. With Chef Garrera's compliments, it's just what the doctor ordered for a celiac's first tooth. The secret is letting the biscuit cool and dry thoroughly before baking a second time. For uniform shape, pipe the dough through a #8 pastry bag without a tip.

Makes 3 dozen biscuits

12	large eggs
1¾	cups vegetable oil
2	cups sugar
5	cups gluten-free baking mix
5	teaspoons baking powder
3	teaspoons gluten-free vanilla extract

1. Preheat oven to 375 degrees. At low speed in electric mixer, mix eggs, vanilla, and oil. Add sugar gradually and mix until sugar is no longer grainy.

2. In a separate bowl, mix baking mix and baking powder together. Add mixture to egg, sugar, and oil mixture, beating at low speed until a thick, but pipe-able, batter develops.

3. Pipe through #8 pastry bag with a 1-inch hole without tip onto parchment-lined cookie sheets about 3 inches apart.

4. Bake 14 to 16 minutes or until golden. Cool 15 to 20 minutes and slice into desired widths.

5. Turn oven down to 250 or 275 degrees and bake biscuits another 15 to 20 minutes. Cool completely.

GLUTEN-FREE BAKING MIX

6	cups white rice flour
3½	cups potato starch
1¼	cups tapioca flour
6	teaspoons xanthan gum

Sift together all ingredients two to three times and use in place of wheat flour. This works well for cookies, cakes, biscotti, and as a thickening agent. Store remaining mixture in a sealed tin for other baking jobs.

Cornmeal Porridge with Dried Fruit

Kay Thompson's irrepressible character Eloise always said, "You have to eat oatmeal, or you'll dry up. Everybody knows that." Yes, there are lots of gluten-free cold cereals and toaster waffles, but the way to start a special day, as we've all been taught, is with a hot breakfast.

Save this hearty and healthy porridge for a cold and stormy, yellow-slicker, stick-to-the-ribs kind of day, then send them out to the school bus. If time is just too precious for a weekday whisking, save this cozy treat for a snowy Sunday morning. It should go without saying that this is the ideal meal to serve two teddy bears on a picnic.

This wonderful and classic porridge comes courtesy of *Gourmet* magazine.

Serves 2

2   tablespoons golden raisins
½   cup yellow cornmeal
¼   teaspoon salt
½   cup milk or gluten-free milk substitute, plus additional to pour into cereal
1   tablespoon unsalted butter, halved
8   dried apricots, cut into small pieces
    Light brown sugar or maple syrup

1. In a small bowl, cover the raisins with cold water and let them stand for 10 minutes. In a medium saucepan, whisk together the cornmeal, ½ cup cold water, and the salt until the mixture is smooth. Add 1½ cups boiling water and the ½ cup milk in a slow stream, whisking all the time.

2. Cook the mixture over a pan of simmering water, stirring often for 10 to 15 minutes, or until the liquid is absorbed and the porridge is thickened.

3. Divide the porridge between two bowls and top it with the butter, the apricots, and the raisins that have been drained of their water. Serve the porridge with sugar or maple syrup and the additional milk to taste.

Blondies

Once upon a time, in the original *Against the Grain*, I nicknamed Beth Hillson's son Jeremy "Kid Cookie." Time flies when you're gluten-free. Now he's a handsome, well-adjusted, and super-bright college student. No doubt there'll be some separation anxiety on both sides, but no freshman care packages from home will be quite like his. Who knows, maybe these blondies will help him meet one of his own—for study dates, of course. They'll pretend to be blasé about these, but that's what they do at this age. When you're not looking they'll devour every morsel. Speaking of not looking . . . sneak one before you break out the bubble wrap.

Makes 16 squares

¾ cup soy flour
¼ cup potato starch
¼ cup cornstarch
¾ teaspoon baking powder
½ teaspoon salt
½ teaspoon xanthan gum
1 stick (8 tablespoons) unsalted butter, softened
1 cup firmly packed light brown sugar
2 eggs
1 teaspoon gluten-free vanilla extract
¾ cup toasted pecans
½ cup semisweet chocolate chips

1. Preheat oven to 350 degrees. Coat a 9-inch square pan with vegetable spray.

2. In a small bowl, stir together soy flour, potato starch, cornstarch, baking powder, salt, and xanthan gum. Reserve.

3. In a medium bowl, beat butter and brown sugar until light and fluffy. Add eggs and vanilla; beat well.

4. Add dry mix and stir to thoroughly combine. Fold in pecans and chocolate chips. Spread evenly into prepared pan.

5. Bake 35 to 40 minutes or until a toothpick inserted into the center comes out with a few moist crumbs sticking to it. Allow to cool completely in pan before cutting into 16 squares.

Rice Pudding

Christina Pirello, whole foods chef and Emmy Award–winning host of the cooking show *Christina Cooks*, proves silky smooth nursery food can be as soul-satisfying as it is good for little ones. This, from *Christina Cooks: Everything You Wanted to Know about Whole Foods but Were Afraid to Ask* (HP Books) is mild enough for a child's budding palate and memorable enough to become a family favorite.

6 to 8 servings

- 4 cups gluten-free vanilla soy milk
- 1 cup almond milk
- 1 cup arborio rice (do not rinse)
- ⅔ cup maple syrup
- 1 teaspoon pure vanilla extract
  Generous pinch of sea salt
- ¼ cup dried currants
- ¾ teaspoon ground cinnamon, plus an extra pinch
- ½ teaspoon ground cardamom
- ½ teaspoon ground nutmeg
- ⅛ teaspoon ground allspice
- ½ cup slivered almonds, toasted
- 3 tablespoons gluten-free granulated sweetener

1. Combine the soy milk, almond milk, rice, maple syrup, vanilla, and salt in a heavy saucepan over medium heat. Cook, stirring constantly, until the mixture boils. Stir in the currants, ¾ teaspoon cinnamon, the cardamom, nutmeg, and allspice; reduce heat to low and cook, covered, stirring often, until the rice is creamy and the pudding thickens, about 1 hour.

2. Place the almonds, pinch of cinnamon, and sweetener in a hot skillet over medium heat and pan-toast just until the almonds are coated. Transfer to a small bowl to cool and set aside.

3. Spoon the pudding into individual bowls or dessert cups and sprinkle with the almonds.

"No More Tummy Aches" Cupcakes

Isabel O'Brian, the heroine of my illustrated children's book, *No More Cupcakes & Tummy Aches*, is convinced that if she doesn't have a birthday cake, she'll never grow up. And if she never grows up, she'll never be tall enough to be a ballerina. What's a celiac parent to do? Bake these Happy Birthday cupcakes with icing as pink as a ballet slipper created by Lee Tobin, a celiac himself and mastermind behind the Whole Foods Market Gluten-Free Bakehouse, and prove to your darling that happy endings aren't only found in storybooks.

The secret to these pretty golden yellow cupcakes is egg yolks. Bright raspberry puree gives the icing its pretty pink color. For a wonderful birthday party, light a candle in each one and let all the children make a secret wish. For those tummies that are lactose intolerant as well, Chef Tobin has offered a dairy-free variation.

Makes about a dozen cupcakes

1½   cups rice flour
1   cup potato starch
½   cup tapioca starch
1   tablespoon plus 1 teaspoon baking powder
1½   teaspoons xanthan gum
½   teaspoon salt
6   eggs yolks
1   cup milk
2¼   teaspoons vanilla
1½   sticks unsalted butter, at room temperature
1½   cups sugar

CUPCAKES
1. Preheat oven to 350 degrees.
2. Combine rice flour, potato starch, tapioca starch, baking powder, xanthan gum, and salt in one large bowl. Set aside. Combine egg yolks, milk, and vanilla in a separate bowl.
3. In a stand mixer or with a hand mixer, on medium speed, cream the butter with the sugar until light and fluffy, 2 to 3 minutes. Add, alternately, the wet and dry ingredients, scraping down the sides of the bowl with a spatula and mixing well to thoroughly combine ingredients.
4. Fill cupcake tins ⅔ full, and bake for approximately 25 minutes, or until golden brown and springy to the touch.
5. When cool, cupcakes can be removed from pan and frosted.

RASPBERRY FROSTING
    One 16-ounce box confectioner's sugar
       1 stick unsalted butter, at room temperature
       2 tablespoons milk
  2 to 4 tablespoons raspberry purée (see below)

1. Combine the confectioner's sugar and the butter in the mixer bowl on low speed.

2. Scrape down sides of the bowl with a spatula, and add the milk.

3. Continue mixing, adding raspberry purée to taste. (More milk and/or puree can be added as desired to achieve the frosting consistency you prefer.)

PURÉE
    One 12-ounce bag of frozen raspberries

1. Thaw the contents of in microwave.

2. When the berries are completely softened, strain through a fine sieve to remove the seeds. Extra purée (and frosting) can be frozen for future use.

Dairy-Free Version
Substitute Spectrum brand palm oil shortening for the butter, and soy or gluten-free rice milk for the cow's milk.

Incredible Edibles

Ask any parent. Not everything that gets into a toddler's mouth is supposed to be there. To be a child is to be tactile, messy, creative, silly, experimental, and free. As long as the medium is gluten-free. Connie Sarros, gifted cookbook author and child at heart herself, makes sure everything that can end up on sticky curious fingers and faces and in mouths is not only safe but fun to play with. The following recipes for play dough, face paint, and bubbles are reprinted with Connie's kind permission, from her bestselling, kid- and parent-friendly *Wheat-Free, Gluten-Free Cookbook for Kids and Busy Adults* (Contemporary Books), and they are sure-fire winners.

Play Dough

This great-tasting play dough can be kept in an airtight container for up to three days.

      1 cup gluten-free peanut butter
     ¾ cup light corn syrup
     ¼ cup honey
    1¼ cups confectioners' sugar
    1¼ cups nonfat dry milk

1. Put the peanut butter, corn syrup, honey, confectioners' sugar, and dry milk in a medium bowl.

2. With your hands, mix the ingredients thoroughly. Do not refrigerate.

Face Paint

Circus clowns, Halloween goblins, rock stars, hobbits, Harry Potter, jugglers, and pirates—face painting is the most fun an imagination can have. Let the kids paint each other or hire a professional to paint them for a memorable party and picture taking. Connie Sarros suggests using her all-purpose flour mixture for this one.

      2 teaspoons solid vegetable shortening
      5 teaspoons corn starch
      1 teaspoon gluten-free flour mixture
    3 to 4 drops of glycerin (available at pharmacies)
           Food coloring

1. Put the shortening, cornstarch, and flour mixture on a large dinner plate. Stir with a small spoon to form a smooth paste. Add 3 to 4 drops of glycerin for a creamy texture.

2. The mixture will now be a wonderful white. You may apply as is. If you wish to color your paint, divide the mixture into several small piles on your dish. Stir 2 drops of food coloring into each pile.

Connie's Gluten-Free Flour Mixture

Makes 5 cups to keep on hand for edible purposes

2½ cups rice flour
 1 cup potato starch flour
 1 cup tapioca flour
 ¼ cup cornstarch
 ¼ cup bean flour
 2 tablespoons xanthan gum

1. Sift the rice flour, potato starch flour, tapioca flour, cornstarch, bean flour, and xanthan gum together in a large mixing bowl.

2. Store the flour mixture in a resealable plastic bag or in the refrigerator until you are ready to bake. If you won't be baking for a week or so, store it in the freezer. When it's time to get cooking, measure the amount you need, and let stand at room temperature for 15 minutes before using it.

Bubbles

Children love bubbles, as do puppies, kittens, and all creatures possessing a playful spirit and a sense of wonder. The clever Ms. Sarros suggests blowing these with a slotted spoon if you don't have an empty spool.

2 cups warm water
 2 tablespoons liquid dish detergent
 1 tablespoon sugar
 1 empty thread spool

1. In a bowl, stir together the water, detergent, and sugar.
2. Dip one end of the spool into the soapy mixture.
3. Blow bubbles through the spool from the dry end.

Bathtub Paint

No more tears at bath time. This toddler-friendly recipe comes to us courtesy of Elaine Monarch and the *Celiac Disease Foundation Newsletter,* Spring 2003. Talk about water color. You may find this one as much fun as your little one. Just make sure you have a handy sponge or rag for quick cleanups, and by all means, involve your bathing beauty in this part. I'm sure Matisse's mother made him clean up, too.

½ cup liquid hand soap
1 teaspoon cornstarch
   Food coloring
   A rag or sponge for cleaning up

1. Mix soap and cornstarch in a container. Pour equally into ice cube trays, each batch making about four cubes. Let your child put drops of food coloring in each cube and experiment mixing the colors.

2. Play to your heart's content. Use the rag or sponge to clean the walls afterward.

Summer Camps: "Hello mudda, hello fadda . . ."

As Shel Silverstein so famously pointed out in his musical postcard from Camp Grenada, summer camp is not always a day at the beach. All parents abandon their children from time to time. Doesn't every well-adjusted adult harbor memories of soggy bunks, one-legged races, s'mores, and crushes on counselors? In *The Lanyard,* Poet Laureate Billy Collins contrasts in perfect deadpan the item every camper makes for his mother against the greater gift of life itself. Guilt is an important part of the camping experience.

Abandoning a celiac child to face paint, ghost stories, and mosquitoes is quite another matter. But thanks to the many groups and associations that organize such things, it is now entirely possible to feel just as guilty sending your darling off to a few weeks of gluten-free marshmallows on a stick as any other parent. Obviously, most of these camps are organized for summer. Some are only a few days, some longer. No matter, they fill up quickly. There's nothing like learning new skills, making new friends, not feeling quite so isolated by your diet, forgetting to brush your teeth, and being homesick with other kids just like yourself.

Bearskin Meadow Camp in California's Kings Canyon National Park is run by the Diabetic Youth Foundation. This camp is primarily for kids with diabetes but is equipped to welcome and cater to kids with celiac disease as well. In addition to children's camps, this organization runs teen and family camps. For dates, rates, and information about financial assistance, www.dyf.org.

Ben's Friends Camp. This annual fling for children and their siblings with CD, ages 8 to 17, is an annual event at Camp Courage in Maple Lake, Minnesota, sponsored by the Twin Cities chapter of R.O.C.K. There is swimming, water-skiing, tubing, canoeing, sailing, fishing, nature hikes, and wagon rides, even an overnight campout. For schedules and rates, call (507) 263-4254, or go to www.couragecamps.org.

Camp Celiac. This annual five-day sleepaway camp for children ages 7 to 16 specializes in canoeing, rowing, swimming, arts and crafts, low ropes, high ropes, group activities, outdoor adventures, and all sorts of fun activities. Follow the Cel-Kids link on the CSA USA Web site to learn more, www.csaceliacs.org.

Camp Kanata, Wake Forest, North Carolina. GIG volunteers prepare gluten-free foods in a separate kitchen while kids learn arts and crafts in the mountains of North Carolina. For more information, www.gluten.net.

Camp Stealth, Vashon Island, Washington. Part of the Campfire Boys and Girls Camp, Seattle's Gluten-Intolerance Group runs this camp in two special sessions for children with CD. Camp information for the following summer is available in early January and places fill up fast. For dates and schedules, go to the GIG Web site, www.gluten.net.

Don't forget to pack the mosquito repellant.

Learn More

Some useful places to find support and information, exchange ideas, and discover you are never alone.

Allergic-Child
Support, information, food advisories, networking, advocacy and chat.
www.allergicchild.com

American Academy of Pediatrics
Physician referrals.
www.aap.org

Cel-Kids of CSA/USA

Support, special events, and summer camps tailored to celiac youngsters and their parents. For a chapter near you, call (877) CSA4CSA or go to www.csausa.com, or see "The Resourceful Celiac," chapter 21.

Crayola

For a list of gluten-free Crayola Products, contact Binney & Smith (800) 272-9652.
www.binney-smith.com

The Feingold Association

Information about the role of foods and synthetic additives in behavior, learning, and health problems.
127 East Main Street, Suite #106
Riverhead, NY 11901
(800) 321-3287
www.feingold.org

Food Allergy and Anaphylaxis Network

Supplies information on common food intolerance, including peanuts.
www.foodallergy.org

Food Allergy Initiative

Advocacy and information on common allergies.
www.foodallergyinitiative.org

GIG

Seattle's Gluten-Intolerance Group sponsors an annual summer camp and special events for parents of children with CD and dermatitis herpetiformis. For information and contacts for an affiliate near you, call (206) 245-6652.
www.gluten.net

Parents of Food-Allergic Kids

Online support.
groups.yahoo.com/group/POFAK

Raising Our Celiac Kids

Founded by Dana Korn, mother of a celiac child, San Diego–based R.O.C.K. provides support, special events, and all manner of small-fry fun. For information about a group near you, go to www.celiackids.com, call (858) 395-5421, or see "The Resourceful Celiac," chapter 21.

Further Reading

No More Cupcakes & Tummy Aches: *A Story for Parents and Their Celiac Children to Share*, by Jax Peters Lowell, illustrated by Jane Kirkwood, foreword by Alessio Fasano, M.D. (Xlibris)

Wheat-Free, Gluten-Free Cookbook for Kids and Busy Adults by Connie Sarros (Contemporary Books)

Just for Fun

The Silly Yak Shirt Company
  Kid-friendly T-shirts
  www.silly-yak.com

PART V

Medical Matters

the doctor will see you now

Never go to a doctor whose
office plants have died.

—ERMA BOMBECK

A fact of modern life: that nice Marcus Welby type who came to your house with a little black bag has gone the way of the Edsel. His replacement (as often as not a she) is overburdened, buried in paperwork, frustrated, frazzled, and threatening to quit medicine altogether. Insurance companies run the show. And the show is not a pretty one. Premiums are rising, services are falling, most good doctors are fed up and an unscrupulous few have contracts with HMOs that actually pay them bonuses for *not* referring patients to the specialists they need. With red tape, co-pays, soaring malpractice premiums, and about fifteen minutes with each patient (if they are to earn enough to make the daily grind worthwhile), it's a wonder the doctor ever gets around to seeing all those people sitting in her waiting room. When you do get in and the physician writes a prescription for this or that, the drug companies put a choke hold on your wallet and take what little money you have left after you've paid your premiums.

It can make a celiac cranky, especially one with interrelated conditions. I've seen it in the support groups I've visited—smoldering, take-no-prisoners, full-tilt boogie, rock-and-roll fury. I don't say this isn't without due cause. Some celiacs have kicked around the medical block for years before being diagnosed. I won't mention any names, but there is a big need for anger management out there.

Before you unleash on your doctor, think of it from her point of view.

Would you give your all to someone who doesn't trust you with a chip the size of Cleveland on her shoulder? Or are you going to give it to someone who's optimistic, open, well-informed, and eager to get well?

Enough said.

Whatever you do, don't waste precious appointment time with a new doctor discussing the old one's missteps. Try not to blame the entire profession for one person's condescension, irritability, or inability to figure you out. If you're fed up with your doctor and haven't found a new one, all I can say is, "Dog bites man once, shame on dog. Dog bites man twice, shame on man." More about that later.

I always give a new doctor my acid test. "Look," I say, "I am a walking medical mystery. I've been ignored, misdiagnosed, hospitalized, trivialized, put-off, pooh-poohed, told to get a good shrink. But I'm stubborn. And smart. And I really need your help. My heart/stomach—you fill in the blank—hurts and what I don't have is another five years to spend on the problem." This is the time to pass along a compliment you've heard about the person along the way. "Dr. So-and-so tells me you are really good at tough cases and I want to work with you to figure it out." The idea is to present a challenge without coming across as belligerent or nutty (the medical term for this is hypochondriacal).

If you're not good at being direct, another strategy is to have your family doctor or internist phone the specialist ahead of your appointment, either to help you get seen faster or to create a sense of urgency about your symptoms. This legitimizes your complaints and lets you off the confrontational hook. I've had great success with this approach recently. At the urging of one doctor, I was seen immediately by another who has a six-month waiting list. By conveying professional concern, my GI doctor got through to a very busy and very smart colleague on my behalf. I got the diagnosis and the medicine I needed a whole lot faster than going it on my own.

Spend a great deal of time finding the right internist or family doctor. This is the person you will see more than any other medical professional. Be clear about what you need and expect from the doctor-patient relationship. If there is the slightest hint of argument or ego, drop that person like a bag of wheat germ and start interviewing other candidates. Book appointments with several other doctors and don't be shy about saying you're "just looking."

Several years ago, I had a medical mystery that stumped many of my doctors and was solved only after a month at the Mayo Clinic in Rochester, Minnesota. I was forced to reconsider my medical relationships upon my return home. Certain people couldn't handle being wrong. Anyone who felt threatened by my Mayo diagnosis was out. Those who were genuinely happy for me

The GI Bill of Rights

1. You have the right to have your symptoms taken seriously.
2. You have the right to insist that diagnostic tests be done, even if the doctor feels they are unnecessary.
3. If you feel you are being denied treatment because of insurance issues, file a complaint with your insurance company and the Better Business Bureau immediately.
4. You have the right to request that a teaching fellow not be allowed to do your procedure.
5. You have the right to a second opinion.

were in. As a result, I now have what the nurses refer to as the "A-list," good and caring people who are happy to consult with one another regarding the management of my health. You can't make an omelet without breaking a few eggs.

You say you need to stay within your insurance company's network? Book appointments with people within that network and use your first impressions to pick the one who is a good fit. Ditto for your GI doctor, and others you need to see with some frequency. If the insurance company keeps you from choosing one of these specialists, ask your internist to refer you to the person on the list who is not only the best one for the job, but the best fit for you— even more reason to develop a good relationship with your primary care physician.

Do's and Don'ts at the Doctor's Office

- **Do remember it's the squeaky wheel that gets the oil.** If you had a test two weeks ago and haven't gotten the results, don't assume everything's peachy because you haven't heard. And don't suffer, either. Phone the office and politely ask (always, always be polite first), "What time today can I expect the doctor to call back with the report?"
- **Do be prepared.** I can't emphasize this enough. If your appointment is tomorrow, get ready today. Even better, give yourself a week or two to make notes. A good way to make the most of every doctor visit and learn more about what your body is or is not doing is to keep a daily

medical journal. List foods consumed, drugs taken, symptoms, bowel movements, twinges, pains, sleep, anything and everything relevant. As you begin to pay attention, patterns will emerge. Those nasty hives or that sharp pain in your gut may mean that you ate too many strawberries or that you shouldn't have polished off a bucket of popcorn in one sitting. Not all diarrhea is malabsorption and not all malabsorption announces itself as diarrhea. Help your doctor to connect the dots.

- **Do stay focused on the big picture.** CD can be protean in its manifestations (as can other conditions), and associated problems can be triggered by a sagging, overstressed or aging immune system. Swollen, painful joints, fatigue, dry eyes, varicose veins, kidney problems, fevers or sweats, dry, cracked skin, and rashes may be unrelated, but they can also be signs of other autoimmune disorders. It's very easy to wander off the path in pursuit of these symptoms. Help your doctor see "the whole you" by being faithful to your journal, by asking questions like "What could this be a symptom of?" Otherwise you could be treated for something that is merely a manifestation of something else.

- **Do read pertinent details from your journal directly to your doctor.** This will help you to avoid forgetting or getting tongue-tied and intimidated by the pressures of a busy office.

- **Do carry a list of all your medications, including vitamins and other supplements, complete with dosages, to every doctor appointment and update your record every time.** It should be standard office procedure for a nurse or a teaching fellow to take this history before your consultation and ask if you are allergic to any medication. I cannot tolerate epinephrine and could have a life-threatening reaction to it. I make sure this is written in huge letters on all my charts, including the dentist's. Taking responsibility can prevent potentially dangerous errors. Always ask if a new medication will work well with existing ones.

- **Do let your doctor know what you expect on this visit.** You'll get more out of a visit if the doctor knows how much time it will take. You will also be seen as considerate with another person's time. Open with "I have six questions today," or, "I've had so many puzzling problems, I've written them all down." A joke may be necessary. "I hope you have six or seven hours today" should elicit a smile and put things in perspective. No matter how you say it, starting out with your agenda will focus your doctor's attention on you, not who needs to be seen next. This technique is so effective, you may find the doctor prompting you, as mine did recently, for the sixth question you forgot to ask.

- **Do ask that a written report be sent to your internist or family practitioner, as well as to you.** This may be the age of specialization, but you've got only one body to work with. The left hand needs to know what the right is doing.
- **Don't complain. Explain.** When issues arise that you feel aren't being covered adequately, photocopy a pertinent article from your support group literature or put your doctor on a mailing list. It's your body. The mechanic should be well informed.
- **Don't let long hours in the waiting room interfere with your consultation.** Always bring some reading material or office work. If the delay is intolerable, don't walk out without letting the doctor know why. It's usually the staff that overbooks and is not considerate of your time, not the doctor. If you do stay and you're simmering about the wait, say so and get it off your chest before you begin your meeting. Chances are the doctor will thank you for your candor and speak to the staff.
- **Don't fall prey to White Coat Syndrome.** This peculiar mix of fear and nervousness can turn patients into quivering blobs of acquiescence. Do try to see your doctor as human and fallible. Visualization can help. Imagine him in his underwear, as a couch potato, passing wind. Picture her struggling with something you do well: ballooning, giving birth to twins, running a marathon, writing a novel.

Which brings me to an important subject . . .

Your Family Doctor, Your Quarterback

When CD and other related problems require treatment by a specialist, like a GI doctor or a rheumatologist or an endocrinologist, your internist or family doctor can be a critical factor in managing them. Never visit a specialist without making sure a copy of the report goes to you and your internist. Nowadays many medical practices charge for photocopying important records and files and some busy practices are so understaffed and overworked they simply do not forward medical records even in response to a physician's request. Getting a copy of a report the day it is presented to you assures no hassles should you decide to seek another opinion, switch specialists, or simply need the information in a hurry. Always ask for a copy of the test results when you see the doctor.

When there is an ongoing situation, visit your family doctor every three to six months or more frequently as the situation warrants and your insurance permits. This way you can discuss the specialist's recommendations, work on strategy together, and know that someone is managing your condition and/or helping to pursue an investigation other than a very busy (read that inaccessable) specialist. Likewise copy your internist on correspondence to your specialist and save a copy for your home file, too.

The more conditions you have, the more important this is. Don't get swallowed up in a medical system that is narrowly defined by specialty and often too shortsighted to see the big picture. You may even be asked to submit to overlapping tests the insurance company may not pay for. You need an interlocutor, a translator, a strategizer, and sometimes even a cheerleader. In short, somebody who can run with the ball.

Use visits with your family doctor to touch base, discuss important findings, decide which avenue to pursue, run down possible leads, and decide what he or she can manage and what must be given over to a specialist. I can't emphasize this relationship enough. When a specialist asks me to submit to a test or a medication I've never heard of, I say "I will check in with Dr. M. and get back to you." If you entrust your care to someone who is smart and likable and who has your interests at heart, you will be repaid with peace of mind.

If you are still uncomfortable being assertive at the doctor's office, ask a family member or close friend to advocate for you, but remember you are giving up your privacy by not taking care of this matter yourself. Choose someone who can ask tough questions without blinking. Resist asking your cousin Arnold whose massive jaw twitches dangerously when things do not go his way.

If it's love at first sight with your doctor, mazel tov. If it's not, never slam a doctor's door without explaining, either in person or in a note, why you are leaving. I would advise against parting shots like, "My brother Vinnie, the malpractice attorney, says . . ."

Better to say, "You seem competent, but I don't feel you are interested in celiac disease" or "I don't feel you are willing to spend enough time with me." And never leave without asking, "Can you recommend someone in your network who can follow me?"

Try to see things from the doctor's point of view. Empathy is what you are asking for from your physician. Give some yourself. Make a comment about how hard it must be to be so overworked and have to follow rules created by insurance company bean counters. Send a thank-you note when something goes well, especially to a person whose specialty doesn't result in a lot of successes. See the person inside the white coat. Be appreciative. And be kind. You'd be amazed at what someone is willing to do for a patient who doesn't see the relationship as adversarial.

A Doctor Checkup

- You can check on virtually any physician's certification in the United States by specialty online via the American Medical Association's Physician Selected www.ama-assn.org.
- Is your physician licensed and board certified? Are there any legal or disciplinary actions taken against him or her? To find out, go to Federation of State Medical Boards at www.fsmb.org. For background and performance, www.physicianreports.com.
- Always ask which hospital your doctor is affiliated with because this is where you'll go if he or she admits you. Check hospital accreditation at the Joint Commission on Accreditation of Healthcare Organizations at www.jcaho.org and click Quality Check.
- Make sure you haven't gotten an appointment with one of the bad apples out there. Public Citizen, a consumer advocacy group listing doctors disciplined by state medical boards and federal agencies in the last ten years, is found at www.questionabledoctors.org.

Realize that sometimes a stony demeanor is a kind of defense. My mother's oncologist was just such a person, a brilliant doctor whose considerable skill was often bested by the cancer he'd made a career of battling. He often had to tell people they didn't have much time.

My mother teased him, told him he ought to take a day off or else he'd get sick and be no help to anybody. She brought him her homemade raspberry jam. I tried to make him laugh, too, but he never cracked. He could not cure my mother's illness, but he found a drug that shrank it down to nothing, giving her four more years with us—good, symptom-free years. By the time the medicine stopped working a heart problem had intervened, and she slipped quietly away. I wrote to Dr. D., not only to tell him that my mother had died but to say that I knew how few thanks he got in his particular line of work, and to express my deep gratitude for those wonderful years of grace he gave her. Well, you know the end of this story. The minute the dour doctor received my letter, he called and we both had a good cry.

Be as human as you want your treatment to be. Who knows? You may even end up with a new friend. You'd be amazed how easy it is to talk to someone you really like.

Ladies and Germs

Some celiacs, especially those of us with serious associated autoimmune conditions like Sjögren's syndrome (see page 378) are particularly vulnerable to germs. If we're not careful, a long wait in a doctor's reception room can make us sicker than we were when we came in.

Look around. Everyone in the room is sick. People are sneezing and coughing with open mouths, spraying germs into the air, which is usually dry and overheated, the perfect medium for spreading bugs. People are blowing their noses, then touching everything around them. And it's not just the patients. A secretary once coughed right into my receipt, then handed it over with the same hand she used to wipe her nose. I asked her to write a new receipt *after* she washed her hands.

How do you avoid getting more than you bargained for? Start thinking like a germ.

Make it a rule never to read a magazine or newspaper in a waiting room. Consider how many sick people have handled that piece of paper. Bring a book or a paper of your own to pass the time. Never sit on a chair that has a discarded tissue on the seat. NEVER pick up a tissue and throw it away.

Try to find a chair in a corner away from the crowd. If that is not possible, check in with the receptionist and tell her you will be in the hall. If the office is willing, ask that you be called on your cell, then go downstairs and have a cup of coffee while you wait.

Try not to use the bathroom. If you must use the facilities, wash your hands carefully and use the paper towel to open the door. Most people think the seat is where the problem lies, but consider the doorknob. Who ever washes a doorknob? If possible, wait until you are called back to where the doctor's offices are and use a toilet not designated for the public.

Keep alcohol wipes in your pocket or purse and use them.

It gets worse when you are sick enough to be admitted to the hospital. In its August 17, 2004, issue, *Time* magazine reports that hospital infections contribute to the deaths of nearly 90,000 patients in the United States each year. A life-threatening bacteria called *C-dificile* commonly affects the elderly with their compromised immune systems. Many times the germ is already on a patient's skin and a needle stick or catheter becomes the vehicle for its swift entry into the body. But more often than not the culprit is a hospital worker who didn't wash his or her hands before touching you. The article goes on to say that hospital staff generally follows the hand-washing rules less than 40 percent of the time. Nurses are more apt to wash than doctors.

So what's a celiac, with a not-so-peak immune system, to do? Do ask any hospital workers who are about to put in an IV or check an incision or do any sort of procedure if they've washed their hands first. If the answer is no, insist that they do so before touching you. Ditto for the person who takes your temperature, blood pressure, or, even more important, your blood in the doctor's office. The trick here is to ask in a nonconfrontational way, maybe even with a little humor: "While you're in the bathroom washing up, would you mind putting a little Ajax in the sink?" Or, if you can't carry something like that off, simply say, "I know I'm weird, but do you mind washing your hands?" Chances are you'll be told you're not weird at all and be thanked for the reminder. The idea is not to turn people off. These are people you want on your side.

Even trickier is asking your doctor if he or she has remembered to wash. The last thing you want to do is strike the wrong note. What I do if I see my doctor hasn't washed up before examining me is to couch my request in the reason for the visit—if I have the flu, I ask with a smile how the patient before me with ebola or SARS is doing and when can I expect to get it. If I'm there for an autoimmune problem with its opportunistic infections, I say something silly like, "If I have to wear a Michael Jackson mask on a plane, you have to wash your hands." Remember that it's all in the delivery. Body language and tone of voice count as much as what you say. A light touch is very important here. The doctor will get your point and be glad you reminded him.

The minute you get home, wash your hands thoroughly.

Testing, Testing, One, Two, Three

If you're reading this book, you may already know you're a celiac. If not, a visit to the doctor may lead to the following blood tests designed to screen for celiac disease and subsequent biopsy. The key here is a gastroenterologist who is familiar with celiac disease and a lab that can interpret the results properly. Remember, to get accurate results, you must be eating gluten.

Blood Tests for CD

These are some or all of the tests your doctor may order:

IgC Antigliadin
IgA Antigliadin
tTG Antigliandin

IgC Tissue Translutaminase
IgA Tissue Transglutaminase
Total IgA

There are also new stool tests said to pick up gluten sensitivity in earlier stages than the blood tests do. Dr. Kenneth Fine of Dallas, Texas, is on the leading edge of this research (www.finerhealth.com), but these tests are not widely accepted by the medical community as yet.

The small bowel biopsy is still the gold standard for a diagnosis of celiac disease. This is a painless procedure conducted under local anesthesia in which the doctor takes a sample of your intestinal villi (fingerlike projections that help a normal intestine absorb nutrients) to examine it for the characteristic flattening and scarring that takes place in response to the insult of gluten. Some people choose not to have this procedure, relying on the results of the blood work for an assumption of celiac disease. Given the fact that the gluten-free diet is for life and the blood work can result in false positives, most GI doctors will press for the definitive biopsy unless there is a reason not to consider it.

Janet Rinehart, chairman of CSA's Houston celiac support group (www .houstonceliacs.org), advises parents in her new patient packet that "children be diagnosed by the blood screening tests plus biopsy taken in the endoscope procedure. It is not sound medical practice or fair to the child to be put on a gluten-free diet without good medical/clinical evidence of gluten sensitivity. If one child is diagnosed in the family, it is an excellent idea for all the others in the family to be screened." She goes on to say, "The antibody blood tests may not be reliable for a child under the age of three, but if the blood tests turn out elevated, there is good evidence to do the endoscope."

Not all parents agree with this advice and face tough diagnostic decisions. All the more reason to consult with a pediatric gastroentolerologist familiar with childhood celiac disease. I do agree that it is unfair to assume a diagnosis. We're talking about the rest of a little person's life here.

My own biopsy was done many years ago, and I've had two more over the course of twenty years, one to confirm healing and the other to rule out a relapse. Now I repeat the blood work as part of my annual GI exam in order to ensure that I am not getting any accidental gluten. It makes good sense. This way you know you are on the gluten-free straight and narrow, and it's comforting to know hidden gluten or any other accidental is not turning up on the radar in any meaningful way.

You do know that it is your responsibility to nag, wheedle, and cajole first-degree relatives (especially those with symptoms) to get tested? Good.

Tests for Associated Conditions

If you've just been diagnosed, it's always wise to spend some time with a registered dietician. Depending on how old you are at diagnosis, it might be years
since you absorbed your vitamins and minerals properly. As a celiac, you may
also be at greater risk for developing certain other disorders (see chapter 16,
"The Seven-Year Itch & Other Associated Conditions"). Talk to your doctor
about making some or all of the following tests part of your annual routine.

CBC or complete blood count
Blood tests to monitor levels of B_{12}, albumin, calcium, vitamin D, magne-
   sium, and zinc
Thyroid functioning
Blood sugar
DEXA or bone density scan

Testing for General Good Health

General health is even more important after you've been sick for a while. Depending on your age, your medical history, and your doctor's inclinations,
other items on the annual checklist may include:

Lipid panel to measure blood cholesterol, including good HDL and bad
   LDL levels
Pap smear
Blood pressure
Mammogram
PSA level and digital prostrate exam
Colon cancer screening
Flu and pneumonia immunizations (when available)
Dental checkups and cleanings
EKG and/or stress echocardiogram of the heart

Define Your Terms

Does your doctor use ten-dollar words when twenty-five-cent ones will do?
Admit it, you pretend you know what the heck he or she is talking about, then
you run home and look it up, only to forget exactly how it was used in the sentence. Even worse, there's no headache like the headache (cephalalgia) you get

trying to make sense of an article on the Internet or in a medical journal where every third word is Greek to you.

Short of carrying a big fat medical dictionary around in your purse or enrolling in a crash course on "med-speak" (that's *after* the class on deciphering the doctor's handwriting), here, with the help of my dog-eared *Mosby's Medical Dictionary*, is a handy translation of some of the common conditions behind the fancy scientific terms that come with an expensive medical education.

Achalisia: A spasm in which the muscle cannot relax, usually the esophagus.

Adenopathy: Swollen glands.

Angina pectoris: Chest pain originating in the heart.

Bruxism: Involuntary grinding or gnashing of teeth.

Cephalalgia: Headache.

Dyspepsia: Indigestion.

Dysphagia: Difficulty swallowing.

Dyspnea: Shortness or breath.

Ecchymosis: A bruise.

Edema: Swelling caused by water retention.

Emesis: Vomit.

Eructation: Belching.

Excipient: A nonmedicinal ingredient in prescription medicine.

Febrile: Having a fever or feverish.

Hyperhidrosis: Excessive sweating (the prefix *hyper* means too much; *hypo* means too little).

Hypertension: High blood pressure.

Hypotension: Low blood pressure.

Intermetatarsal neuritis: Pain and numbness in the toes.

Lesion: Wound, sore or infected patch of skin.

Lipid: Fat.

Myalgia: Muscle pain.

Myocardial infarction: Heart attack.

Nephrotoxic: Poisonous to the kidneys.

Nocturia: Peeing a lot at night.

Oncologist: Doctor who treats cancer.

Onychomycosis: Nail fungus.

Paronychia: Hangnail.

Pityriasis sicca: Dandruff.

Postprandial somnolence: Sleepiness after a big meal.

Rhinitis: Inflammation of the mucous membranes of the nose.

Steatorrhea: Fatty diarrhea common in celiac disease.

Stomatitis: Mouth infection.

Syncope: Loss of consciousness, fainting, blackout.

Pallor: Pale skin.

Paresthesia: Numbness, tingling, or pins-and-needles sensation.

Pathogenesis: The mode of origin or development of a disease.

Pruritus: Itching.

Purpura: Purplish skin discoloration caused by bleeding under the skin.

Purulent: Infection containing pus.

Rhinorrhea: Runny nose.

Tetany: Muscle spasms, twitches, and cramps.

Tinea pedis: Athlete's foot.

Ventilation: Breathing.

Vertigo: Dizziness.

Villi: Fingerlike projections in the intestine involved in CD.

Xerosis: Dry, itchy skin.

Look Who's in the Hospital

Celiac disease rarely requires hospitalization, short of a same-day procedure or two. So why are we talking about hospitals? Because you are human. Celiac tonsils have to come out, as do ruptured appendixes. Babies have to get born, gallbladders removed, and every celiac has to eat, in hospital or not.

According to Webster's, the word *hospitality* is a noun meaning "hospitable treatment, reception, or disposition." One would think such treatment would be dispensed at the hospital. One would think.

The good news is your stay probably won't be long. With insurance companies refusing to let even the frail and the elderly check in the night before a procedure, sending people home with tubes and shunts, staples and things best taken care of by trained professionals, it's a wonder they just don't do surgery in the parking lot. Hard enough to be dignified with a piece of threadbare cotton flapping open in the back, but getting a dinner tray piled high with turkey stuffing and glutenous gravy is enough to make a sick person sicker.

Of course, you packed your phone book, a list of prescription medications, vitamins and supplements, along with dose and frequency, cosmetics, reading material, playing cards, alarm clock, and slippers (with no-slip soles), and a nice robe for hallway strolling. Now that you're a celiac, you can add a restaurant card and/or any one of the support group pamphlets explaining your condition to give to the nurse, to the kitchen, to the dietician, and to the hospital director, if you're so inclined. The fact of the matter is you still may get nothing safe to eat.

Why? Why does the nurse wake you up to give you a sleeping pill? Why are you sent home when you are still sick? Why is the sky blue?

—➤

Okay. Open that overnight bag and add a few gluten-free energy bars, a few slices of gluten-free bread (ask if you can keep it in the fridge at the nurse's station) and a couple of gluten-free heat-and-serve dinners to nuke at the nurse's station (again, ask first). Be considerate. Don't expect to load up their fridge. Have a spouse or a friend bring fresh supplies every day. Oranges, bananas, apples, takeout, and gluten-free snacks are always much better than bland steamed food on a hospital tray.

But you're not in the hospital to eat. You're there to get something taken care of. You won't starve if you order soft-boiled or cooked eggs. These are hard to mess up on as long as they're real. Ask first.

Plain baked potatoes are usually safe, too. Ditto for steamed vegetables. Not tasty, but a safe choice. Most hospital kitchens have cream of rice cereal. And that's not a bad way to go for a few days. Cottage cheese is boring, but it will fill the bill for a short time.

Ask about snacks like applesauce, gluten-free yogurt, and fruit cups. And, of course, there's always room for Jell-O.

Don't assume you have to stick to the spaces allotted on the menu checklists. Write all over them. Make requests. Order ice cream by brand. Ask for extra juice, gluten-free cereal, fruit.

Forget the chips, candy bars, and the Fritos. You're in the hospital, for goodness sake.

Do express your dietary concerns to your doctor. He or she may have some pull with dietician or may be able to arrange a visit from the dietician on duty.

Be patient. The better you are at explaining your diet, the better your chances of getting the kitchen to listen.

Take advantage of the patient advocate in your hospital. This is the one who will express your needs to hospital staff in terms they can understand. Bear in mind, it is this person's job is to help you negotiate all aspects of the hospital experience in a way that doesn't open the hospital up to legal action.

Be the first in your support group to ask that a volunteer bring you gluten-free food. Some of the local groups are considering this wonderful service to members, especially those with no family to assist them.

Rx Meds—Yours or Theirs?

I understand why the hospital insists on giving you their medications. It makes sense for them to control something they could be held accountable for should there be a mistake. If you are determined to take your own drugs to the hospital, ask your doctor to write an order allowing you to do so and bring them in their original bottles (forget the little weekly dispenser). Give your medicine to the nurse with dosage instructions so they are dispensed back to you properly.

If you choose to take the generic version offered by the staff, ask them to look up the ingredients in their pharmacy before giving them to you. Nurse's stations have a reference for the doctor to check before ordering your medication. I recently went over every one of my husband's meds with his cardiologist before a duplicate was given. It was not difficult. It helps to know which brand name and which generic is gluten-free to make the hospital process smoother (see chapter 17, "Rx For Health").

Doctors pop in and out as needed. Understand that the nurse controls everything that happens to you. If the nurse is afraid to feed you because you've made the gluten-free diet sound impossible and dangerous if not complied with to the letter, you may not get any food at all.

Make friends with this person. Bond. Be a good patient and be considerate of someone who is doing the work of six people these days. Be appreciative of special treatment. Like everything else, with few exceptions, you will get back what you give.

Gluten Isn't the Only Accident That Can Happen in the Hospital

With hospital staffs cut down to the bone, more mistakes are happening even in the best institutions. In the old days, when one person did one job, there was a good failsafe procedure and usually a non-sleep-deprived person checking on the residents during a long tour of duty. Someone without a two-day beard was careful to make sure your X rays were right-side up on the light box, so the surgeon didn't take out the wrong kidney or replace a perfectly good knee. There were enough nurses to actually take care of the patients. Today, according to a study by the Washington, D.C., Institute of Medicine, as many as 98,000 people die each year as a result of medical errors. Coffee nerves, no sleep, no back-up.

The best way to protect yourself is to assume nothing is going right. I've already talked about hospital infections and the importance of proper hand washing, but there's much more you can do to minimize your risk than to engage in germ warfare. One of the best ways to defend yourself is to learn how to distinguish between a student, a first-year resident, senior resident, attending physician, and consultants and those lay workers who are often mistaken for medical or nursing personnel. People are supposed to wear name and job identification tags. If you don't see one, ask.

"So what's your job here?" is as good as any opener, offered in a friendly way. Always ask the person in your room what they are about to do. Often, this is enough to make them realize they're on automatic pilot.

True story: when I was hospitalized many years ago for the symptoms of celiac disease, my roommate was a wonderful Italian grandma from South Philly in a cast up to her hip. Like many women of her generation who actually scrubbed their front stoops, she grumbled about our bathroom not being up to her standards. She open her purse, pulled out a bottle of Windex and a spray can of disinfectant, thumped over to the bathroom and started cleaning.

"What happened to your leg," I asked, too weak to get up and help.

She shrugged. "Nothing. I'm here for my gallbladder and they just put me in a cast."

I was incredulous that she let them do it.

Just then two sheepish residents walked into our room. "Mrs. Angelini?" one of them called out nervously.

My roommate stuck her head out of the bathroom.

"I knew you two would be back," she said, thumping over to her bed to let them take off the cast that belonged to another patient.

Always, always, always ask the person who is about to do something to you what exactly he or she is going to do and why it's being done. Ask if your doctor has approved. This focuses an otherwise tired professional. And don't save your questions for the juniors. Ask your surgeon what she's doing, too. If she says, "I'm removing a neuroma [tiny benign nerve tumor, usually caused by wearing high heels] from between your toes," ask her which foot.

I actually did have this procedure done and I folded the good foot under my body before I fell asleep. I was so careful to make sure everyone knew which foot was being cut, the OR nurse teased me mercilessly. "That's right, it's your left," she'd say, winking at the surgeon. I was not at all amused and apparently continued to mutter about this while under sedation.

The moral of the story? Murphy's Law is still is in effect. What can go wrong *will* go wrong.

If you're scared and in pain on the way in and woozy and sleepy afterward, make sure you have someone with you who isn't.

People in the know who don't want to be quoted tell me never to opt for an elective procedure at the end of the week. Something goes wrong and everybody who can help is either swatting tennis balls or on the golf course. Another bad time to schedule anything is late June and early July. That's when the green (in more ways than one) first-year residents show up at the teaching hospitals. Wait until they find out where the defibrillators are.

Are You Still Here?

Sometimes checking *out* of a hospital is as dangerous to your health as checking in. More often than not, the insurance company—not your doctor—decides when you leave the hospital. Or the insurance company overrules your doctor. You don't want to know how many people return to the emergency room after being released the day before. This happened to my husband after his heart attack.

Not a full day after being released from the hospital, he experienced severe chest pain and we wound up in the emergency room waiting for him to be readmitted. Three hours later, I got up and went over the central desk. In the most even tone I could manage after sitting in a hard chair for what seemed like an eternity, I said, "Okay, it's late and I'm tired. I'd like to know whom I need to sue for releasing my husband too soon after his heart attack—the hospital, the doctor, or the insurance company." You can't believe how fast a room materialized. You don't know how many losing fights with bean counters your doctor had before he or she wrote your release order. It's hard to fight every single ruling every time. You have to help your doctor be tough by being tough yourself.

"Am I well enough to go home so soon?" is a valid and important question. It alerts the doctor to the fact that you know the difference between being discharged and being *ready* to be discharged.

For bedside reading on negotiating the finer points of gluten-free hospitalization:

CSA Patient Pamphlets
www.csaceliacs.org

Celiac Disease Foundation
Guidelines for a Gluten-Free
Lifestyle
www.cdf@celiac.org

Gluten Intolerance Group
GIG Hospital Guide
www.gluten.net

A List of Celiac-Savvy Doctors and Medical Centers

The best way to find a doctor in your area who is familiar with celiac disease is to talk to other celiacs. Asking your local support group for a recommendation comes with many benefits, not the least of which is that this person has been vetted by many others in your situation. When you are talking within "the family," you can be candid about personality, location, insurance affiliation, hospital association, etc. My own physician received so many new patient forms with Jax Lowell written in the space reserved for "referring doctor," he just gave up and become the consulting physician for the Philadelphia group.

The good news is that more and more fine doctors are devoting themselves to CD. Centers are opening all over the country, not only for the care and treatment of patients but for research in diagnostic and genetic testing and improving the quality of the gluten-free life. The average time between displaying symptoms and getting to diagnosis is shrinking, and I wouldn't be surprised to learn there's a pill or a patch on the drawing board right now that will render gluten as harmless as house dust. Here are a few of the best people and the best places.

Who's Who

Obviously, this is a partial list, a representative sampling of doctors from around the country. More and more wonderful people are specializing in and treating celiac disease. I have had firsthand experience with only three of these fine professionals, and would trust them with my life. The rest come highly recommended by celiacs themselves and by support groups around the country. All of these physicians are gastroenterologists unless otherwise noted.

Thomas J. Alexander, M.D.
18161 West 13 Mile Road, Suite B-1
Southfield, MI, 48076
(248) 647-4100

Jeffery M. Aron, M.D.
2330 Clay Street, 6th Floor
San Francisco, CA 94115
(415) 600-3700

Craig A. Aronchick, M.D.
Hospital of the University of
Pennsylvania Department of
Gastroenterology
230 West Washington Square, 4th
Floor
Philadelphia, PA 19146
(215) 829-3561

Dorsey Bass, M.D.
Pediatric Gastroenterology and
Nutrition
Lucile Packard Children's Hospital
at Stanford University Hospital
Room 116, MC 5731
Palo Alto, CA 94304
(650) 723-5070

Stuart Berezin, M.D.
Pediatric Gastroenterology
Westchester County Medical Center
Valhalla, New York
(914) 594-4610

David Borislow, M.D.
1260 South Greenwood Avenue,
Suite E
Clearwater, FL 33756
(727) 443-2920

Catherine Petroff Cheney, M.D.
Beth Israel Deaconess Medical
Center
Division of Gastroenterology and
Hepatology
330 Brookline Avenue
Boston, MA 02215
(617) 667-1846

Carl Dezenberg, M.D.
Pediatric Gastroenterology &
Nutrition Associates
3196 South Maryland Parkway,
Suite 309
Las Vegas, NV 89109
(702) 791-0477

Joseph DiAntonio, M.D.
2999 Princeton Pike
Lawrenceville, NJ 08648
(609) 882-2185

Anthony J. DiMarino, M.D.
Chief, Division of Gastroenterology
Director, Jefferson Digestive Disease
Institute
Thomas Jefferson University
Hospital
132 South 10th Street, Suite 480
Philadelphia, PA 19106
(215) 955-2728

David E. Elliot, M.D.
Director, Celiac Disease Clinic
University of Iowa Health Care,
4611 J.C.P.
200 Hawkins Road
Iowa City, IA 52242
(319) 356-4901

Myron Falchuck, M.D.
Gastroenterology at Beth Israel
Deaconess
110 Francis Street, Suite 8E
Boston, MA 02215
(617) 632-8623

Alessio Fasano, M.D.
Associate Professor of Pediatrics
Department of Pediatric
Gastroenterology and Nutrition
Director, Center for Celiac Research,
University of Maryland
22 South Green Street,
Room N5-W70
Baltimore, MD 21201
(410) 328-0812
afasano@umaryland.edu

Kenneth Fine, M.D.
Finer Health Entero Labs
10851 Ferguson Road, Suite B
Dallas, TX 75228
(972) 686-6869
email@enterolabs.com

Charles Gerson, M.D.
80 Central Park West
New York, NY 10023
(212) 496-6161

Gary Gray, M.D.
Professor of Medicine
Stanford University Medical Center
269 Campus Drive, CC SR 3115;
MC 5187
Stanford, CA 94305
(650) 725-6457

Peter H. R Green, M.D.
Director, Celiac Disease Center
Columbia-Presbyterian Medical
Center
161 Fort Washington Avenue
New York, NY 10032
(212) 305-5590
pg11@columbia.edu

Stefano Guandalini, M.D.
Director, University of Chicago
Celiac Disease Program
5839 South Maryland Avenue
MC 4065
Chicago, IL 60637
(773) 702-7593
Michelle Melin-Rogovin, Program
Director

Ivor Dennis Hill, M.D.
Professor of Pediatrics
Doctors Hospital
Medical Center Boulevard
Winston-Salem, NC 27157
(336) 716-3009

Sanford L. Herold, M.D.
University of Pennsylvania Medical
Center
Wright-Saunders Building, Suite 218
39th and Market Streets
Philadelphia, PA 19104
(215) 662-8900
herolds@mail.med.upenn.edu

Stephen Holland, M.D.
1828 Bay Scott Circle, Suite 112
Naperville, IL 60540
(630) 357-4463
www.napervillegi.com

Karoly Horvath, M.D., Ph.D.
Associate Professor of Pediatric
Gastroenterology and Nutrition
University of Maryland
22 South Green Street
Baltimore, MD 21201
(410) 328-0812
khorvath@peds.umaryland.edu

Ciaran P. Kelly
Associate Professor, Harvard
Medical School
Director, Celiac Center at Beth Israel
Deaconess Medical Center
330 Brookline Avenue, DA-601
Boston, MA 02215
(617) 667-1272
ckelly2@bidmc.harvard.edu

John Kerner, M.D.
Pediatric Gastroenterology
Lucia Packard Children's Hospital
Stanford, CA 94304
(650) 723-5070

Allen M. Lake, M.D.
Maryland Pediatric Group
10807 Falls Road, Suite 200
Lutherville, MD 21093
(410) 321-9393

Keith Laskin, M.D.
Main Line Gastroenterology
Paoli Memorial Medical Building 3,
Suite 333
255 West Lancaster Avenue
Paoli, PA 19301
(610) 644-6755

Alan Leichtner, M.D.
Division of Pediatric GI/Nutrition
The Children's Hospital of Boston
300 Longwood Avenue, Hennewell
Ground
Boston, MA 02115
(617) 355-6058

Mark DeMeo, M.D.
Associate Professor of Medicine
Rush Presbyterian St. Luke's Medical
Center
1653 West Congress Parkway
Chicago, IL 60612
(312) 942-5861

Joseph Murray, M.D.
Director GI Center, Mayo Clinics
Mayo Building West 19
200 First Street S.W.
Rochester, MN 55905
(507) 284-2511
joseph.murray@mayo.edu

L. Henry Pham, M.D.
2206 East Villa Maria
Bryan, TX 77802
(979) 776-4600

Michelle M. Pietzak, M.D.
Chidren's Hosptial of Los Angeles
Division of Pediatric
Gastroenterology, MS 78
4650 Sunset Boulevard
Los Angeles, CA 90027
(323) 669-2181
mpietzak@chla.usc.edu

Cynthia Rudert, M.D.
Pediatric Gastroenterology
555 Peachtree Dunwoody Road,
Suite 312
Atlanta, GA 30342
(404) 943-9820

William Santagelo, M.D.
Baylor University Medical Center
3600 Gaston Avenue, Suite 809,
Barnett Tower
Dallas, TX 75246
(214) 818-0948

Michael Shapiro, M.D.
Medical Plaza II, Suite 101
10290 North 92nd Street
Scottsdale, AZ
(480) 657-3400

Ted Stathos, M.D.
Rocky Mountain Pediatric
Gastroenterology
9224 Teddy Lane, Suite 200
Lone Tree, CO 80124
(303) 869-2121

Theodore Stein, M.D.
Cedars Sinai Medical Group
200 North Robertson Boulevard,
Suite 300
Beverly Hills, CA 90211
(310) 385-3506
steint@csmns.org

John R. Stroehlein, M.D.
Anderson Cancer Center
1515 Holcomb Boulevard, Unit 436
Houston, TX 77030
(713) 794-5073

Jerry S. Trier, M.D.
Brigham & Women's Hospital
75 Francis Street
Boston, MA 02215
(617) 732-5824

Ritu Verma, M.D.
Section Chief, Gastroenterology
and Nutrition
Children's Hospital of Philadelphia
Philadelphia, PA 19104
(215) 590-1680

Wilfred Weinstein, M.D.
UCLA Digestive Disease Center
10833 Le Conte Avenue
Los Angeles, CA 90095
(310) 825-1597

Leonard B. Weinstock, M.D.
10287 Clayton Road, Suite 200
St. Louis, MO 63124
(314) 997-0554
www.specialistsingastro.com

Learn More

For more celiac-friendly doctor referrals in your area, contact your local or national support group (see chapter 21, "The Resourceful Celiac").

Antibody Testing

IMMCO Lab/Diagnostic Testing
www.immocodiagnostics.com

Prometheus Laboratories
5739 Pacific Center Boulevard
San Diego, CA
(888) 423-5227
www.prometheuslabs.com

Web Sites

Information gathering can never replace a face-to-face meeting with your doctor, but it can make that meeting more productive. For general medical information from reliable resources, try the following Web sites:

MayoClinic, www.mayoclinic.com. This site offers the latest medical news and health articles from the venerable Rochester, Minnesota, institution. Sign up for e-mail on subjects of interest.

Medlineplus, www.medlineplus.gov. This government-operated site (U.S. National Library of Medicine) offers encyclopedic background on all diseases and conditions, including definitions of medical terms and referrals to organizations that deal with specific illnesses. It is also helpful for searching for the top doctors in each field.

WebMD, www.webmd.com. This easy-to-navigate site guides you from general information to more specific links to possible causes and treatments.

Apples are gluten-free. One a day may keep the you-know-who away.

the seven-year itch &
other associated conditions

If you want to make God laugh, tell him your plans.

—*Peters family saying*

Many years ago, my husband began to exhibit bizarre personality changes and abrupt mood swings. He knocked about from endocrinologist to psychiatrist to internist for years, each time getting a piece of the puzzle, but never the entire picture. In the age of specialization, no one looked at the whole person, only at his or her area of expertise, to solve the mystery of why an otherwise gentle human being had turned suddenly into an irrational and angry person. As many men do, the patient submitted to a few cursory tests in each discipline, then gave up in disgust (this, too, was a symptom). In the end, it was decided hypoglycemia or low blood sugar caused the moods, a condition he had suffered from for many years. No one had the time or the inclination to coddle him into going further.

I *did* have the time and I had the best reason in the world, so I turned to the *Merck Manual*, my trusty, dog-eared physician's reference. It was slow-going, painstakingly slow. I, too, wanted to quit many times—mind-numbing medicalese is not my idea of relaxing bedtime reading—but I slogged on. After referencing and cross-referencing, comparing his symptoms to any number of conditions and coming to many dead ends, I narrowed my suspicions down to early senile dementia (not likely at the age of forty), or to a brain tumor in the temporal lobe where behavior, among other important functions, resides. Presented with the information I'd gathered, my husband's doctor ordered a CT scan (MRI was not readily available then). Soon after, he placed us in the capable hands of the brilliant and brave surgeon who removed from my husband's head an especially pernicious and slow-growing brain tumor called an astrocytoma. That was twenty years ago last month. Would my husband be here today if I hadn't done the homework? We'll never know.

While it's true there is no substitute for good medical care and there are many dangers involved in self-diagnosis, nobody has a better reason for sticking with a mystery than you or the person who loves you. Love helps, but it is dogged, pit bull-on-your-pant-leg tenacity that gets the job done. Especially now, when all you can reasonably expect is fifteen or twenty minutes of the doctor's attention. You can hope for a referral to the specialist you know you need, or even better, a good clinic like Mayo, Cleveland, or Johns Hopkins, but there are no guarantees. Many of today's doctors are too overworked, over-scheduled, and often too stressed to connect the dots. Like it or not, this is now your job.

As I surf around the various celiac bulletin boards and chat sites online, one newly diagnosed celiac complains of chest pain and wonders if the drug company has added gluten to the formula for her prescription medicine. Another writes that "I'm tired all the time and I have a rash across my nose and cheeks." She struggles to remember every microscopic ingredient of every meal in the last month. While it's true that some people react in odd ways to hidden grains—bones ache, eyes sting, energy levels lag, joints hurt, skin erupts and blisters, glands swell, mouths ulcerate—gluten isn't always the culprit.

Yes, I know it's overwhelming to have to tackle another mystery, but the simple fact is CD predisposes us to other immune conditions, diseases, and syndromes, many quite difficult to diagnose even by the experts. It's important to know the symptoms and signs of these associated problems, some of which develop over months and sometimes years, while others are immediately obvious. It's also crucial to know what kind of specialist to seek and what kinds of tests to expect. It's tricky, I know, getting to the right person in the age of managed care (should I say *mis*managed care?). But if you can be specific about which kind of specialist you need to see and why; if you are able to present your symptoms in the context of how they relate to CD; *and* you insist on it, you've got a better shot at a referral. As with all conditions, the earlier you get a diagnosis and begin treatment, the better off you are.

At a recent CSA conference, Dr. Peter Green, director of the Columbia Celiac Disease Center in New York, said, "It should be shouted from the rooftops that early diagnosis of CD is protective." The longer we are exposed to gluten, the higher our chances for developing an associated autoimmune disease. All well and good, but we're not living in the age of routine screening for CD. At least, not yet. What do we do in the meantime? We get our families tested as soon as possible and we arm ourselves with as much knowledge as we can.

Not everyone is as stubborn as I am, as assertive with professionals, or as good at plowing through complicated information. I am not a doctor, nor am I an expert on any of these conditions. I am not suggesting that you will develop any of the conditions described in this chapter any time soon. Some of us do, many of us won't. My purpose here is to provide a quick profile of each of the conditions believed to be related to celiac disease, who diagnoses them, what tests will confirm them, and how and where to turn for more information and support. In the increasingly narrow world of health care choices, knowledge has never been more powerful or more crucial.

You'd think having to live on a strict gluten-free diet would be enough for anybody. We get as much as we can carry. Sometimes more. But you knew that.

Here, from my faithful *Merck* and other professional sources, and with expert guidance from the physicians who reviewed the following sections, I've done a bit of the research for you. Let's start with the "seven-year itch."

Dermatitis Herpetiformis

To paraphrase the *Merck Manual*, DH, as it is commonly called, an intensely itchy, blistering, burning skin rash is, literally, the skin's reaction to gluten. It has driven more than one celiac to distraction. According to Dr. John Zone, professor of dermatology at the University of Utah, 100 percent of DH patients are celiacs.

DH usually starts off gradually. Tiny red bumps appear across the elbows, knees, back, buttocks, and scalp and often on the face and neck with tiny blisters on the surface of the lesions. There is burning. And itching. Incessant scratching often causes the blisters to open and crust over, obscuring the original outbreak and creating new injury.

Dermatitis herpetiformis may be mistaken for eczema, psoriasis, and various other forms of dermatitis, which is why it's important to find a dermatologist who is familiar with the condition and its relationship to celiac disease. Short of that, help the doctor to connect the dots—or the bumps, in this case. Provide a context for suspicion by informing the doctor that there is, or may be, celiac disease lurking in the background.

After examination of the lesions, the dermatologist most likely will ask permission to take a small specimen for biopsy, usually from an area near the outbreak, but not directly on it. After freezing the area, the tissue will be sent to a lab to be examined for antibodies within the skin, specifically IgA granules, which are diagnostic of DH.

It is critical for the lab your doctor uses to be familiar with DH. Specimen kits are available to patients and their doctors from the University of Utah, Immunodermatology Laboratory, which specializes in DH.

Often strict adherence to the gluten-free diet is enough to keep DH under control. In some cases, drugs like dapsone or sulfapyradine are given for a short time to relieve the itch. It's important to know that these medications come with potentially serious side effects—including liver damage, kidney stones, and lowering of white and red blood cell counts with long-term use. If you are given one of these drugs, you should expect to be asked to have a CBC (Complete Blood Count) and liver functioning tests done from time to time in order to monitor organ functioning. If you are not asked to have this blood work done, it would be wise to request it.

If dapsone and sulfapyradine are used correctly and monitored by a physician who understands the potential side effects, it can produce complete improvement of the skin symptoms in greater than 90 percent of patients. These drugs have no effect on the surface of the intestine skin.

Many celiacs with DH avoid drugs altogether and use over-the-counter and home remedies to soothe the itch. One person I know wears gloves to bed in order to minimize the damage from scratching. Others take long soaks in the bathtub followed by a thick slather of rich skin creams like Eucerin, Neutrogenia, Bag Balm, et al. Some swear by bath oils, bathing in lukewarm water, Aveeno oatmeal baths, Epsom salts baths, saltwater soaks, and many use mild body washes instead of soap. Others report that drinking plenty of water, taking omega-3 fatty acids and flaxseed oil all help. Still others are convinced humidifiers and various anti-itch gels, including old-fashioned calamine lotion, do the trick.

What works for one person may not work for another.

If you're reading this, you already know you are a celiac, but I would advise sharing this with any relatives who might be at risk for CD and who complain of intense itching and ugly, blistered skin. DH, I am told, often appears in the absence of gastrointestinal symptoms.

John J. Zone, M.D.
Professor and Chairman
Department of Dermatology
University of Utah School
    of Medicine
30 North 1900 E., 4-B, 454
Salt Lake City, UT 84132
(801) 581-2955

Dr. Marc Grossman
Clinical Professor of Dermatology
Columbia University
New York, New York
(914) 946-1101

For other doctors specializing in dermatitis herpetiformis, contact:

American Academy of Dermatology
930 North Meacham Road
Schaumberg, IL 60173
(847) 330-0230
www.aad.org

For specimen kits and skin testing information:

University of Utah
Immunodermatology Laboratory
(866) 266-5699
www.uuhsc.utah.edu/derm/immunoderm

Osteoporosis

As we age, osteoporosis is a problem many of us will face, especially those diagnosed with celiac disease as adults. According to *The Merck Manual*, "osteoporosis is a generalized progressive diminution in bone tissue mass, causing skeletal weakness, even though the ratio of mineral or organic elements is unchanged in the remaining normal bone." This is really a fancy way of saying osteoporosis is a thinning of the bones that can result in pain, a loss of height, and fractures of the hip, spine, and other bones.

There is drug-induced osteoporosis, typically caused by corticosteroid use, smoking, barbiturates, and blood thinners. There is endocrine osteoporosis, which occurs in hyperthyroidism, hypogonadism, diabetes mellitus, and other glandular conditions. And there is a kind of osteoporosis celiacs should take a special interest in, which falls into the category of miscellaneous osteoporosis and can be induced by anything from prolonged periods of weightlessness, such as found in space travel (or sitting on our fannies in front of a computer every day for hours on end) to kidney and liver failure and malabsorption syndrome.

Malabsorportion: this is the ten-dollar word for what happens when the intestine is injured in celiac disease. Nutrients can't get through. We may be taking our calcium and vitamin D (*and* faithfully doing our weight-bearing exercise), but as celiacs we may not be absorbing enough of each to keep our bones healthy, or we may be coming from too far behind to catch up. The longer CD goes without diagnosis, the higher the risk of developing osteoporosis. In fact, very often celiac disease is discovered only after we seek treatment for our aching bones. If ever there was a case for getting blood tests for family members that may be at risk for CD, it's this insidious and potentially disabling condition.

Osteoporosis may be silent for many years, often doing nothing more than causing a low-level ache. By the time pain sets in or fractures occur, the condition is usually advanced.

There are two ways to seek a diagnosis of and treatment for osteoporosis. One is through a rheumatologist and the other is through an endocrinologist (my own bias is toward the latter). Either should rule out osteomalcia (a softening of the bones usually caused by a vitamin D deficiency) and other metabolic diseases of the bone as part of your workup.

You may be issued a jug with a stinky chemical in the bottom and asked to use it to collect your urine for twenty-four hours. It's inconvenient (you must keep this on ice or in the refrigerator between uses), but it is the way to find out if you have any other problems with calcium.

The Merck Manual further tells us that standard X rays are not sensitive enough to reveal osteoporosis until 30 percent of bone has been lost. The Dual Energy X-ray Absorptiometry (or DEXA) scan is a brief, painless test that measures the density of the spine and hip and is the gold standard for detecting osteoporosis or osteopenia, a condition that occurs before full-blown osteoporosis sets in.

Anyone with long-standing celiac disease should insist on a DEXA. Depending on the results and your age, a follow-up every year to measure improvements is wise. I am told by an expert in the interpretation of these test results that it's important to have this test on the same machine each time. Different scanners may interpret or measure results differently, making it difficult to compare results from year to year.

Calcium, magnesium, and vitamin D supplementation, coupled with a gluten-free diet rich in calcium, may arrest bone loss or even help to reverse it. In other cases, drugs like Fosomax, Actonel, Miacalcin (a calcitonin-salmon nasal spray), or Evista, an estrogen-based drug that mimics estrogen's beneficial effect on bone density, are prescribed. There is a downside to everything, and many of these drugs, while highly effective, come with risks and contraindications. Some side effects are more serious than others and new research concerning the consequences of estrogen supplementation makes the decision even harder. All medications should be considered, not only for their gluten-free status but also for their effect on your particular condition or conditions, given your family history and health. All are prescriptions that should be taken under a doctor's supervision.

The National Academy of Sciences recommends the following daily intake of dietary calcium and vitamin D for healthy Americans:

Calcium		Vitamin D	
0–6 months	210 mg/day	0–50 years	200 I.U./day
7–12 months	270 mg/day	51–70 years	400–600 I.U./day
1–3 years	500 mg/day	71 years plus	600–800 I.U./day
4–8 years	800 mg/day		
9–18 years	1,300 mg/day		
19–50 years	1,000 mg/day		
51 years plus	1,200 mg/day until menopause		
51 years plus	1,500 mg/day after menopause		

Note: These figures apply to the general population. Newly diagnosed celiacs often need to take higher doses of calcium, vitamin D, magnesium, and other minerals in order to make up for years of not absorbing these important bone-building elements. Supplementation and/or correction of any deficiency should be undertaken with your doctor's supervision.

A Word about Vitamin D

The National Institutes of Health tell us vitamin D is vital for proper absorption of calcium and other minerals. The best source for this vitamin, which the body stores in the fat cells against a rainy, dark day, is exposure to direct sunlight (glass interferes with vitamin D absorption, so sitting in front of a sunny window won't help). But don't think you have to fry yourself to a crisp. Approximately 20 minutes exposure without sunscreen in the morning or afternoon, when ultraviolet rays are the least damaging, should do the trick.

Few food sources besides cod liver oil (ugh), eel (double ugh), salmon, mackerel, sardines, and other oily fish provide vitamin D. Some foods are fortified with vitamin D, but many of these are cereals and cereal bars that are not gluten-free. Most people absorb enough vitamin D during the summer to last through the winter, but long hours indoors at computers and use of sunscreens have cut down on sun exposure. Add to this the absorption difficulties in people with celiac disease and it's wise to have vitamin D levels (as well as other vitamin and minerals) measured. There is a dark side to taking too much vitamin D. Excessive amounts can cause nausea, loss of appetite, weight loss, and serious muscle weakness, so it's best to have your doctor prescribe the dose that's right for you and monitor your progress from time to time.

For more information, contact:
The National Osteoporosis Foundation
P.O. Box 930299
Atlanta, GA 31193
(877) 868-4520
www.nof.org

Addison's Disease

Rumors abound in the celiac community that John F. Kennedy was an undiagnosed celiac. Given his Irish heritage and the fact that in childhood he suffered from severe gastrointestinal distress and weight and growth problems, it's a fair guess. As an adult, abdominal pain, migraines, weight loss, and osteoporosis plagued him. Over the years and during his presidency, he was extensively and quietly evaluated at major medical centers in Boston, New Haven, and New York, as well as by the Mayo Clinic. Among his multiple diagnoses were ulcers, colitis, spastic colitis, irritable bowel syndrome, and food allergies.

Imagine what a gluten-free Camelot would have done for awareness of celiac disease. We'll never know. What we do know is that among his many problems, JFK suffered from Addison's disease, a chronic, insidious, and rare insufficiency of the adrenal glands that can be associated with celiac disease.

To paraphrase *The Merck Manual*, Addison's disease is an endocrine disorder caused by atrophy of the adrenal cortex, most likely by an autoimmune process, resulting in insufficient product of an important hormone called cortisol. In the absence of cortisol, insufficient carbohydrate is formed from protein and hypoglycemia (low blood sugar) and diminished liver function result. This leads to serious neuromuscular weakness. Resistance to infection, stress, and trauma is diminished because of reduced adrenal output.

Symptoms of Addison's disease include weakness, fatigue, low blood pressure, and increased pigmentation, which is characterized by tanning of both exposed and unexposed portions of the body, especially on pressure points (bony areas), skin folds, and scars. Black freckles appear over the forehead, face, neck, and shoulders and often bluish-black discoloration appears on the lips, mouth, rectum, vagina, and other mucous membranes. Addison's can cause a decreased tolerance to cold. Dizziness and fainting attacks can occur, as can weight loss, dehydration, vomiting, and diarrhea. There also may be some abnormalities on the EKG (electrocardiogram).

If Addison's is suspected, a referral to an endocrinologist is crucial. Blood levels of sodium and potassium and BUN (a measurement of kidney function) will be taken. Cortisol levels are measured and tests for adrenal insufficiency may be ordered. A substance called cosyntropin is injected and cortisol is measured at 60 minutes. People with Addison's disease have low cortisol values that do not rise in response to cosyntropin.

Other tests that may be ordered are WBC (white blood count) and fasting blood glucose. X rays may be ordered to examine the heart, to look for calcifications in the adrenal glands, and to screen for kidney or lung problems.

Addison's is a serious disease, but with carefully monitored substitution of the missing or insufficient hormones by an endocrinologist, the prognosis is excellent.

For information, support, and referrals, contact:
The National Adrenal Disease Foundation
505 Northern Boulevard, Suite 200
Great Neck, NY 11021
(516) 487-4992
www.medhelp.org/nadf/

Systemic Lupus Erythematosus (SLE)

According to the Lupus Foundation, lupus is "a chronic inflammatory disease that can affect various parts of the body, i.e., skin, joints, blood, and kidneys." The body's immune system normally makes antibodies to protect against viruses, bacteria, and other foreign materials. These foreign materials are called antigens. In an autoimmune disorder such as lupus, the immune system loses its ability to tell the difference between foreign substances and its own cells and tissues. The immune system then makes antibodies directed against "self." These antibodies, called auto-antibodies, then react with the "self" antigens to form immune complexes. The immune complexes build up in the tissues and can cause inflammation, injury to tissues, and pain.

For most people, lupus is a mild disease affecting only a few organs, but for others it can cause serious and even life-threatening problems. Lupus can begin abruptly with fever, resembling an acute infection, or it may develop insidiously over months or years with episodes of fever or malaise. The National Institutes of Health tells us the most common symptoms are painful or swollen joints, unexplained fever, skin rashes, and extreme fatigue. The Lupus Foundation adds to the list the classic "butterfly" rash across the cheeks and nose (this rash, resembling the markings of a wolf, *lupus* in Latin, is how the disease got its name), anemia, kidney involvement, pleurisy or pain in the chest on deep breathing, skin photosensitivity to sun or UV light, hair loss, abnormal blood clotting problems, Raynaud's phenomenon (fingers turning white and/or blue in response to cold), low blood counts (white cells, red cells, platelets), seizures, and mouth or nose ulcers.

When someone has many symptoms and positive blood test results, the rheumatologist has few problems making a correct diagnosis and initiating treatment. But more often than not, lupus shows itself over time with vague, seemingly unrelated symptoms like achy joints, fever, fatigue, or pains. Lupus can be mistaken for other types of arthritis, fibromyalgia, chronic fatigue, rosacea, and that great catchall diagnosis, stress. It takes tenacity on the part of the patient and patience on the part of the doctor when lupus is suspected. Often the picture forms over a period of months or years.

Blood tests for lupus include the LE (Lupus Erythematosus) cell test. This was the first diagnostic test for lupus, but is rarely done nowadays because of its lack of sensitivity.

The ANA or immunofluorescent antinuclear antibody test is more sensitive for lupus than the LE cell prep test. Virtually all people with lupus will have a positive ANA. On the other hand, a positive ANA by itself is not diagnostic, since the test may also be positive in individuals taking certain medications, in other connective tissue diseases (scleroderma, Sjögren's, rheumatoid arthritis, autoimmune thyroid disease or Hashimoto's thyroiditis, infectious mononucleosis), and chronic infectious diseases like leprosy, malaria, and liver disease.

Other helpful laboratory tests are ones that measure the complement levels in the blood. Complement is a blood protein that, with antibodies, destroys bacteria. If the total blood complement is low or the specific C3 or C4 complement values are low and the person has a positive ANA, some weight is added to a diagnosis of lupus. Low C3 or C4 in people with positive ANA may also point to lupus kidney disease or active disease in other organs.

Blood tests that measure individual antigen antibody reaction are also helpful. The anti-DNA antibody test, the anti-SM and the anti-RNP, the anti-Ro (SSA), and anti-La (SSA) will most likely be done.

If a skin rash is present, a biopsy may be performed to assist in the diagnosis.

A test may be positive one time and negative the next. The disease may be active one time, quiescent another. While no one test is diagnostic, all results are considered for diagnosis.

The bottom line: Lupus is elusive.

While a cure has not yet been found for lupus, management includes non-steroidal anti-inflammatory drugs (NSAIDs) and drugs like Tylenol for joint and muscle pain. For serious inflammation, corticosteroids may be used. Short treatment periods are recommended to avoid serious side effects. Anticoagulants may be required for people with recurrent blood clots. And antimalarials like chloroquine (Aralen) or hydroxychloroquine (Placquenil) are prescribed for skin and joint systems. Since these can have rare but serious consequences for the eyes, an eye exam is suggested before beginning a course of antimalarials. A yearly or twice-yearly follow-up with the opthamologist is a sensible precaution. Anticancer drugs (methotrexate, azothioprine, or cyclophosphamide) are also used in patients with life-threatening manifestations. As always, gluten-free status must be considered along with the potential risks of these medications.

For more information, doctor referrals, research, support, and subscriptions to the magazine, *Lupus Now*, contact:

Lupus Foundation of America
2000 L Street NW, Suite 710
Washington, DC 20036
(202) 349-1155
www.lupus.org

Sjögren's Syndrome

Sjögren's syndrome, also known as sicca syndrome, is defined as a chronic, autoimmune, inflammatory rheumatic disorder, and as yet experts can't say what causes it. It's characterized by dryness of the mouth, eyes, and other mucous membranes, musculoskeletal pain, and fatigue. It shares overlapping features with other autoimmune or connective tissue disorders, including rheumatoid arthritis, lupus, and scleroderma. Sjögren's syndrome is the second most common autoimmune rheumatic disease after rheumatoid arthritis. Ninety percent of Sjögren's patients are female.

Translation: Unlike lupus which attacks *all* of the body's organ's, Sjögren's mainly attacks the exocrine glands, those glands that produce moisture (tears, saliva, etc.) for normal functioning of the eyes, mouth, digestive and respiratory tracts, skin, and vagina. In Sjögren's, the exocrine glands are invaded by lymphocytes and are gradually destroyed. Sjögren's may be primary, which means it occurs in a previously healthy individual, or secondary, which means it can also develop in an individual with a preexisting connective tissue problem like rheumatoid arthritis.

Symptoms of this serious, annoying, but rarely fatal condition include a dry, gritty, or burning sensation in the eyes due to decreased tear production, dryness of the mouth like cotton mouth, and whole-body dryness (the feeling that one is turning into a tumbleweed). Sjögren's may cause difficulty talking, chewing, or swallowing; a sore or cracked tongue; a change or a loss of taste or smell; increased dental decay; joint pain; digestive problems, dry nose, dry lungs, recurring respiratory infections, dry skin, swollen salivary glands, fatigue, and light sensitivity. In rare cases, experts say, the lymphocytic infiltration may spread to the internal organs and lead to serious complications from inflammation of the lungs, kidneys, or central nervous system.

Lymphoma risk in Sjögren's is forty-four times that of the general population. Combined with the lymphoma risk associated with undiagnosed celiac or noncompliance with the gluten-free diet, there is no better incentive for celiacs to stay on the straight and narrow. Other problems associated with Sjögren's are Raynaud's phenomonon (cold-induced color changes of the hands and feet caused by painful constriction of small vessels), corneal damage, accelerated tooth decay, and salivary duct stones. This condition can cause liver disease, pancreatitis, sensory neuropathy, kidney problems, and alopecia. Dryness of the respiratory tract can lead to chronic lung infections and pneumonia.

Sjögren's syndrome is difficult to diagnose and is best managed by a rheumatologist. Like CD, the average time from onset of symptoms to diagnosis is about six years. A good opthamologist and a knowledgeable dentist also play important roles in this condition. The former conducts diagnostic tests and periodically evaluates the eyes for outer surface damage and the latter attends to the problems caused by a lack of saliva.

The Sjögren's Syndrome Foundation's new patient FAQ lists the following blood tests to expect when you're seeking a diagnosis:

ANA (Anti-Nuclear Antibody)—as in lupus, the presence of ANA in your blood is not diagnostic, but is a marker for the presence of autoimmune reaction.

SS-A (or Ro) and **SS-B** (La)—about 70 percent of Sjögren's patients are positive to SS-A and approximately 40 percent are positive for SS-B. These antibodies may also be found, though less often, in lupus.

RF (Rheumatoid Factor)—many Sjögren's patients have a positive RF just like people with rheumatoid arthritis. That is why one disorder is sometimes confused with the other.

ESR (Erythocyte Sedimentation Rate)—this test measures inflammation. An elevated ESR may indicate an inflammatory disorder like Sjögren's.

Igs (Immunoglobulins)—this test measures blood proteins, which may be elevated in Sjögren's and other immune system diseases.

An opthamologist may be asked to conduct all or some the following:

Schirmer Test—measures tear production, which is reduced in Sjögren's.

Rose Bengal and **Lissamine Green**—corneal staining is used to diagnose dry spots on the surface of the eye.

Slit-Lam Exam—may show a slow or reduced volume of tears or mucous filaments that can sometimes form as a complication of dry eyes.

Other tests that may be ordered:

Saliometry—measures the amount of saliva produced during a certain period and reflects parotid salivary gland function.

Sialography—is an X ray of the salivary-duct system performed after injecting contrast into the duct.

Lip biopsy—confirms lymphocytic infiltration of the minor salivary glands. A 15-minute procedure requiring local anesthesia, this is the most specific test for Sjögren's.

Once pinpointed, Sjögren's management often requires comprehensive care. For the mouth, this includes fastidious dental hygiene and frequent cleanings. Frequent sips of water and sugar-free mints and gum stimulate salivary flow. Artificial tears and saliva (yes, there is such a thing) help ease symptoms of dry mouth and eyes. Household humidifiers, periodic naps, medications that reduce joint pain, avoidance of sugary food and drinks, alcohol in any form (i.e., mouthwashes), rinses, even the wearing of gloves to avoid vessel constriction (especially when shopping in the supermarket freezer case) are all ways to accommodate and reduce symptoms. Frequent slathering with emollient creams help manage dry skin.

Drugs that decrease salivary secretion, such as decongestants and antihistamines, should be avoided. Ditto for sunbathing, as many Sjögren's patients develop photosensitivity. Relocation to the desert should be reconsidered.

There are two drugs available to stimulate saliva flow: pilocarpine (Salagen) and cevimeline (Evoxac). Although only FDA-approved for dry mouth, published studies suggest these drugs may help dryness in other body parts as well.

Antimalarials like those used in lupus have shown promise in treating fatigue, joint pain, muscle pain, and swollen glands. The eyes must be checked periodically for rare but serious side effects. Corticosteroids are reserved for disabling pain, fatigue, or serious internal organ involvement. In the worst cases stronger immuno-suppressants may also be used.

Is there a cure? No.

The Sjögren's Syndrome Foundation puts out a newsletter called *The Moisture Seekers* that is full of tips, conference news, the latest research and support. *The Sjögren's Syndrome Handbook* (3rd edition, 2004) is a valuable resource.

Sjögren's Syndrome Foundation
8120 Woodmont Avenue, Suite 530
Bethesda, MD 20814
(301) 718-0300
www.sjogrens.org

Diabetes Mellitus

Mosby's Medical Dictionary defines diabetes mellitus as "a complex disorder of carbohydrate, fat, and protein metabolism that is primarily a result of a deficiency or complete lack of insulin secretion by the beta cells of the pancreas or resistance to insulin."

The Expert Committee on the Diagnosis and Classification of Diabetes Mellitus of the American Diabetes Association describes the various types of diabetes: "Type 1 Diabetes includes patients with diabetes caused by an autoimmune process and who are dependent on insulin to prevent ketosis," which Mosby's further defines as "an abnormal accumulation of ketones in the body as a result of excessive breakdown of fats caused by a deficiency or inadequate use of carbohydrates, characterized by ketonuria, a loss of potassium in the urine which can lead to life-threatening ketoacidosis, coma, even death."

According to the National Diabetes Information Clearinghouse (NDIC), type I diabetes (formerly called juvenile diabetes or brittle diabetes or insulin-dependent diabetes) is caused when the beta cells of the pancreas no longer make insulin because the body's immune system has attacked and destroyed them. Symptoms include frequent thirst and urination, extreme hunger or fatigue, weight loss, sores that heal slowly, dry itchy skin, loss of feeling or tingling in the feet, and blurry vision. Treatment includes taking insulin shots or using an insulin pump, making wise food choices, exercising regularly, and controlling blood pressure and cholesterol.

Given the autoimmune nature of the condition, this form of diabetes is believed to be associated with CD and, in fact, Dr. Markku Maki of Finland (as reported by the Michigan chapter of CSA/USA in their newsletter) estimates that 5 percent or more of people with type 1 diabetes may have celiac disease.

But that doesn't let us off the hook. Obesity, sedentary lifestyle, and a steady diet of fast and processed foods and humongous portions of fat, sugar, and calories are contributing to a virtual epidemic of type 2 diabetes, even among young children. Celiacs, in particular, may be prone to this problem, because of the high fat, sugar, and carbohydrate contents of many gluten-free breads, cakes, and cookies.

The NDIC further tells us that type 2 diabetes, formerly called adult-onset or non-insulin dependent diabetes, is the most common form of diabetes. People can develop type 2 diabetes at any age—even during childhood. This form of diabetes usually begins with insulin resistance, a condition in which fat, muscle, and liver cells do not use insulin properly. At first the pancreas keeps up with the added demand by producing more insulin. In time, however, it loses the ability to secrete enough insulin in response to meals. Obesity and inactivity increase the chances of developing this type of diabetes, as do high levels of cholesterol and high blood pressure.

Gestational diabetes is another form of diabetes that may occur in the third trimester of pregnancy. It may be a sign of latent diabetes or it may disappear with the birth of the child.

All forms of diabetes require the care and monitoring of an endocrinologist. Periodic eye exams, cholesterol-lowering medications and diet, as well as frequent foot examinations and care on the part of an experienced podiatrist can go a long way to avoid serious complications.

Like celiac disease, proper nutrition is everything. Combining the gluten-free and diabetic diets won't be easy, but it will result in better health.

For diabetes information, diet, and management and support:

American Diabetes Association
www.diabetes.org

National Diabetes Information Clearinghouse
1 Information Way
Bethesda MD 20892
(800) 860-8747
www.diabetes.niddk.nih.gov

Thyroid Disease

The thyroid gland, as described by *Mosby's Medical Dictionary*, is "a pea-sized, ductless gland at the front of the neck that is part of the endocrine system and which secretes the hormone thyroxine (T4) and triiodothronine (T3), an iodine-containing compound, as well as produces the hormone calcitonin." These substances are essential to normal body growth, normal metabolic rate, carbohydrate catabolism (the bodily process of breaking down carbohydrates for energy storage and heat production), skeletal maturation, i.e., growth in infancy and childhood, and cardiac rate, force, and output. Thryroid hormones promote central nervous system development and the synthesis of many enzymes essential for muscle tone and vigor. In other words, it's a small but important pea-sized gland.

Hyperthyroidism (*hyper* meaning "too much") or Graves' disease is characterized by *The Merck Manual* as an "overproduction of these hormones resulting in rapid heart rate, sweating, moist skin, tremors, bulging eyes, increased sweating, palpitations, fatigue, increased appetite and weight loss, frequent bowel movements, insomnia, and atrial fibrillation or sudden, fast heart rhythm." A qualified endocrinologist will measure the levels of thyroid hormone and treat this condition with drugs that will inhibit and normalize the release of what is over-produced. The right dosage comes from careful monitoring of thyroid hormone and adjusting doses accordingly.

Hypothryroidism (*hypo* meaning "too little") or myxedema is just the opposite. Too little thyroid hormone in circulation can contribute to a dull facial expression, hoarse voice, slow speech, puffiness and swelling around the eyes, cold intolerance, drooping eyelids, sparse, coarse, and dry hair and coarse, dry, scaly, and thickened skin. Weight gain is another sign of hypothyroidism, as is forgetfulness and other evidence of intellectual impairment (the "brain fog" celiacs often complain of may be related to hypothyroiditis). There are often deposits of carotene on the palms of hands and soles of feet, and macroglossia or enlargement of the tongue. Undiagnosed myxedema can lead to seizures or coma. Hypothyroidism is thought to be an autoimmune disease, related to celiac disease, and often occurs as a prelude to Hashimoto's thryroidititis. Lifelong supplementation with thryoid hormone compensates for the deficiency and, again, is carefully monitored for the correct amount.

Hashimoto's thryroiditis, or autoimmune thyroiditis, is a chronic inflammation of the thyroid gland with lymphocytic infiltration much like the exocrine gland destruction in Sjögren's and the salivary glands. Symptoms often take the form of a painless enlargement of the gland or fullness in the throat.

When the doctor examines the gland, it is usually not tender and it is smooth, firm, and more rubbery in consistency than a normal thryroid. Other forms of autoimmune disease are common in people with Hashimoto's, including Addison's disease, diabetes, hypoparathyroidism, and yes, celiac disease.

Treatment for Hashimoto's thryroiditis is straightforward, with a lifelong replacement of thryroid hormone.

For doctor referrals and information, contact:

The American Association of Clinical Endocrinologists
1000 Riverside Avenue, Suite 205
Jacksonville, FL 32204
(904) 353-7878
www.aace.com

Lymphoma

Whew. Just writing the word gives one pause. Okay. Let's face the fear head-on. We've all been told there is an association between undiagnosed celiac disease and increased risk from lymphoma or adenocarcinoma, in particular T-cell lymphoma of the small intestine.

According to the Lymphoma Research Foundation, there are more than thirty subtypes of lymphoma. These consist of five types of Hodgkin's lymphoma which arise from abnormal white cells that spread along the lymph nodes, as well as organs outside the lymphatic vessels. Lymphoma also includes twenty-four types of non-Hodgkin's lymphoma, a more common form that starts in the spleen or in lymph tissue found in organs like the stomach or small intestine.

While we are assured by the foundation that most people who have the following complaints will not have lymphoma, anyone (especially any celiac) with persistent symptoms should be examined to make sure lymphoma is not present. These are chills, painless swelling of the lymph nodes, fever, night sweats, unexplained weight loss, lack of energy, and itching. The development of anemia, low blood albumin, or recurring steatorrhea in a previously healthy celiac should prompt further investigation in the form of blood work, CT scanning of the abdomen, and, in some cases, a segment of the bowel obtained surgically under anesthesia through a laparoscope in order to examine the excised tissue for proliferation of T cells. The doctor best suited to pursue an investigation of this kind is a gastroenterologist with a specialty in oncology.

An article in the *American Journal of Clinical Nutrition* suggests that in diagnosed celiacs, malignancy may appear as a return of malabsorptive symptoms or a surgical emergency associated with obstruction, perforation, and sometimes, bleeding. The same article goes on to say the risk for developing lymphoma diminishes with duration and compliance with the gluten-free diet and that malignancy rarely occurs before forty years of age. Patients diagnosed as children and who are compliant have a lower risk of malignancy.

However, a more recent article in the *American Journal of Medicine,* reporting on a study conducted at New York–Presbyterian Hospital between 1981 and 2000, concludes that "the risk of non-Hodgkin's lymphoma among its study subjects persisted despite a gluten-free diet." Also observed was an increased risk of small intestinal adenocarcinoma, esophageal cancer, and melanoma.

So what's a celiac to do? Follow your gluten-free diet religiously, have frequent checkups, and insist that other first- and second-degree relatives get tested for celiac disease. My own unprofessional opinion is this: Be smart, be aware of the symptoms, but don't obsess about it.

For more information, contact:

The Lymphoma Research Foundation
8800 Venice Boulevard, Suite 207
Los Angeles, CA 90034
(800) 500-9976

In New York:
111 Broadway, 19th Floor
New York, NY 10006
(800) 235-6848
www.lymphoma.org

Beyond being forewarned and forearmed, we simply can't worry. Doctors tell us stress contributes to many illnesses, including cancer. All the more reason to eat well, exercise, take our vitamins, keep our fat and sugar and calorie intake low (whether gluten-free or not), maintain a healthy weight, and pat ourselves on the back for getting our celiac disease diagnosed.

Whatever you do, don't tell God your plans.

Learn More

American College of Rheumatology
1800 Century Place, Suite 250
Atlanta, GA 30345
(404) 633-3777
www.rheumatology.org

National Institute of Arthritis and
Musculoskeletal and Skin Diseases
National Institutes of Health
U.S. Department of Health and
Human Services
1 AMS Circle
Bethesda, MD 20892
(301) 495-4484
www.niams.nih.gov

Medic Alert Foundation
International
2323 Colorado
Turlock, CA 95381
(209) 668-3333
www.medicalert.com

rx for health

One pill makes you larger, and one pill makes you small,
And the ones that mother gives you, don't do anything at all.

—GRACE SLICK
"White Rabbit"

Prescription prices are going through the roof, research and development departments of pharmaceutical companies rival the CIA for secrecy and dirty tricks, not to mention allegations of price fixing and all around socking it to the consumer. Big Pharm is not the most forthcoming of industries. Like dry cleaners and funeral directors that do a brisk business regardless of the economic climate, drug companies provide products that all of us need at one time or another and some of us won't be able to live without. Talk about a captive audience.

CD is not something that requires medication. But even the healthiest celiac is going to have to pop a cold pill, take an antibiotic, get his cholesterol down, build up her bones, fight an infection, get out of the dumps, stabilize his blood sugar, soothe an upset stomach, prevent a pregnancy, and soothe a bad cough. Most likely, the older we get, the more medicine we'll need. (You know this is happening when your prescription medicines take up more room in your suitcase than your clothes.) I hate to say it, but even the rare celiac who abuses prescription medicine needs to know if there's gluten in whatever he or she is abusing, unless, of course, the idea of self-destruction on two fronts is doubly appealing.

In the search to root out gluten, the medicine cabinet can be a daunting challenge. Reading food labels is difficult, but deciphering drug labels is even harder. To compound the problem, the old-fashioned neighborhood druggist who mixed his own pills and could tell you what was in every one has gone the way of the buffalo. Huge chain pharmacies dispense prescription medications directly from manufacturers and often cannot (and will not) give you any more information than what is printed on the product literature sheet, itself a blinding exercise in reading miniscule print. With intra-company piracy a billion-dollar business, requests for drug company formulas are routinely met with suspicion. One "consumer relations" person needed the approval of three people before giving me her company's Web address.

Nevertheless, you must persevere, either by using one of the sources for gluten-free medications listed in this chapter or phoning the drug company yourself, a frustrating but necessary evil. Remember that even if you choose to buy one of the available and often reliable gluten-free drug guides, the information is only as good as the day it was verified. If you do get a drug company on the phone and you find a willing ear, try to resist ranting about their excessive profit margins or the strength of their lobby in Washington. Stay focused. You're trying to find out about gluten. Count to ten if you must before you make the call.

Sometimes a drug maker will list certain ingredients on the label as "unspecified" because to disclose them would be giving away trade secrets. While the manufacturer won't reveal these proprietary ingredients, they should be able to tell you if gluten is involved. I emphasize the word *should*. I firmly believe the key to getting the information you need lies in your approach. Honey will get you a lot more than vinegar.

How to Win the War on Drugs

Start out by telling all your doctors and your pharmacist that you are a celiac and what that means in terms of medications. And don't forget the dentist. Do not assume the word *celiac* will ring a bell.

Arm yourself with a short description of the problem, either from this book or from your support group or one of the sources listed in chapter 21, "The Resourceful Celiac," and explain how it can pertain to over-the-counter and prescription medicine. Write it on an index card, make copies, and leave one with each of your health care providers, along with your contact information, to keep as a permanent record in your file.

It's always a good idea to make a list of drugs you may be required to take at some future date, let's say in the event of a sinus infection, flu, or other serious illness requiring an antibiotic. Investigate their gluten-free status before you have to take one. Anticipating problems and planning for them are great ways to make sure everyone is on the same page when and if the time comes.

Next, go through all your existing medications and verify that they are gluten-free, either by using one of the guides listed in this chapter, checking in with your support group, or phoning the manufacturer yourself. This is a good time to clean out the medicine chest and pitch out all expired medicines like the Cipro you've been hoarding since the anthrax scare and the eyedrops you can't remember why you saved. Don't overlook the baby aspirin, as well as vitamins and any other supplements or over-the-counter medications you may be taking. Review even the most innocuous-sounding stuff and switch to a gluten-free brand if necessary.

Before you fill any new prescriptions, ask the pharmacist to give you the product insert. Even better, ask her to check all ingredients for you.

When you do verify that a brand name drug is gluten-free, don't forget to have the doctor specify "brand name necessary" on the prescription.

Periodically check your maintenance medications to make sure their gluten-free status remains unchanged.

If you notice a difference in the color or look of a particular medication you take, call the company right away. The company may have reformulated the drug, which in turn means you have to check for gluten all over again. If you take a generic drug, it may mean a different manufacturer is making your medication. To be on the safe side, ask your pharmacist with each refill if the same company is still making the generic medication you're taking.

Always use the same pharmacy if you can manage it. Be nice. Smile. Tell a joke or two. Give out Halloween candy. Develop a relationship with the people who are filling your prescriptions. This way they won't feel put out when you ask them to call the manufacturer of a particular medicine and check on its gluten-free status for you or, if necessary, fight with the insurance company for you. (Most insurance companies don't get that celiacs must have gluten-free medications.) If the pharmacist knows what you need, he or she can be an important advocate. Show your appreciation. People are much more likely to help if they know they have all your business and you show your appreciation from time to time.

Another way to avoid a drug problem is to find a good compounding pharmacy that can prepare gluten-free medications for you. These people are not on every corner, but they're not entirely impossible to find (I've listed a few at the end of this chapter) and most offer mail-order services. Specially compounded medications and gluten-free vitamins and supplements cost a bit more, but they're well worth it in terms of peace of mind.

WARNING: DO NOT SWALLOW
WHILE TAKING THIS MEDICATION

What exactly is it that's going down with that glass of water? Just as you study a new medication's information sheet for possible reactions, contraindications, side effects, overdose, etc. (you do, don't you?), now you must become equally familiar with the names for the starches, fillers, sweeteners, coloring and suspension agents, and other strange-sounding and possibly glutenous ingredients that make prescription and over-the-counter medications palatable. One way to do that is to buy a *PDR* (*Physicians Desk Reference*), a doorstop of a book listing all the package inserts that are included with prescription medication. Go to the section on inactive ingredients and familiarize yourself with those ingredients that may hold the potential for trouble.

Glutenfreedrugs.com, a Web site run by Steve Plogsted, a celiac with a Ph.D. in pharmacology, lists the following inactive or excipient ingredients as gluten-free. Please note I did not say chemical-free or free of substances you might be reluctant to touch, much less swallow.

Benzyl alcohol is made from benzyl chloride from tar oil, not gluten.

Cellulose (methylcellulose, hydroxymethylcellulose, or microcrytalline) can be made from plant fiber, woody pulp, or chemical cotton, but not gluten.

Cetylalcohol is a substance derived from spermaceti, the waxy substance from the head of the sperm whale. Gluten sounds almost palatable by contrast.

Croscarmellose sodium is an internally cross-linked sodium carboxymethylcellulose for use as a disintegrant in pharmaceutical formulations.

Dextrans are sugar molecules.

Dextrins result from the hydrolysis of cornstarch by heat or hydrochloric acid.

Dextrates are a mixture of sugars resulting from the hydrolysis of starch.

Gelatin is gotten from boiling the skin, connective tissue, and bones of animals. Ugh.

Glycerin can be made in the following ways: saponification of fats and oils in the manufacturing of soaps; hydrolysis of fats and oils through pressure and superheated steam; or fermentation of beet sugar molasses in the presence of large amounts of sodium sulfite or from propylene, a petroleum product—none of which involve gluten.

Glycerols are obtained from fats and oils as byproducts in the manufacture of soaps and fatty acids.

Glycols are products of ethylene oxide gas.

Iron oxide is just that, rust used as a coloring agent.

Mannitol is a sweetener derived from monosaccharides.

Polysorbates come from a chemically altered sugar called sorbitol.

Povidone or crospovidone are synthetic polymers.

Sodium lauryl sulfate is a derivative of the fatty acids of coconut oil.

Stearates are derived from stearic acid, a fat that occurs as a glyceride in tallow and other animal fats and oils, as well as some vegetables, and is made by hydrogenation of cottonseed and other vegetable oils.

Titanium dioxide is a chemical not derived from any starch source. It's used as a white pigment.

Triacetin is a derivative of glycerin.

Silcon dioxide is a dispersing agent made from silicon.

Sister Jeanne Crowe, Pharm. D., R.Ph, and Nancy Patin Falini, M.A., R.D., tell us in their *American Journal of Pharmacology* article, "Gluten in Pharmaceutical Products," that only those medications that come into direct contact with the intestinal tract, i.e., tablets, capsules, syrups, oral solutions, and rectal suppositories, must be checked for possible sources of gluten. Medications that are injected, delivered as transdermal skin patches, or inhaled (as long as the medicine is not swallowed) will generally not cause a problem for the celiac patient.

Ingredients That Should Arouse Suspicion

Starch. This binding agent can be made from corn, potatoes, wheat, rice, or tapioca and its origin may not be readily identifiable on the label. Unidentified starch requires further investigation. In an article reported in the newsletter of the Houston Celiac-Sprue Support Group, Mr. Plogsted tells us that starch is the single most suspicious source of gluten in medication. If a particular drug does not contain starch, chances are really good, 99.9 percent, that it will be gluten-free as well.

Pregelatinized Starch. This, too, may be derived from wheat starch, cornstarch, or tapioca starch.

Dextrimaltose. This is a mixture of dextrin and maltose produced by the enzymatic action of barley malt and corn flour. Any presence of barley malt in the manufacturing process makes this ingredient highly suspicious.

Flour, Gluten, Dusting Powder. The first two should be obvious, but dusting powder from an undisclosed source can be trouble. Verify with the manufacturer before using.

Malt, Malt Syrup. These ingredients are derived from barley and are often used in the making of other inactive ingredients like dextrimaltose.

Not Likely to Contain Gluten, but Ask Anyway

Dextrin. Although wheat starch can be used in the manufacture of dextrin, most dextrins manufactured in the United States are corn-based and gluten-free.

Maltodextrin. Maltodextrin found in medication is *almost always* derived from corn starch and therefore gluten-free.

Caramel Color. Almost all caramel color produced in the United States is gluten-free. However, imported products containing caramel color should be checked. A good idea is to use "dye-free" medications.

Drug companies have to go through an enormous amount of red tape and expense to change a formulation after FDA approval, so if you do find a gluten-free medication, chances are very good that it will stay that way. That is not to say you can be complaisant, just don't be paranoid.

But what about cross-contamination?

Mr. Plogsted says, emphatically, don't worry about it. Drug companies are bound by federal regulation to use one room and one production line to manufacture one product. All equipment is stainless steel, everything is sterilized, and sophisticated ventilation systems eliminate any chance of airborne contamination. These places are "more sterile than an operating room," he says. If only we could get big food processors to follow the same rule.

In Case of an Emergency

If you find yourself hospitalized with a serious infection and have not been able to verify the gluten content of a particular antibiotic, request that you be given the drug intravenously until a safe substitute can be found. Get well. Argue with the insurance company later.

Celiac-Savvy Drug Companies

According to the Crowe-Falini study, only 5 of the 100 pharmaceutical companies that responded to their survey said they had a policy of making gluten-free products. Many more believe their products to be gluten-free, but cannot guarantee it. To compound the problem, most companies will only verify a particular product that is on the market, but may not be able to comment on future production because they claim no ability to verify the gluten-free status of raw materials from their suppliers. This buck-passing is common in the food industry and it leaves a celiac wondering if a product really isn't safe or if the company is simply covering its rear end with this legal hedge.

So what are you waiting for? Get on the phone. Turn on the computer. Here are some of the companies who claim all or some of their products are gluten-free.

Abbott Laboratories	(800) 441-4987	www.abbotcom
Bristol Myers Squibb	(800) 321-1335	www.bms.com
*Eli Lilly	(800) 545-5979	www.lilly.com
Merck	(800) 672-6372	www.merck.com
Roche	(800) 526-6367	www.rocheusa.com
Ross	(800) 551-5840	www.ross.com
Roxanne Labs	(614) 276-4000	www.roxanne.com
Schwarz Pharma	(262) 238-5400	www.schwarzusa.com
Wyeth-Ayerst Labs	(800) 999-9384	www.wyeth.com

*ELi Lilly claims all their products are gluten-free

Common Sense Check

If you're having chest pain, DO NOT refuse to take a nitroglyerin until you're sure that particular brand is gluten-free. If you're having a heart attack, gluten should be the last thing on your mind. FYI: sublingual tablets and transdermal patches made by Mylan Pharmaceuticals and EON Laboratories are gluten-free. Those made by Pfizer are not.

America's Favorite Drugs

We do love our Lipitor. This cholesterol-lowering medication made by Pfizer belongs to the class of drugs called statins, and according to www.rxlist.com, Lipitor is #1 on the bestseller list of most prescribed medications in the United States. It is not gluten-free—most of Pfizer's products are not. Maybe they're doing so well they don't need celiacs.

Herewith, the top prescription medications and how they stack up in the gluten department as described in *A Guide through the Medicine Cabinet* by Marcia Milazzo and pharmacist Steve Plogsted's Web site, GlutenfreeDrugs .com. Remember, as with food, ingredients and manufacturers can change at any time. Always verify for your own situation and recheck periodically.

Lipitor	Pfizer Pharmaceuticals	Not gluten-free
Synthroid	Abbott Laboratories	Gluten-free
Atenolol	Mylan Pharmaceuticals	Gluten-free
Zithromax	Pfizer Pharmaceuticals	Not gluten-free
Amoxicillin	Apothecon, Novapharm, Teva	Gluten-free
Furosemide	Mylan Pharmaceuticals	Gluten-free
Hydrochlorothiazide	Mylan Pharmaceuticals	Gluten-free
Norvasc	Pfizer Pharmaceuticals	Not gluten-free
Lisinopril	EON Labs	Gluten-free
Alprazolam	Mylan Pharmaceuticals	Gluten-free
Zoloft	Pfizer	Not gluten-free
Toprol-XL	Astra Zeneca	Not gluten-free
Zocor	Merck	Gluten-free
Premarin	Wyeth Pharmaceuticals	Gluten-free
Prevacid	Tap Pharmaceuticals	Gluten-free
Zyrtec	Pfizer Pharmaceuticals	GF syrup only
Levoxyl	Monarch Pharmaceuticals	Not gluten-free
Triamterene	Barr Laboratories and Mylan Pharmaceuticals	Both gluten-free
Celebrex	Pfizer Pharmaceuticals	Not gluten-free
Ambien	Sanofi	Gluten-free
Allegra	Aventis Pharmaceuticals	Gluten-free
Cephalexin	Mylan Pharmaceuticals and Ranbaxy	All but capsules Gluten-free
Nexium	Astra Zeneca	Not gluten-free
Fosamax	Merck	Gluten-free
Viagra	Pfizer	Not gluten-free
Cialis	Eli Lilly	Gluten-free

Lactose Alert

· ·

Many celiacs are intolerant of lactose as well as gluten. For some, this condition is temporary until the gut heals, and for others it is a permanent fact of life. Lactose is a common filler in prescription medication; if you take a drug containing lactose every day, several times a day, you're looking at a lot of lactose. The same rules apply to gluten. Do your homework.

Glutenfreedrugs lists the oral contraceptives Alesse, LoOvral, Nortrel, Ortho Cyclen, Ortho Novum, and TriPhasil as gluten-free.

Prescription-Speak

Most doctors are usually too busy to tell you on the spot what's in a given drug (*if* they know). So why is it they always have time to scribble instructions for taking it in arcane code (Latin for "I'm smarter than you") known only to other doctors and pharmacists?

It has always struck me as ironic that the very people whose lives depend on taking a medication properly are the same ones who aren't in on the secret. You don't have to be a celiac to see what little sense this makes. With a little help from the School of Pharmacy, herewith a once and for all state-of-the-art unscrambling of common abbreviations and notations found on prescription pads, medicine bottles, tubes, sprays, dispensers, etc. So you will never scratch your head again.

aa: of each
a.c.: before meals
ad: up to
a.d.: right ear
ad lib.: at pleasure, freely
a.m.: morning (we knew that)
amp.: ampule
aq: water
a.s.: left ear
ASA: aspirin

ATC: around the clock
a.u.: each ear
b.i.d.: twice a day
BM: bowel movement
BP: blood pressure
BSA: body surface area
c.: with
cap: capsule
CHF: congestive heart failure
dil.: dilute

disc or D.C.: discontinue
disp.: dispense
div.: divide
d.t.d.: give of such doses
DW: distilled water
D5W: dextrose 5% in water
elix.: elixir
e.m.p.: as directed
et: and
ex aq.: in water
fl or fld: fluid
ft.: make
g. or Gm. or g: gram
gr. or gr: grain
gtt.: drop
H: hypodermic
h. or hr.: hour
HA: headache
HBP: high blood pressure
HC: hydrocortisone
h.s.: at bedtime
HT: hypertension
ID: intradermal
IM: intramuscular
inj.: injection
IV: intravenous
IVP: intravenous push
IVBP: intravenous piggy back
LCD: coal tar solution
M.: mix
m2 or M2: square meter
mcg. or mcg: microgram
mEq: milliequivalent
mg. or mg: milligram
ml. or ml: milliliter
mOsm or mOsmol: milliosmol
MS: morphine sulfate
N & V: nausea and vomiting
NF: national formulary
NMT: not more than

noct.: night
non rep. or N.R.: do not repeat
NPO: nothing by mouth
N.S. or NS: normal saline
½ NS: half-strength normal saline
NTG: nitroglycerin
O: pint
o.d.: right eye
oint.: ointment
o.l.: left eye
o.s.: left eye
o.u.: each eye
o2: both eyes
p.c.: after meals
p.m.: afternoon, evening
p.o.: by mouth
p.r.n.: as needed
pulv.: powder
q: every
qd: every day
qh: every hour
qid: four times a day
R: rectal
R.L. or R/L: No. this is not Ralph Lauren, it's Ringer's Lactate.
Sig.: write on label
SL: sublingual
SOB: shortness of breath
sol.: solution
s.o.s.: if there is need
ss.: one-half
stat.: immediately
subc or subq or s.c.: subcutaneously (under the skin)
sup.: suppository
susp.: suspension
syr.: syrup
tab.: tablet
tal.: such

tal. dos.: such doses
tbsp: tablespoonful
tid: three times a day
tiw: three times a week
top: topically
TPN: total parenteral nutrition
tr.: tincture
tsp.: teaspoonful
U or u: unit
u.d. or ut dict: as directed
ung.: ointment

URI: upper respiratory infection
USP: United States Pharmacopeia
UTI: urinary tract infection
VS: vital signs
w/: with
WBC: white blood cell count
w/o: without
X: times
y.o.: year old
ZnO: zinc oxide

Take an ASA and call me in the A.M.

Gluten-Free and Compounding Pharmacies

College Pharmacy
3505 Austin Bluffs Parkway,
Suite 101
Colorado Springs, CO 80918
(800) 888-9358
www.collegepharmacy.com

Compounded Solutions in
Pharmacy, LLC
Michael Roberge, R.Ph.
179 Main Street
Monroe, CT 06468
(203) 268-4964
www.compoundedsolutions.com

Freeda Vitamins
36 East 41 Street
New York, NY 10017
(800) 777-3737
www.freedavitamins.com

Gluten-Free Vitamins
514A North Western Avenue
Lake Forest, IL 60045
(847) 615-1209

Pine Pharmacy
Alfonse Muto, R.Ph.
1806 Pine Avenue
Niagra Falls, NY 14301
(800) 355-1112
www.pinepharmacy.com

Pioneer Nutritional Formulas
Chewable Vitamins and Minerals for
Adults & Children
(800) 458-8483
www.pioneernutritional.com

Stokes Pharmacy
639 Stokes Road
Medford, NJ 08055
(800) 754-5222
www.stokesrx.com

For a compounding pharmacy in your area, contact:

International Academy of Compounding Pharmacists
P.O. Box 1365
Sugarland, TX 77487
(800) 927-4227
www.iacprx.org

Gluten-Free Drug Information, Guides, Web Sites, Software

Clan Thompson Gluten-free Prescription Drug Database, Guide to Over-the-Counter Drugs, available from www.clanthompson.com.

Drug Facts and Comparisons, (800) 223-0554, www.drugfacts.com.

A Guide through the Medicine Cabinet by Marcia Milazzo (2004), available from the author at P.O. Box 1306; Medford, NJ 08055; (609) 953-5815, www.celiacmeds.com.

Gluten-Free Drugs, an Internet guide to gluten-free prescription and over-the-counter drugs, researched by Steve Plogsted, Ph.D. in pharmacology, www.glutenfreedrugs.com.

The Physicians' Desk Reference (Thompson Healthcare)
Prescription Drug and Over-the-Counter editions
P.O. Box 10689
Des Moines, IA 50336
(515) 284-6782
www.pdrbookstore.com

Internet Drug Index, www.rxlist.com. Drug information, side effects, ingredients, alternatives to prescription medications, health updates.

If after all your research, you're still not sure something you're taking regularly is safe or not, Consumer Labs, an independent laboratory, will test vitamins, minerals, supplements, and nutritional products for quality and ingredients, www.consumerlab.com.

And While We're in the Drugstore . . .

Over-the-counter drugs, vitamins, minerals, toothpaste, stomach remedies, cough syrups, pain remedies, allergy medications, antidiarrheals, laxatives, decongestants, cold and flu remedies, digestive enzymes, lip balms, and nasal sprays all have to be investigated for gluten. Really boring when you've thrown your raincoat over your pajamas to run out in the middle of the night and get a bottle of decongestant for your little celiac or yourself. Not a good time to start phoning manufacturers. Educate yourself now, before you have to make a midnight run.

The same rules apply to over-the-counter medications as do for prescription drugs. Inactive or excipient ingredients are used in these products to sweeten, color, suspend, or otherwise make palatable and may be hidden sources of gluten. Always, always, always call the company to verify, and if you are buying the generic brand, let's say Rite-Aid versus the brand name to save some money, make sure you ask the pharmacist or company rep to verify that the cheaper alternative is gluten-free.

The following over-the-counter preparations from *A Guide through the Medicine Cabinet* and glutenfreedrugs.com have been declared gluten-free by their manufacturers at this writing. Remember, the operative phrase is "at this writing." Bear in mind that many drugs deemed Not Gluten-Free are listed that way because their manufacturers could not (or would not) verify their ingredients. Keep trying; as manufacturers begin to recognize we're a big and growing market, this will get easier.

The following products have been declared by their manufacturers as gluten-free:

Advil
Advil Cold and Sinus
Afrin
Aleve
Alka-Seltzer Gold
Bufferin—all products except
    Bufferin regular 325 tablets
Centrum Kids Complete Rugrats
    Vitamins
Cepacol Mouthwash in Original and
    Mint
Citrucel
Dristan 12-hour Nasal Spray

Dristan Cold Multi-Symptom
Ensure and Ensure High
    Calcium
Enfamil and Enfamil Human Milk
    Fortifier
Freelax
Fleet Phospho Soda Flavored and
    Unflavored
GenTeal Eye Drops
Herplex
Immodium
Kaopectate
Lacrisert

Milk of Magnesia Concentrate
Motrin IB caplets
Motrin Children's Oral Suspension
Nature Made Vitamins and
  Supplements—all except those
  that are naturally not gluten-free
NyQuil
OcuHist
Pepto-Bismol
Robitussin Cold & Congestion
  Caplets
Robitussin Cold & Severe
  Congestion liqui-gels

Robitussin Honey Cough Drops
  (Almond and Honey, Herbal and
  Honey, Honey Citrus, and Honey
  Lemon Tea)
Salinex Nasal Mist
Tom's of Maine toothpaste
Tums
Tylenol cherry infants' oral drops
Tylenol extended relief caplets
Tylenol PM extra-strength gelcaps
Visine A
Xylocaine dental anesthetic
  ointment

To name a few.

Making Up Isn't Hard to Do

According to the FDA, cosmetics can be anything from mascara to tooth-paste, nail polish to deodorant sprays. Unlike drugs, which are strictly regulated and tested before being marketed for human consumption, cosmetics are not required to undergo approval before being sold to the consumer, though they must display ingredients on any package intended for sale. The active ingredient or chemical that makes the product effective must be listed first, followed by a list of inactive ingredients in order of decreasing quantity. By law, cosmetic companies are not required to substantiate claims or conduct product testing, but if safety has not been voluntarily substantiated, the product label must state this with "Warning! The safety of this product has not been determined." You won't see a warning like this on your Adobe Sunrise blusher or your Arrest Me Red lipstick any time soon.

The ingredients in cosmetics are tough to understand, and that's by design in a highly competitive industry. One way to bone up on the definitions and trade names for the stuff you're putting on your skin is to slog through *The International Cosmetic Ingredient Dictionary and Handbook*, published by the Cosmetic, Toiletry, and Fragrance Association. It's available at public libraries or at the Office of the Federal Register, www.gpoaccess.gov. Phone calls to cosmetic companies may be helpful, but alas are not always satisfying. In the "secrecy and obfuscation department," these people are better than the CIA.

Image is really what sells a cosmetic (I'll look like Halle Berry if I use this lipstick; I'll have a Tom Cruise smile with this toothpaste, etc. etc.) and these elusive promises are impossible to regulate. How could you possibly back up a promise like "Your Wind Song Stays on His Mind"? While cosmetics advertising is full of suggestion and innuendo, it's also riddled with legal hedges like "helps to reduce the surface look of fine lines" and "coats each hair with luminescent bubbles to create the temporary appearance of healthier hair." Toothpaste X boldly displays EXTRA WHITENING, but in the fine print, we do not find bleach, only extra abrasives to work on stains. These are loopholes you could drive a truck through. Buying this stuff is mostly about impulse, slick packaging, and nonverbal association. Why do you think cosmetics counters are always near the front door in department stores? Sometimes it's just impossible to resist the promise of perfect skin and shining tresses. Nothing to be ashamed of, we all buy into it from time to time. As long as the product is safe and free of gluten, we could do worse with our discretionary or, as the industry likes to think of it, aspirational spending.

Do personal products really need to be gluten-free?

Yes and no.

Many celiacs, especially those suffering from dermatitis herpetiformis, report reactions to foundations, facial moisturizers, hand lotion, sunscreen, shampoos, conditioners, lip balm and body creams, and especially those containing wheat germ oil. Dr. John Zone of the University of Arizona Department of Dermatology, in his presentation at the annual conference of the Celiac Disease Foundation, said it is impossible to get a gluten reaction from products absorbed by the skin, that is, topical. And yet many celiacs are skeptical. They wonder why, if prescription patches allow systemic medication to be absorbed this way, then why not gluten in external preparations? It's a good question, and the answer lies in the size of gluten molecules, which are too big to be absorbed through the skin. (For the official answer, see page 66.)

All well and good, but why do so many celiacs report reactions—everything from rashes to brain fog? Well, it may not be the gluten they're reacting to. The FDA reports that nearly a quarter of those questioned (non-celiacs) in a 1995 cosmetics survey responded "yes" to having suffered an allergic reaction to foundations, moisturizers, and eye shadows. That's a pretty large group. Celiacs are often sensitive to many substances besides gluten. If you agree that our immune systems aren't quite normal to begin with, it makes sense that we suffer from airborne allergies, chemical sensitivities, and often do not do well with products containing fragrance and chemicals.

An allergic response can take many forms—from mild and immediate irritation and redness to scaly, flaking, and itchy skin, outright hives, and, in rare cases, more dire reaction like anaphylaxsis (peanut oil is an ingredient used in cosmetic products). The point is, you don't have to be a celiac to have a reaction to a cosmetic, unless of course it contains gluten and you've swallowed some inadvertently.

Frugality can pose a problem, too. More often than we care to admit, the product we are using has been sitting in a drawer for over a year and is well past its prime. The bacteria in makeup that's gone off can cause even a cow's hide to break out.

When there *is* a gluten reaction, it is usually because a gluten-containing product, while not intended for internal use, has found its way into our systems in odd ways. Lipstick and lip balms, for example, end up in the stomach with each meal, lick of the lips, or through kissing and other romantic behavior (see "Sex and the Celiac," page 289). We touch our faces, then put our hands in our mouths. Soaps and shampoos get in our eyes and mouths. A common problem for celiacs is hand lotion. With sticky hands, we wipe crumbs off the counter or handle bread. Before we know it, we're getting gluten and we're not even having a meal.

A commonsense approach is to view cosmetic advertising and packaging claims with a healthy dose of skepticism. Don't take what these companies say as absolute truth. Use the product, by all means, but make no assumptions about one brand's purity or its imperviousness to allergic reaction over another brand. The *Celiac Disease Foundation Newsletter* lists some of the more common terms that consumers should be aware of. Familiarize yourself:

Natural. The implication here is that ingredients that come from nature, and hence are good and pure and safe, generally don't include anything chemical or produced synthetically. Then again, there are plenty of things in nature that could cause a nasty reaction.

Hypoallergenic. Scrawling this word across a label conjures the idea that this product is less likely to cause an allergic reaction than any other or that it has been formulated to rule out the possibility. Ditto for the terms "dermatologist-tested" or "allergy-tested" or "non-irritating." There is absolutely no substantiation required for these claims.

Alcohol-Free. This means the product doesn't contain ethyl or grain alcohol, but it doesn't mean you won't find other fatty alcohols like cetyl, stearyl, cetearyl, or lanolin.

Fragrance-Free. You'd think this means the product has absolutely no smell. Not so. Fragrance is often added to cover up unattractive odors given off by certain ingredients. Not so that the nose knows, but it's there.

Shelf Life or Expiration Date. Most people think this is important only in terms of food. Makeup that's gone off is more likely to cause a reaction

---

Gluten-Free Skin-Softening Tip

Fill a bowl with pure jojoba oil and nuke for 30 seconds, then soak your hands up to the wrists for about 10 minutes, says Bernadette Brescia of Brescia Salon in Philadelphia. Oil from jojoba is similar to your own sebum, so your hands will readily soak it up, leaving smooth skin minus the goo. Good for a non-greasy scalp massage, too.

---

than makeup that's fresh. Incidentally, the date on the label refers to conditions and use that are ideal. When was the last time you stored your nail polish in the refrigerator? Any makeup that's gotten clumpy or thick, turned color, separated, or otherwise congealed should be pitched out immediately.

Cosmetics Companies

Before you powder, paint, puff and fluff, moisturize and glamorize, do your homework. It may be the perfect shade of tangerine, but if it's the "kiss of death," who needs it? Here's a directory of our favorite cosmetics companies. Some are more forthcoming than others, and that old food company trick of supplying you with a list of what isn't gluten-free is rampant here. (Who do they think they're kidding?) If you're not good at cold-calling, go to www.delphiformus.com and click into the archives for the gluten-free status of your favorite products. But remember, as always, information that is dated is not information that is necessarily good. How are we ever going to increase awareness of celiac disease without telling somebody what we need?

If you use a particular product regularly (or your lover does and there's a lot of smooching going on), check, check, check, and check again. While you're at it, ask them why they always discontinue our favorite colors.

Almay
(800) 992-5629
www.almay.com

Avon
(800) 210-5758
www.avon.com

Did You Know?
. . . .

In ancient times, Japanese women were called *nuka-bijin*, or bran beauties, because they rubbed their faces with rice bran to cleanse their pores. Sounds like a celiac's revenge to me. Rice is so nice to us in so many ways. You go, kabuki girl.

Aveda
(886) 823-1425
www.aveda.com

Blistex Lip Balms
(630) 571-2870
www.blistex.com

Bobbi Brown
(646) 602-7800
www.bobbibrown.com

Bonne Bell
(800) 321-1006
www.bonnebell.com

Burt's Bees
(800) 849-7112
GF and non-GF list of products
available
www.burtsbees.com

Chanel
(800) 550-0005
www.chanel.com

Chapstick/Wyeth Consumer
Healthcare
(888) 797-5638
www.chapstick.com

Clinique
(646) 602-7800
www.clinique.com

Cover Girl
(800) 832-3012
www.covergirl.com

Dermal Therapy
   (Moisturizers for diabetics,
Sjögren's syndrome patients, and
others with severely dry skin)
(800) 668-8000
www.dermaltherapy.com

Ecco Bella Natural Cosmetics
(877) 696-2220
www.eccobella.com

Elizabeth Arden
(800) 755-7301
www.elizabetharden.com

Estée Lauder
(888) 378-3359
www.esteelauder.com

Kiss My Face
(845) 255-0884
www.kissmyface.com

Lancôme
(800) 526-2663
www.lancome.com

L'Oréal
(800) 322-2036, cosmetics
(800) 631-7358, hair products
www.loreal.com

Mac
(646) 602-7800
www.mac.com

Mary Kay
(972) 687-5577
www.marykay.com
   (Ask for their "Consumer Guide
to Cosmetic Ingredients")

Max Factor
(800) 832-3012

Maybelline
www.maybelline.com

Merle Norman Cosmetics
(800) 421-2060
www.merlenorman.com

Neutrogena
(800) 480-4812
www.neutrogena.com

Origins
(800) 674-4467
www.origins.com

Prescriptives
(646) 602-7800
www.prescriptives.com

Revlon
(800) 473-8566
www.revlon.com

Do-It-Yourself Lip Balm

½ teaspoon beeswax
1 teaspoon pure cocoa butter
1 teaspoon almond oil

In a double boiler, melt all ingredients, pour into a small round tin and
let harden. Pucker up.

Shiseido
www.shiseido.com

Stila
(646) 602-7800
www.stila.com

Gluten-Free / Allergy-Free /
Earth-Friendly Personal Products

BeautiControl
   Cosmetics, skin care, and spa products
   Designed by Caryn McClain, beauty and image consultant and celiac
(770) 214-8314
cmmclain@bellsouth.net
www.beautipage.com/
makeoverbycaryn

Earth Friendly Baby
(802) 425-4300
www.earthfriendlybaby.com

Kathy's Family Personal Care Products
(866) 634-0008
www.kathys-family.com

Naturelle Cosmetics
(800) 442-3936
www.naturalbeauty.com

Nu Skin
   GF skin care and makeup
   Represented by Stacy LaRoche
1225 Park Avenue, NY 10128
(212) 534-2059
www.nutritionalscanner.com

Pure & Basic
(800) 432-3787
www.pureandbasic.com

Shop by Diet
www.shopbydiet.com
(630) 355-4840

Sierra Soap
(530) 626-5197
www.sierrasoap.com

Vermont Soapworks
(866) 762-7482
www.vermontsoap.com

Learn More

To research other eco-friendly, animal cruelty-free products, go to *www.SaffronRouge.com*, a Web site devoted to organic and earth compatible cosmetics made with a minimum of preservatives.

   Now go powder your nose. But don't forget to clean the sink:

Non toxic Cleaning Products

Allen's Naturally
(800) 352-8971
www.allensnaturally.com

BI-O Kleen
(360) 576-0064
www.bi-o-kleen.com

Environne
(800) 869-5942
www.environne.com

Lifekind, Inc.
(800) 284-4983
www.lifekind.com

Trader Joe's
(781) 433-0234
www.traderjoes.com

Supermarket Brand Toothpastes, Powders, Mouth Washes, Rinses

Church & Dwight
(800) 786-5135
www.churchdwight.com

Colgate Palmolive
300 Park Avenue
New York, NY 10022
(800) 221-4607
www.colgate.com

Procter & Gamble
6071 Center Hill Road
Cincinnati, OH 45224
(800) 543-7270
www.pandg.com

PART VI

This Is Bigger Than Me

amazing grace

God, I thank thee that I am not as other men are.

—JOHN 18:11

Every Thanksgiving, we leave our downtown loft and drive through an avalanche of falling leaves along the Schuylkill River, into the red and orange blaze of Philadelphia's suburban Main Line. On the way, we gush over the postcard perfection of this bastion of camel-hair coats, black Labrador retrievers, and red Jeeps, entertaining ourselves with the "what if we lived here" game and knowing perfectly well we are urban dwellers down to the ground. We love the ethnic tumble of the city. We can't imagine having to drive everywhere, of not being steps away from a good restaurant or a new play and the café around the corner where painters and writers come up for air and a bit of gossip after a day's work, sipping coffee and making a stand against anonymity. Still, we are drawn, as on no other day, to the neat white pickets and dark hills, wood smoke drifting up from pumpkin-studded porches.

At Bryn Mawr College and the Victorian turrets of the Baldwin Academy, we turn into Jack and Barbara's driveway. Here with these cherished friends, in the bucolic hush of their pretty cul-de-sac, the most American of holidays unfolds in the same way, give or take a canapé or two, as it has for almost twenty years.

The meal hasn't changed much, and that's the way we like it—turkey, of course, gravy and stuffing, and sweet potato casserole, green beans, velvety potatoes mashed with butter and cream, and homemade cranberry sauce—simple American food. Good silver and candles give the room and those gathered around the gleaming table a sheen lacking on lesser occasions. Minutes before we gather around and clasp hands for our host's blessing, a ramekin of gluten-free stuffing appears to the right of my plate. It is joined by a pitcher of gravy made with cornstarch. Next, a gluten-free dinner roll arrives, unbidden, on my bread plate. These gifts do not call attention to themselves, they are given quietly and with deep affection. As Jack ticks off our blessings and burdens, gains and losses, triumphs and tragedies, some years better or worse than others, I bow my head and offer my silent thanks for the evidence of what sets me apart in this family circle—not as sick, but as someone well loved.

As children, most of us are taught that it's better to give; we learn that self-effacement is superior to self-gratification. But our gluten-free diet forces us to receive, something many of us are not very good at doing. It teaches us to ask for help, to accept that our happiness and well-being depend on the kindness of others, and to know we are part of something much larger than ourselves. The ability to communicate our needs to others and to be grateful for the response is a form of intimacy and trust, within which lies the seeds of our own generosity.

I look back on the years after diagnosis, and I am thankful for a lifetime of wonderful food prepared with love—the pasta ordered for my visits, the gluten-free waffles stocked for my breakfasts, the surprise birthday cakes and pizzas, and also for the sensitivity they have inspired in me. Without my own restrictions, I might not have been as determined to find lactose-free ice cream for my friend Marty or peanut-free foods for Michele, or sugar-free treats for Susan. I might not have been as conscientious about creating a pepper-free zone for Jane or so aware of Tina's mushroom phobia and Tom's aversion to tomatoes. If it were not for being a celiac, I might not have become as mindful as I am of cholesterol, and salt, and fat, and carbohydrates, and vegetarian issues in planning dinners and lunches for my nutritionally challenged tribe. I have only to look around my own table, see the pleasure on my friends' faces, and know the meaning of the Golden Rule.

If we let it, living without gluten can sharpen our instincts about what gives us pleasure. Thanks to my restrictions, I know what I like and what isn't worth the effort. I am forever marked with indelible memories. I remember the gluten-free pizza on a Venetian street I will never find again and the bakery in California with chocolate-dipped almond paste macaroons. Indochine rice wrappers will never be as good as they were in an exotic corner of Paris on a perfect spring night. Instead of restricting me, my diet has reinforced my belief in serendipity and confirms my suspicion that the universe gives us what we need the second we need it. Having a never-ending supply of something dulls the thrill of discovery. Some foods are meant for the moment, not for the freezer.

Unlike many Americans who eat on the run and rarely have time to think about what they're ingesting, those of us who are gluten-free are forced to go "against the grain" of our very culture. We can't eat on the fly. We must plan our nourishment, taking our time in choosing a food that will please us and be safe for us to eat. If we're smart, we avoid overprocessed "dead" foods in favor of vibrant flavored ones—fresh cheeses, ripened fruit, fragrant rice, and vegetables bursting with garlic and good olive oil, a cake made with ground almonds and chocolate. In so doing, we reclaim our health and rediscover anticipation, a calorie-free indulgence practically extinct in our fast-paced and artificial world. Shared meals are a connection to the people we love most— and because I have to think about them more than most, those times are more alive for me.

On a subzero night this winter, my husband and I dined with another couple at Django, one of our favorite restaurants (see their recipe for Goat Cheese Cake with Lemon Curd on page 141). As is the custom there, I was given a special menu with little hearts marking all the dishes the chef had determined, through his many thoughtful questions about my diet as well as my food preferences, were safe for me. I adore his scallops, but it was downright frigid and there was a big heart next to a delicious and cozy sounding pheasant cassoulet.

It was freezing. And I was torn.

"I thought this dish always contained bread crumbs," I said, nibbling the warm chickpea socca bread made just for me. The idea of a bread crumb–free cassoulet made my mouth water.

"I did, too," said the server. "But if Bryan put a heart on it, it must not."

"Cassoulet it is," I said, trusting these people completely. "I can have scallops anytime."

A few minutes later the chef's wife, Aimee, came out of the kitchen, beaming. "We didn't want to influence your choice," she said, "but we made one order of cassoulet without bread crumbs just in case you ordered it."

Let me say that again in case you missed it: *Just in case I ordered it.*

I struggled for a moment, fighting tears. I felt privileged, cared for, and cosseted, sorry for people who, by virtue of their ability to eat everything, would never know the joy of being the recipient of this kind of generosity.

Every year I count among my blessings the bakers, chefs, support group leaders, lobbyists, scientists, and physicians who give us their passion, their dedication, and food, glorious food. This year I will remember Phyllis Brogden, a woman who blessed us all with her deep devotion and tireless energy, a good and kind friend to every celiac.

Recently, I had a yen to make crab cakes and popped around the corner to Mr. Ritt's Bakery for some gluten-free bread crumbs (now there's a reason to give thanks). As I was chatting with the manager, a family of five from Seattle walked in. The husband picked up a copy of one of my books and waved it at his newly diagnosed wife. "I'll buy this for you if you promise to read it," he said.

"If she promises to read it, I promise to sign it," I chimed in, enjoying their surprise at running into the author. After a good laugh, they asked where in the neighborhood they could find a celiac-friendly restaurant. I gave them the address of a place nearby where the chef makes a magnificent salmon and pasta dish with olives and capers, as well as directions to a health food store where they could purchase some gluten-free pasta to take to the restaurant.

At this, the manager reached into the grocery bag he had stashed behind the counter and pulled out the package of pasta he had purchased for his own dinner.

"*Bon apetito,*" he said, offering them his purchase.

We all know that stuff like this does not happen every day. We know that not everyone is kind and we have the scars to prove it. But the way I see it, bad treatment is an opportunity as well. The fastest way to see what a person is made of is to ask for special treatment. Sad and disappointing as it is, I've purged from my life, or given a less important place, to those who can't or won't give me what I need, who feel diminished somehow if they cater to another. I am grateful for this, too. Toxic relationships with selfish people are far more dangerous in the long run than gluten or wheat.

〜

There is a newly vociferous toddler at Jack and Barbara's table this year. He will bang his spoon, gum his apple pie, and give us his own garbled benediction. "Gooden frwee!" he will screech, proud of his new ability to parrot my delight in discovering his mother has made a pumpkin cheesecake Aunt Jax can eat. And eat it I will, coming back for seconds with all the attendant guilt the holiday demands. Treats are just that, meant to be enjoyed down to the last heavenly morsel.

We have much in common, this child and I. My plate has been rendered free of gluten, his of the slightest whiff of peanuts. The fireplace stands cold in deference to our mutual asthma. He is about to learn what it has taken me a lifetime to know: that to be given less is the fastest way to find out how much more we can be.

We are loved, this child and I. And we know it. We only have to look down at our plates and around this happy table to see tangible proof. This is what grace is. It's an amazing feeling. I wouldn't trade it for all the pizza in the world.

A Gluten-Free Thanksgiving

Whether you go to friends and family or stay put and prepare the feast yourself, Thanksgiving can be the most satisfying holiday for the gluten-free, provided everybody knows the parameters. Since this is not the holiday to dine with strangers, I'm going to assume you've already shared your dietary restrictions with your family and close friends. If not, you must do so right away. Why? This is not the day to sit in the corner. If anyone expects you to, they are wrong. This is the day we go to any lengths to make others happy.

Remember that many commercial turkeys like the Butter Ball brand are pre-basted or injected with flavorings that may contain gluten. Ordering a fresh, unadulterated turkey in advance of the holiday will not only taste great, it will guarantee no nasty surprises. If you've been invited elsewhere, don't forget to talk turkey with your hosts well before it's time for them to buy the bird. As soon as you accept the invitation, have this conversation. Considering how long a 25-pound gobbler takes to thaw, the week before Thanksgiving may already be too late.

At my house, everyone eats gluten-free stuffing. No one has ever noticed the difference, nor would they care if they did. But many of you like to make two kinds and that's fine. No matter what kind of stuffing you prepare, always bake it outside the bird. This way you can be sure of not getting a stray bread crumb with your meat and be confident that it has baked long enough to ward off salmonella or some other nasty microbe that can contaminate undercooked stuffing, especially those containing eggs. And, of course, you do know a good thermometer stuck into the fatty part of the thigh will register the safe internal temperature of 165 degrees Fahrenheit. And always, always give a thorough washing to utensils, cutting boards, and any kitchen surfaces that come in contact with raw poultry, including your hands. But you knew that.

Your centerpiece taken care of, herewith a glorious meal for which to give thanks.

Classic Gluten-Free Bread Stuffing with Crisp Sage Dressing

With a few clever accommodations and a generous heart, tradition does not have to give way to special diet considerations. This classic savory stuffing comes from Torte Knox chef and cooking teacher Rebecca Reilly, author of *Gluten-Free Baking: More Than 125 Recipes for Delectable Sweet and Savory Baked Good, Pies, Quick Breads, Muffins, and Other Delights* (Simon & Schuster) and has appeared in *Living Without* magazine. Make it your own by adding wild mushrooms, dried fruits, apples, cranberries, lightly toasted nuts, fresh shucked oysters, or cooked gluten-free sausage. And enjoy it for years to come.

Serves 10 to 12

    4 cups gluten-free bread, cut into little cubes and lightly toasted
    4 plus 2 tablespoons unsalted butter or margarine, divided
    1 cup quarter-inch diced onion
    1 cup quarter-inch diced celery
    ⅓ cup quarter-inch diced carrot
    16 large fresh sage leaves
    ⅛ teaspoon fresh grated nutmeg
    1 pinch dried thyme leaves
    ½–¾ teaspoon coarse salt
    24 grinds fresh black pepper
    ¾–1 cup broth (gluten-free vegetable or chicken)

1. Put the bread cubes into a mixing bowl. Melt 4 tablespoons of the butter in a small skillet. Sauté the onion, celery, and carrot until tender. Then lightly mix in the vegetables with the bread.

2. Using the same skillet, melt the remaining 2 tablespoons of butter. Toss in the sage leaves. Over medium heat, brown the butter. The butter will be ready when it has a nutty smell and the sage leaves begin to crisp and brown. Remove the sage leaves and place them on a paper towel to drain.

3. Pour the brown butter over the bread mixture. Chop the sage leaves and lightly mix in with the bread and vegetables. Season with nutmeg, thyme leaves, salt, and pepper. Use just enough broth to moisten the stuffing. If you insist on stuffing it inside the bird, leave the mixture on the dry side. For a separate baked side dish, make it a bit moister.

4. Transfer stuffing to an ovenproof casserole and bake at 350 degrees until browned on top.

"Give Thanks" Gluten-Free Gravy

Serve this, as my friend Barbara does, in a pretty gravy boat. Save the rest for hot open-faced turkey sandwiches on gluten-free bread.

Makes about 2 cups

- 4 tablespoons hot turkey drippings
- 4 tablespoons cornstarch
- 2 cups gluten-free turkey or chicken broth
  Salt and pepper, to taste

1. Whisk together drippings and cornstarch. Gradually add broth, stirring constantly over medium-high heat until smooth and simmering.

2. Season to taste with salt and pepper. Serve in individual gravy boat.

Cassidy Family Sweet Potato Casserole

This is one of those family favorites we can't imagine Thanksgiving without. We like ours just fine without the marshmallows, but if you simply can't manage without their gooey sweetness, make sure the brand you buy is gluten-free.

Serves 8

- 2 pounds sweet potatoes, cooked and mashed
- 1 cup granulated sugar
- ½ teaspoon salt
- ½ cup milk
- 2 eggs
- 1 teaspoon gluten-free vanilla extract
- ⅓ stick butter or margarine, melted

TOPPING
- 1 cup brown sugar
- ⅓ stick butter or margarine, softened
- 1 cup chopped pecans

1. Preheat oven to 350 degrees. Mix sweet potatoes, granulated sugar, salt, milk, eggs, vanilla, and melted margarine. Pour into greased ovenproof casserole dish.

2. Mix topping ingredients and sprinkle on top of sweet potato mixture.

3. Bake for 35 to 40 minutes.

Native Corn Bread

This was not always the land of plenty. Native Americans not only helped the white settlers to plant corn, they taught them how to survive. Legend has it food stores were so low and starvation so imminent that first terrible winter in Jamestown, that every man, woman, and child were allowed only five kernels of corn each day. Those who lived to see that first harvest honored the memory of those who perished by including five kernels of corn in the feast. The first symbolizes the harvest, the second God's love and care, the third family, the fourth friends, and the fifth freedom. Rebecca Bunting, who is part Native American, has converted this savory corn bread from an Abenaki formula for her cookbook, *Sumptuous and Savory without Gluten or Wheat*. Be sure to check your source for cornmeal, to make sure there is no cross-contamination from wheat.

Makes 1 loaf

½ cup butter
2 cups cornmeal
1 cup GF flour mix
1 teaspoon salt
2 teaspoons baking powder
½ teaspoon baking soda
1 tablespoon dry yeast
3 tablespoons sugar
2½ cups lukewarm buttermilk

1. Preheat oven to 350 degrees.

2. Place butter in 10 to 12-inch cast-iron skillet and put in oven until butter melts.

3. Combine dry ingredients in large mixing bowl. Add buttermilk and blend well.

4. Pour batter into hot buttery skillet. Cover with lid or foil and let rise in warm place 20 to 30 minutes.

5. Remove cover and bake for 30 minutes until lightly browned. Serve warm.

REBECCA BUNTING'S GF FLOUR MIX
- ⅔ cup brown rice flour
- ⅔ cup tapioca flour
- ⅔ cup potato starch
- 3 tablespoons cornstarch
- 1 tablespoon xanthan gum

Combine and use as substitute for flour when baking. Store in tightly sealed container.

Count Your Blessings Pumpkin Cheesecake

Who needs pie when you've got this heavenly finale to a perfect Thanksgiving dinner adapted from a recipe that has been in the Cassidy family as long as anyone can remember. Make it for your own guests or bring it to another table. Forget to mention it's gluten-free—wait for everyone to taste theirs, then take a healthy slice. Watch them drop their forks and attempt to save you from yourself.

Serves 8

CRUST
- 1½ cups gluten-free cracker crumbs
- ½ teaspoon ground ginger
- ½ teaspoon cinnamon
- ⅓ cup melted butter or margarine

FILLING
- 1½ pounds (three 8-ounce packages) GF cream cheese, softened
- 1 cup granulated sugar
- ¼ cup brown sugar
- One 16-ounce can GF pumpkin purée
- 2 eggs
- One 5-ounce can evaporated milk
- 2 tablespoons cornstarch
- 1 teaspoon cinnamon
- ¾ teaspoon nutmeg

TOPPING

    2 cups sour cream

  ¼ cup sugar

      Vanilla extract

1. Preheat oven to 350 degrees.

2. Combine crust ingredients and press into bottom and slightly up sides of greased 9-inch springform pan. Bake for 8 minutes. Allow to cool while making filling.

3. For filling, beat cream cheese and sugars together until fluffy. Beat in pumpkin, eggs, and evaporated milk. Add cornstarch and spices and beat well.

4. Pour into crust. Bake for 60 minutes or until edge is set.

5. Combine topping ingredients and spread over warm cheesecake.

6. Return to oven and bake an additional 5 minutes.

7. Cool on wire rack. Store in refrigerator until ready to serve.

Christmas

My husband is British and more than slightly eccentric. The truth is, he is a living tribute to going "against the grain." This is never more evident than at Christmastime when the fact that he's been an American citizen for more years than we can count is conveniently forgotten. Dinner is always a standing rib roast (except for one year when it was a goose and the fire department had to be summoned). There is Yorkshire pudding, haricots verts, field greens studded with walnuts and pears, steamed plum pudding with hard sauce, and a round of Leicestershire cheese. To complete the picture, there are Christmas crackers, those little explosive devices stuffed with silly hats, toys that get lost in the rug, and jokes even a kindergartner would find puerile. You haven't lived until you've seen grown people in paper hats playing silly sods over dessert and coffee.

Years ago, when I had more strength and less time, I spent hours trying to create a gluten-free version of the dense and floury plum puddings of yore, steaming the thing in a *bain marie* and generally making a mess of things. The result was a pudding that weighed more than a small child and pleased no one, including me. Nowadays, I pick up an imported, store-bought pudding and a little jar of hard sauce and save my appetite for something far more memorable.

Nigella Lawson's Proper Christmas Trifle

First, allow me to be absolutely clear about one thing. Nigella Lawson doesn't bite. Not only does she not bite, she is generous, warm, witty, and one of the most passionate chefs on the planet. And yes, she is drop-dead, movie-star gorgeous. Best-selling author of the outrageously successful *Nigella Bites: How to Be a Domestic Goddess* and *How to Eat: The Pleasures and Principles of Good Food,* regular food columnist for the *New York Times,* and wildly popular star of the Style Network cooking show, *Nigella Bites,* you'd think she'd be at least a little bit snooty. On the contrary.

We are advised to use lots of jam, lots of custard, lots of sponge soaked in orange liqueur or pound cake in a pinch (gluten-free, of course), lots of cream, and our best and biggest crystal bowl, but not to get so fancy that we end up with something "posturingly elegant." Indulgent, but not pretentious is the key here. "A degree of vulgarity," Ms. Lawson tells us, "is requisite in the proper English trifle." Besides, this is Christmas, after all.

With Connie Sarros's sponge cake from *Wheat-Free, Gluten-Free Dessert Cookbook* (Contemporary Books), we can only ask ourselves how a dessert this rich and sinfully gooey could possibly be considered a trifle.

Serves 8 to 10

2½   cups light cream
      Zest and juice of 1 orange
½   cup Grand Marnier
¼   cup Marsala
One   8-inch sponge cake
10   heaping teaspoons best-quality raspberry or boysenberry jam
4   cups ripe raspberries
8   egg yolks
½   cup superfine sugar
2   cups heavy cream
½   cup flaked almonds
1   orange
½   cup sugar

1. Pour the light cream into a wide, heavy-bottomed saucepan, add the orange zest—reserving the juice, separately, for the moment—and bring just to the boil. Remove from heat and set aside for the orange flavor to infuse.

2. Mix together the Grand Marnier, Marsala, and the reserved orange juice and pour about half of it into a shallow soup bowl, keeping the rest for replenishing halfway through. Split the sponge cake horizontally. Make little sandwiches of the sponge and dunk each one, first one side, then the other, into the booze in the bowl. Arrange the alcohol-saturated slices at the bottom of the trifle bowl. When the bottom of the bowl is covered, top with the fruit and put in the fridge to settle.

3. Bring the orange-zested cream back to the boil, while you whisk together the egg yolks and sugar in a bowl large enough to take the cream. When the yolks and sugar are thick and frothy, pour the about-to-bubble cream into them, whisking as you do so. Wash out the saucepan, dry it well, and return the custard mixture, making sure you disentangle every whisk-attached string of orange zest.

4. Fill the sink with enough cold water to come about halfway up the custard pan. On medium to low heat, cook the custard, stirring all the time with a wooden spoon or spatula. With so many egg yolks, the custard should take hardly any time to thicken (and it will continue to thicken as it cools), about 7 minutes. If it looks as if it might be about to boil or bread, quickly plunge the pan into the sink of cold water, beating furiously until the danger is averted. When it's cooked and thickened, take the pan over to the sink of cold water and beat robustly, but calmly, for a minute or so. When the custard's smooth and cooled, strain it over the fruit-topped sponge and put the bowl back in the fridge for 24 hours.

5. Not long before serving, whip the heavy cream till thick and, with a spatula, smear it thickly over the top of the custard. Put it back in the fridge. Toast the flaked almonds by tossing them in a hot, dry frying pan for a couple of minutes, and remove to a plate until cool.

6. Squeeze the orange and pour the juice into a measuring cup, and measure out an equal quantity of sugar, usually about ½ cup. Pour the orange juice into a saucepan and stir in sugar to help it dissolve. Bring to the boil and let bubble until you have a thick, but still runny, caramel. If you let it boil too much until you have toffee, it's not the end of the world, but you're aiming for a densely syrupy, sticky caramel. Remove from heat when cooled slightly, dribble over the whipped cream; you may find this easier to do teaspoon by teaspoon. You can do this an hour or so before you want to eat it. Scatter the toasted almonds over the top before serving.

CONNIE SARROS'S GLUTEN-FREE SPONGE CAKE

6 eggs, separated
½ teaspoon cream of tartar
1½ cups sugar
½ cups water
1 teaspoon GF vanilla
1½ cups gluten-free flour mixture
Pinch of salt

1. Preheat oven to 325 degrees and butter a 9 × 13-inch baking pan.
2. Beat the egg whites with cream of tartar until stiff peaks form.
3. In a small saucepan over medium heat, cook the sugar and water until it threads. Watch carefully, this takes only a few minutes.
4. Slowly pour the sugar water over the egg whites, beating constantly.
5. In a small bowl, beat the egg yolks until thick; add the vanilla and fold into egg white mixture.
6. Pour mixture into the buttered pan, and bake for 35 to 40 minutes or until a toothpick inserted in the center comes out clean.
7. Cool and reserve for the trifle.

CONNIE SARROS'S GLUTEN-FREE FLOUR MIXTURE

Makes 5 cups

2½ cups rice flour
1 cup potato starch flour
1 cup tapioca flour
¼ cornstarch
¼ cup bean flour
2 tablespoons xanthan gum

1. Sift the rice flour, potato starch flour, tapioca flour, cornstarch, bean flour, and xanthan gum together in a large mixing bowl.
2. Store the flour mixture in a resealable bag. Refrigerate up to 1 week or freeze.

Lee Tobin's Gluten-Free Fruit Cake

In the days of Christmas yore, before CD got in the way of my frenzied holiday baking, I concocted my own variation of Craig Claiborne's famously moist and spicy fruitcake and practically burned out my electric mixer whipping up dozens for our annual tree-trimming party. At the end of the evening, a basket stood at the door and each guest was given one of these fragrant loaves. At home, we toasted and buttered slices for breakfast, served them as is with omelets, crumbled it over ice cream and spread small squares with cream cheese for nibbling with drinks and wrapped another to take for a hostess gift. A great moan went up among our friends when word of my diagnosis got around. "No more fruitcakes," the gang wailed collectively. Well, not until now.

This is as close to my old favorite as they come; in fact, it may just be better. Do not mistake this dense cake for those sorry bricks studded with embalmed fruit in grotesquely unnatural colors. Rich with healthy dried fruit, held together with a pinch of gluten-free flour, the secret to this fragrantly spiced and moist cake is apple juice and applesauce. This will start a tradition, mostly likely, one you will be expected to uphold year after year. Here with permission from Whole Foods Market chef Lee Tobin, three festive fruitcakes to wrap for presents and one to keep for yourself.

Makes 4 one-pound loaves

- 1 cup dried apples, chopped
- ¾ cup dried apricots, chopped
- ¾ cup halved dates (Note: Do not buy previously chopped date pieces, as these are often rolled in oat flour.)
- ⅓ cup currants
- ⅓ cup raisins
- ⅓ cup dried cranberries
- ½ cup apple juice
- ½ cup pecans, chopped
- 1 cup soy flour
- ½ cup potato starch
- 1 teaspoon xanthan gum
- 2 teaspoons baking powder
- 1 tablespoon cinnamon
- ½ teaspoon nutmeg
- ½ teaspoon allspice
- 1 stick unsalted butter
- ½ cup sugar
- 3 eggs
- 1 cup applesauce

1. Combine the apples, apricots, dates, currants, raisins, and cranberries in a large bowl. Heat the apple juice just to a boil and then pour over the fruit. Mix well and let sit overnight at room temperature.

2. Preheat oven to 350 degrees. In a large bowl, stir together the pecans, soy flour, potato starch, xanthan gum, baking powder, cinnamon, nutmeg, and allspice. Set aside.

3. Cream together the butter and sugar. Add the eggs, one at a time, to the creamed mixture, scraping the sides of the bowl with a spatula to ensure proper mixing. Add the dry ingredients alternately with the applesauce. Finally, mix in the fruit.

4. Divide the thick batter evenly between 4 greased loaf pans. Bake for approximately one hour, or until the center of a loaf passes the toothpick test (comes out clean).

Optional decoration: Heat ½ cup of corn syrup and brush it over the cakes; sprinkle toasted pecans and dried cranberries on top for a festive look.

Passover

Passover should be considered National Celiac Day. In keeping with the tradition of unleavened bread, Jewish bakeries everywhere make cookies, cakes, breads, and kugel with potato flour, cornstarch, and absolutely no gluten. The year I was first diagnosed a Jewish friend gave me a box of iced cookies and I'm sure I ate them all before the Pesach candle was out. Still, the heart and soul of Passover is matzoh, which does contain wheat, and Beth Hillson gives us her own family's gluten-free version of this seder centerpiece, the symbolic flat bread that was made for the flight out of Egypt.

Beth Hillson's Gluten-Free Matzoh

Makes one large or 3 generous matzohs

1 cup of all-purpose Gluten-Free Pantry baking mix
1 egg
4 tablespoons of water

1. Preheat oven to 425 degrees.
2. Mix ingredients in an electric mixer on high speed for about 20 seconds until it forms a dough ball.

3. Spray two sheets of plastic wrap with vegetable spray. Sandwich dough between sheets of plastic and roll out very thin (the thinner the better).

4. Pierce it with a fork in the same pattern as regular matzoh and place in the oven on parchment paper for 18 minutes. Let cool on the paper.

Note: Baking mix is available by mail from the Gluten-Free Pantry and at specialty stores. (See chapter 5 for details.) Or experiment with any of the mixes found in this book.

Joe Garrera's Hamantaschen

What's a nice Italian boy doing making a Passover cookie? Celiacs of every persuasion will be grateful to master baker Garrera for this buttery holiday delight. While the name may be a mouthful, these traditional Passover treats shaped like a three-cornered hat fall somewhere between a cookie and cake. The secret to these sticky sweet treats is poppyseed or prune filling found in the kosher section of the supermarket. Raspberry jam makes a delicious filling as well.

Makes about 2 dozen

¾　cup sugar
2½　cups gluten-fee flour mix
½　teaspoon salt
½　pound butter, cut into small chunks
1　egg
1　jar of prune or poppy seed spread or raspberry jam
1　teaspoon gluten-free vanilla or almond extract
　About ½ cup milk, enough to brush the tops of cookies

1. Preheat oven to 350 degrees. Mix all sugar, flour mix, and salt in an electric mixer bowl and mix at low speed, adding small chunks of butter until a mealy texture develops. Add egg and vanilla or almond extract, beating until a soft dough clings together. Chill 1 to 2 hours.

2. Place dough between two pieces of plastic wrap and roll until dough is uniformly ¼-inch thick. Using a glass or 3-inch cookie cutter, cut dough into 3-inch circles.

3. Place ½ teaspoon of jam in the center of each circle and pinch into three corners, so a triangle is formed. Brush with milk or milk substitute.

4. Bake 10 to 15 minutes. Let cool completely, 20 to 30 minutes.

Joe Garrera's Gluten-Free Baking Mix

Makes approximately 11 cups

6 cups white rice flour
3½ cups potato starch
1¼ cups tapioca flour
6 teaspoons xanthan gum

1. Sift 2 to 3 times and substitute for wheat flour for cookies, cakes, biscotti, and as a thickener.

2. Store unused portion in airtight container.

Amen.

how many celiacs does it take to change a label?

Be the change you wish to see in the world.

—MAHATMA GANDHI

There are many reasons to join an organization. First, when we are newly diagnosed, we need to look into the faces of people who understand what we're going through. Even better to learn from those who are ahead of us and to see in their healthy bodies and vibrant energy evidence that we will feel better. It is in their steady companionship that we receive proof that we will not only eat again, we will eat with gusto and take a deep pleasure in the everyday joys of the table and of family and friends. It's good to know we are not alone.

As we become more confident in our gluten-free ways, we veterans renew our membership to give back some of what we received when we were afraid, lost, and alone. We stuff new-patient packets with tasty samples of life after diagnosis, we answer questions that are now as basic to us as second nature, we trade cooking tips and give hugs, we honor those who gave so selflessly and well. Those of us with an activist streak walk for awareness, lobby for labeling legislation, share the latest research with our doctors and hospital dieticians, and push for more funding. We challenge food and drug companies to do better, and help them see the profit potential in us as a market. We write letters to newspapers, pitch articles to magazines and popular TV shows, and work with restaurants to show them what it means to cook us gluten-free meals. Some of us write books to educate, entertain, and raise awareness in the wider world. We look forward to our newsletters, knowing there is always something new to learn or, even better, to eat. For those of us in small towns and rural areas, just knowing we are part of a caring network of knowledge-able and like-minded souls can make all the difference.

Joining a group can be as intimate as sitting around the kitchen table with bighearted friends; it can be as energizing as being part of a grassroots activist movement, or it can be as anonymous as writing a check. It depends on the group and what you want to get out of it.

Like all big families, celiacs don't always agree. About what to eat. About what to put on a food label. About what standards for the gluten-free diet should apply. Some believe the Canadian-American gluten-free diet is correct, while others lean toward its European cousin, which allows wheat starch. No group officially sanctions the eating of oats, but some accept them off the record in moderation as long as the source can be declared free of contamination. Some accept that the distilling process renders grain alcohol, vinegar, and vanilla extract free of gluten molecules, while others say the jury is still out.

To further complicate matters, there isn't one national celiac organization. Unlike most other diseases and conditions, which, typically, are represented by a single association with a constellation of local support chapters, the celiac community offers a dizzying array of choices. Each comes with its own newsletter, each with a slightly different philosophy and personality, each with its own idea of what comprises the gluten-free diet and what food labels should say in the future.

When I was diagnosed with Sjögren's last year, I encountered no such confusion. I joined the Sjögren's Syndrome Foundation, which publishes a quarterly magazine called *The Moisture Seekers* (a title that conjures hordes of thirsty people crawling across the Sahara toward a mirage of Niagara Falls) which lists local chapters all over the country. I dutifully attended one of their meetings and, after toying briefly with the idea that these people badly needed a good laugh in the form of a book written by me, I decided to take care of myself first and think about it some more. For now, I've got a few like-minded Sjögren's buddies with whom to share coping strategies, and I see my doctor, a leading researcher in the field, regularly. Beyond that, I attend the national conference, take my medicine, get enough rest, use eye-drops, add my annual check to the search for the cure, read my magazine cover to cover, and I'm done.

Celiac disease is not like that. Celiac support meetings are not dreary affairs full of sob stories because celiac disease isn't about prognoses and flare-ups, medicine and side effects. It is as much about food as it is about science.

For many of you, a support group meeting will be the first time you eat something that doesn't make you sick. It may be the first time you realize the diet isn't so bad after all. You may find your palms sweating at the sight of pie, cookies, bread, and pretzels gathered at the vendor tables. You will catch yourself praying the brownie samples hold out long enough to get to you. You will learn which exotic-sounding flours will work as wheat-flour substitutes in your old baking recipes and which bread maker bakes the best loaf. You will learn, via the grapevine, which products not to waste your money buying. With three squares and a few snacks every day for the rest of your life, the right support group can be your cooking buddy, shopping guide, and test kitchen, as well as your advocate to the wider world.

Many of those who run groups do so out of a need to make sure no one else suffers or feels as isolated as they once did. Several years ago, I received a letter from an eighty-year-old widow who had just been diagnosed with CD. She had no idea what to do, nor was it easy for her to get out to the store at her advanced age. I enlisted the aid of Phyllis Brogden, who ran CSA's Philadelphia support group until her death this spring. Within days, Phyllis had organized the woman's shopping for her, had samples of gluten-free food shipped to her home, arranged a consultation with a dietician, and got her a ride to the meeting.

There are many other celiac angels waiting in the wings. There is Elaine Monarch, busy founder of the Celiac Disease Foundation in Los Angeles, who always has time to take the call of a stranger's sick son. Cynthia Kupper of GIG is a registered dietician who wasn't satisfied asking the restaurant industry for gluten-free menus, she's helping to design them for chains like Outback and PF Chang's. Dana Korn, the mother of a celiac child, transformed her own fears into a national network called Raising Our Celiac Kids and became a positive force for a whole generation of little celiacs. Alice Bast founded the fledging National Foundation for Celiac Awareness because she is determined that no one should have to bear the tragic reproductive consequences of undiagnosed celiac disease as she did. Diane Eve Paley, Mary Schluckebier, and Janet Rinehart, executives of the huge national organization CSA, never stop working for their local support groups. They make time to answer questions, take phone calls, track down food companies and guide their friends and neighbors through the growing maze of choices available to the celiac today. And there is Annette Bentley, who pushed and prodded and persevered at a time when no one had even heard of celiac disease, founding the American Celiac Society Dietary Support Coalition, one of the earliest lobbies for medical research and grant funding for blood screening.

Many of these people were diagnosed in the dark days of bananas and rice and made do with gluten-free food that had all the taste appeal of wood glue.

Some suffered greatly, and a few were left for dead before their mystery illness was solved. All had every reason to be glum, but instead they took Mahatma Gandhi's words to heart—they became the change they wished to see in the world.

These are passionate, committed, and highly opinionated people who have dedicated themselves to bettering the quality of life for those of us with CD. It's what makes them so dogged in their determination, so fierce in their protection, and it's also what makes some of them so skeptical of nutritional science which virtually left celiacs to their own devices for decades. All would agree that celiacs should speak with one voice and agree on one standardized diet. Deciding exactly what constitutes that diet and and whose voice it shall be is another matter entirely.

The aforementioned committed, opinionated, and involved people may also explain why CD claims two months of the year. National Digestive Diseases Week, a time for medical experts all over the world to get together to discuss the important issue of human plumbing, takes place in May. This is why many celiacs here and abroad attempt to draw attention to this condition in May. May is also national osteoporosis month, which is an interesting coincidence because so many undiagnosed celiacs end up with osteoporosis. Spring is a great time to walk, run, bike, swim, party, play, write their congressperson, have a gluten-free block party, show off awareness T-shirts, hats, silly sweatshirts, and stick HONK IF YOU'RE A CELIAC stickers to their car bumpers without getting too cold or wet.

However, there is another school of thought that says there's nothing like a crisp day in fall to do these things without working up a sweat. To members of CSA, October is Celiac Awareness Month and has been for over thirty years. Maybe it's because of the cooler weather, but most likely it is because this is when the group holds its national conference.

Both sides of the argument think the other is redundant and silly. I say, the more often we call attention to CD, the better. Besides, there are bigger fish to fry. Without bread crumbs, of course.

On balance, this is a small price to pay for all the good these groups have done. But as the larger world takes more notice of our condition, presenting a united face is critical if we are to be taken seriously by the medical community, the government, and those who manufacture our food. Kathie Cavanaugh, the quietly independent leader of three Pennsylvania groups affiliated with no national organization, is waiting for the day the entire celiac community is united under one national umbrella. "A girl can dream," she quips. Until such time, she goes her own way, supporting her members, while arguing, cajoling, and lobbying for the day there is one gluten-free diet all celiacs can easily follow.

There is such a movement afoot. The National Gluten-Free Diet Project, in concert with the American Dietetic Association and the ADA group, Dieticians in Gluten Intolerance Diseases, consisting of dieticians from the United States and Canada, has been created to review current science and nutritional research with the goal of forming consensus on a standardized diet. According to Shelly Case, R.D., coauthor of the celiac section of the *Manual of Clinical Dietetics* of the American Dietetic Association and Dietitians of Canada, the team will survey the needs and concerns of all support groups and deliver a single legitimate resource with supporting data designed to dispel confusion, one that can be embraced by professionals and patients alike.

Until such time, educate yourself and decide with your doctor what the best way is to follow the gluten-free diet for your particular condition. Shop around before choosing an organization. Attend a meeting or two to get a sense of its spirit, its collective personality, what foods it allows, what foods it doesn't, and, most important, why. A good fit is important, but so is geography. No point in joining a club with no support network in your area.

Attend an annual educational conference hosted by each of the national groups. There is no substitute for the wealth of medical knowledge, cooking instruction, and coping strategies that can be acquired in a few short days at one of these things, usually in a terrific city with three gluten-free catered meals every day. The food alone is a luxury worth attending for. I did just that many years ago, after my own diagnosis. With each conference, you may find yourself learning something new or, more to the point, be ready to hear something you haven't been open to previously. At one such meeting, during a presentation by an expert on genetics, I experienced a lightbulb moment that spared my first cousin even more heartache in his quest to solve a medical mystery related to CD. Just recently, in a darkened auditorium at the National Institutes of Health, I understood why my mother had the health problems she did, why her cancer came back after so many years. There are many reasons to attend these big meetings, not the least of which is spending a few days with like-minded people without having to worry about eating. But in the end, you have to go home and live on the diet for the rest of your life. Being part of a group that is willing to give you the kind of support you need and the disease the public attention it deserves is well worth the trouble it takes to find it.

Herewith, a quick sketch of each of the main organizations serving celiacs in the United States and Canada (for a list of local chapters and contacts for each of the national organizations, see chapter 21, "The Resourceful Celiac"). Consider a big chunk of your homework done.

U.S. National Organizations

Celiac Disease Foundation

Founded in 1990 by the dynamic Elaine Monarch, a former "banana baby" and diagnosed celiac since 1981, the national Celiac Disease Foundation is based in L.A.'s San Fernando Valley, with over 3,000 members all over the country. As per its mission statement, CDF provides support, information, and assistance to those affected with celiac disease and/or dermatitis herpetiformis and works to increase awareness of these diseases in the general public. As an organization, CDF uses its considerable clout, as well as its founder's irrepressible passion, to press for better food and drug labeling and physician awareness, and works closely with professionals in the pharmaceutical, medical, and research communities.

The Celiac Disease Foundation advisory board boasts an international group of experts. Alessio Fasano, M.D., of the University of Maryland; Ivor D. Hill, M.D., of Doctors Hospital in Winstem-Salem; Mayo Clinics' Joseph Murray, M.D.; John Zone, M.D., of the University of Utah; Michelle M. Pietzak, M.D., of the University of Chicago Center for Celiac Research; and Peter Green, M.D., director of the Columbia Celiac Disease Center, are among the notables. Under the guidance of this eminent team, CDF forms a bridge between the scientific community and the improvement in the quality of life for celiacs, working hard to make its membership aware of all the newest scientific and clinical advancements and helping to put this information into a practical, actionable context.

CDF puts out the quarterly *Celiac Disease Foundation Newsletter*, which gives its members articles on the latest research, product news and warnings, professional conferences, prescription and over-the-counter drug information, dining out, traveling, personal stories, recipes, new products, and other issues pertinent to the gluten-free life. Through the efforts of its board, CDF hosts symposia, offers a long list of books and articles, and sponsors many events that benefit celiac research, awareness, and government lobbying efforts. With its roots in California, CDF has formed a support network all over the country and has joined in partnerships with other groups, including Seattle's Gluten Intolerance Group and Raising Our Celiac Kids (R.O.C.K.) to create a grassroots effort it calls CDF Connections, furthering its mission to create awareness in the general public as well as in the physician community. A not-for-profit organization, CDF sponsors all kinds of fun events and benefits to raise money for lobbying efforts, awareness and research, both clinical and nutritional. Contributions are tax deductible. CDF holds an annual conference, usually in the Los Angeles area, in May. Membership is paid in annual dues.

Celiac Disease Foundation
13251 Ventura Boulevard
Studio City, California
(818) 990-2354
www.celiac.org

CSA

The old cliché about necessity being the mother of invention has never been truer. Frustrated by the lack of gluten-free food and even the barest scrap of information about celiac disease, the late Pat Murphy Garst of Des Moines, Iowa, marched into her kitchen almost thirty years ago and began to bake her own breads and cakes and cookies. When she developed a recipe that pleased her, she photocopied it and added it to the collection that would become the first gluten-free cookbook, a homemade, spiral-bound volume called *Gluten-Free Cooking*. In December of 1977, she contacted every person who bought her little book and with twelve members and donations totaling a whopping $75, the Mid-Western Celiac Sprue Association was born. By the end of February 1978, there were 41 members representing 11 states, forming the basis for what eventually became CSA/USA and now simply CSA, the largest non-profit national celiac organization in the United States, claiming over 9,000 members in 95 chapters and 55 resource units across the country.

With patient support still at the heart of its mission, the CSA of today solicits and awards grant money for research through its Research Grant Program. It provides to its members the newest scientific and research data and information relating to celiac disease and dermatitis herpitiformis, maintains a member Web site and publishes *Lifeline,* a quarterly newsletter filled with recipes, research, and personal articles, and publishes the annual *CSA Gluten-Free Product Listing*. CSA offers a referral service to help newly diagnosed celiacs find local support groups, maintains a hotline for member questions (877-CSA-4-CSA), and hosts an annual educational conference. The organization offers to its dues-paying members a library of cookbooks, audiotapes, pamphlets, dining cards, and educational materials.

In addition to its adult chapters, CSA offers support for families, children, and teens through Cel-Kids Network and sponsors Camp Celiac, an annual summer camp in Rhode Island.

Despite its size and reach across America, the tone of this organization is still decidedly folksy—"No WBRO [wheat, barley, rye, oats] is the way to go" is its slogan, and its gluten-free diet philosophy, the strictest of all the groups, is zero tolerance. CSA works for meaningful, verifiable, and consistent food ingredient labeling, supports ELIZA gliadin testing of products labeled "gluten-free," and believes the word *wheat* in the current congressional labeling bill is too vague to be of help to those who must avoid all sources of gluten. Membership dues are paid annually and a national education conference is held in October.

CSA
P.O. Box 31700
Omaha, NE 68131
(402) 558-0600
www.csaceliacs.org

Gluten Intolerance Group

Founded in 1978, this Seattle-based national organization, also known as GIG, is home to the creator of the *Gluten-Free Gourmet* cookbooks, beloved author Bette Hagman. With official branches and affiliate partner groups all over the United States, GIG's emphasis is on current nutrition information and education. The group states its mission thusly: "To increase awareness by providing current, accurate information and education, as well as support to persons with gluten intolerance diseases such as celiac disease and dermatitis herpetiformis, their families, health care professionals and the general public."

According to their charter, GIG Partners "embrace and support the mission of Gluten Intolerance Group for the good of all persons with gluten intolerance diseases." GIG states that by partnering with other organizations, they can work more effectively toward national unity, an important goal of the organization. Unity is necessary to be respected and heard by manufacturers and leaders that influence decisions affecting our health care and food regulation. GIG and its Partners believe the celiac community must "Speak with One Voice."

Programs supported by this group's mission include New Patient Packets and the *GIG Quarterly Newsletter* with articles on the gluten-free diet, nutrition advice, recipes, book reviews, product information, and the latest nutritional and medical research. GIG sponsors a summer kids' camp, an integrated program for children ages 7 to 18, and runs educational meetings, sponsoring visiting lecturers on CD and DH for patients, health care professionals, and the general public. Their annual educational conference is a multi-program event for dieticians, physicians, and the general patient population.

Gluten Intolerance Group is very strong on advocacy involvement and legislative reform and is involved in the education of governing bodies responsible for research funding and regulation. The group has worked in tandem with the American Celiac Task Force to press Congress for the passage of the first gluten-free food labeling bill. Tandem Tracks for Celiacs is billed as "a cycle adventure from Canada to Mexico" to raise awareness for CD.

GIG's president, Cynthia Kupper, a registered dietician, has taken advocacy straight to the restaurant industry and through her efforts and consultation theme restaurants like P.D. Chang's, Outback, and others are offering gluten-free menus.

Gluten Intolerance Group states they are a 501 (c) (3) nonprofit organization funded by private donations, including the Combined Federal Campaign, United Way Designated Giving, Employer Matching Funds, and proceeds from membership and the sale of products and educational materials. GIG also relies on private contributions that are tax deductible and 85 percent of their revenue is used to support membership programs. Membership is by dues and an annual May conference is held in the Seattle area.

Gluten Intolerance Group/GIG
15110 10th Avenue S.W., Suite A
Seattle, WA 98166
(206) 246-6652 / fax: (206) 246-6531
www.gluten.net

Raising Our Celiac Kids (R.O.C.K.)

R.O.C.K. started thirteen years ago, as all worthwhile organizations do, to fill a need that had been largely ignored. Danna Korn's story is not so different from those of so many parents of celiac kids. Her little boy Tyler suffered from severe chronic diarrhea, his belly was painfully distended, and his usually sunny disposition turned moody, whipsawing between lethargy and tantrums. Doctors tracked down possible causes, missing what was clearly celiac disease, a condition still thought to be rare at the time, and the family sweated out tests for cystic fibrosis, cancer, and other terrible blood diseases. By the time a definitive diagnosis was made, Tyler's mom was worn out, but grateful this was a condition managed by diet.

And so began the isolation, overwork, and heartbreak so many parents experience trying to help their little ones negotiate the birthday parties, the trick-or-treats, snack time at school, and all the problems posed by babysitters, grandparents, school chums, all the while encouraging them to feel as normal as possible. There were support groups for adults, but none addressed the special needs of children and the burden of such a diet on stressed-out, overworked moms and the rest of the family. Like most loving parents, Danna wrote to food manufacturers, made countless lists of gluten-free foods, bought herself a bread machine, talked to teachers and friends and neighbors, and got pretty good at making sure her darling had safe food. This is where an average mom became decidedly unaverage.

Raising Our Celiac Kids was born in San Diego, in order to make sure no other family suffered the isolation, exhaustion, and fear the Korn family had experienced. Word spread and a decade later, through the founder's advocacy and cheerleader spirit, R.O.C.K. is now a huge nationwide grassroots effort. Meetings still take place at parks and other venues where kids can picnic and play and members are asked to bring "kid food." There are parties, potlucks, walks, runs, and bike rides for awareness. Members range in age from one year to preteen, and sharing experiences is encouraged.

Toddlers point to their bellies and proudly report that it doesn't hurt anymore. Older children discover they are not "nerdy" or "weird" and make friends that last well beyond the difficult years. There is a special teen group in the making to help youngsters (and their parents) cope with the burden of the gluten-free diet and life in general at this awkward and rebellious age.

Parents, too, learn they are not alone and share information and resources, giving them the confidence and reassurance they need to know they are doing the best they can for their children. Children on casein-free diets are welcome, as is any family on the gluten-free diet for any reason.

R.O.C.K. is not a nonprofit, but rather an upbeat club in which membership is free.

Raising Our Celiac Kids R.O.C.K.
c/o Danna Korn
3527 Fortuna Ranch Road
Encinitas, CA 92024
www.celiackids.com

Canadian National Organizations

Canadian Celiac Association/
L'association Canadienne de la Maladie Coelique

Whether in English or *en français,* this is the national celiac association of Canada. With over 15,000 members across the length and breadth of Canada, there are 26 affiliated chapters and 21 satellite groups across British Columbia, Alberta, Saskatchewan, Manitoba, Ontario, Quebec, Nova Scotia, Prince Edward Island, and Newfoundland, and in cities and towns large and small. While this group is bilingual, the organization is the best example of what can happen when celiacs speak with one voice to an entire country.

Founded in 1972 by two celiacs from Kitchener, Ontario, for the sole purpose of providing support and sources for gluten-free food to others in a similar position, the mission of the Canadian Celiac Association has never wavered. As stated on its Web site, the CCA is "a national organization dedicated to providing services and support to persons with celiac disease and dermatitis herpetiformis through programs of awareness, advocacy, education, and research." The Canadian Celiac Association is incorporated under the Canada Corporations Act and is a registered charity with Revenue Canada.

The purpose of the CCA is to assist its affiliated chapters and to represent their members' needs on the national level, which includes raising awareness of CD among health care professionals and the public, and provide reliable and up-to-date information on the gluten-free diet through newsletters, availability of gluten-free products, and relevant literature.

The Canadian Celiac Association consults with government and the food and drug industries of Canada about gluten-free foods, research, and other interests of Canadian celiacs. It encourages and funds research and offers reduced rates to their membership on conference registration and the purchase of educational books and materials.

CCA receives financial support through grants from Health Canada, and the Trillium Corporation has funded its public awareness campaign. Dues and charitable donations are received from members and private donors.

Every celiac in Canada is on the same page. Food alerts are posted on the CCA's Web site, but perhaps the most telling advantage of such a unified approach to celiac disease are these step-by-step instructions (posted on the Web site) in case of a food reaction caused by mislabeling or cross-contamination.

1. Immediately follow your emergency treatment plan. (This is a plan you and your doctor have decided is best for you in the event of an accidental or otherwise ingestion of gluten.)
2. Do not throw out any remaining portion of the offending food. Wrap and save it, along with the label and package.
3. Contact the nearest office of the Canadian Food Inspection Agency (CFIA) for advice. Report the type of reaction (i.e., vomiting, hives, diarrhea, etc.). If requested to do so, give CFIA the remaining portion of food, along with the label and package for laboratory testing.
4. You may report the reaction to the food manufacturer. The company may want code numbers so that it can investigate. If the company offers to pick up the remaining food, tell them the CFIA will be doing this.

A further note to the members: If the CFIA tests the food and finds that mislabeling and contamination has occurred, CFIA will contact the manufacturer. In some cases, the food has to be recalled.

Imagine the FDA contacting an American food company to possibly recall a product that has caused an unsuspecting celiac to become sick. Granted, ours is a culture that panders much too much to the corporation at the expense of the individual, but in Canada this is what can be accomplished when the government hears one strong voice, loudly and clearly. We have much to learn from our neighbors to the north.

Canadian Celiac Association
5170 Dixie Road, Suite 204
Mississauga, Ontario L4W 1E3
(904) 507-6208 or (800) 363-7296
www.celiac.ca

Advocacy

American Celiac Task Force

Formed in March of 2003, this organization is not a support group but rather a coalition of representatives from the celiac community who have come together to accomplish a single task. That task was and is to lobby Congress and to rally celiacs everywhere to petition for the passage of a food labeling bill that would make following the gluten-free diet in the United States safer and easier.

The task force is made up of leaders in celiac disease research, among them founder Alessio Fasano, M.D., University of Maryland Center for Disease Research; Joseph Murray, M.D., Mayo Clinic GI Center; Stefano Guandahni, M.D., of the Chicago Celiac Disease Program; and Peter Green, M.D., Celiac Disease Center at Columbia University. Support group and industry leaders include the American Celiac Society, Celiac Disease Foundation, Gluten Intolerance Group, Dietary Specialties, Bob & Ruth's G/F Travel Club, Ener-G Foods, Gluten-Free Living, Gluten-Free Pantry, *Living Without* magazine, and Prometheus Laboratory.

In 2004, a Senate committee chaired by Senator Edward Kennedy (D-MA) and Senator Judd Gregg (R-NH) and by unanimous consent, put S. 741, "The Minor Use and Minor Species Animal Health Act of 2004" (the MUMS Act) to a Senate vote. The measure requires the top eight allergens (peanuts, tree nuts, eggs, milk, soybeans, shellfish, fish, and wheat) to be listed on food labels by their common or usual name, or by source or ingredient. The bill further requires the Secretary of Health and Human Services to propose rules to "define and permit the use of the term gluten-free on food labels by their common or usual name, or by source or ingredient."

One year later, on March 8, 2004, the bill was passed and sent to committee in the House of Representatives where it became House bill H.R. 3684, the "Food Allergen Labeling and Consumer Protection Act"—a better title, in my opinion. In June of 2004, the House Committee on Energy and Commerce voted to put S. 741 to a House vote, rather than take the time to reconcile H.R. 3684 with S. 741, a process requiring additional votes by the House and Senate.

On August 5, 2004, President Bush signed the Food Allergen Labeling and Consumer Protection Act into law, requiring mandatory labeling of the above mentioned allergens in all food products manufactured in the United States.

The findings section of the act refers to celiac disease as an "immune-mediated disease that causes damage to the gastrointestinal tract, central nervous system and other organs." It also makes note of the "multicenter, multiyear" study which estimates that the prevalence of celiac disease in the general U.S. population is at "0.5 to 1 percent of the general population."

It further states that "2% of adults and 5 to 10% of infants and young children suffer from food allergies and, each year, roughly 30,000 individuals require emergency room treatment and 150 individuals die because of allergic reactions to foods."

This did not happen by accident. In eight short months, 10,000 letters were written and countless telephone appeals were made. Celiacs lobbied Congress and families told their stories on the Senate floor, proof that we can speak with one voice when we are moved to do so.

I sincerely hope that by the time this book is published, this congressional act is in force with the full compliance of all food manufacturers, and we are well on our way to mandatory disclosure of gluten in all products. But, as we all well know, anything can happen in politics. Section 6.A of the act states that "any person may petition the Secretary [of Health and Human Services] to exempt a food ingredient described in section 201 (qq)(2) 20 from the allergen labeling requirements of this subsection"; 6.B says, "The Secretary shall approve or deny such petition within 180 days of receipt of the petition or the petition shall be deemed denied, unless an extension of time is mutually agreed upon by the Secretary and the petitioner."

Further down in 6.E., we read "The Secretary shall promptly post to a public site all petitions received under this paragraph within 14 days of receipt and the Secretary shall promptly post the Secretary's response to each."

In other words, vigilance is required to make sure there is no dilution or corporate modification of this important first step in gluten-free labeling..

No matter, this is a giant step on the road to safer foods and not only wheat-free, but gluten-free labeling. Soon we will have a way of knowing if a food product contains wheat, the most ubiquitous of the glutenous grains used in mass-produced foods.

There is much more work to do. Beyond a gluten-free aisle in every supermarket and specialty food store, my own wish list includes wider public screening, lobbying of the insurance industry for prescription-paid, gluten-free food (current standards of reimbursement do not take into account a disease that is entirely managed by food) and that must be changed. Food *is* the medicine.

And while I'm at it, why not a government subsidy of medically required gluten-free food, especially in poor and rural communities and among those on Social Security and fixed incomes for whom expensive mail-order products are out of the question? And there is the need for inclusion of the Hispanic and African-American celiacs, and government-supported programs for schools, the elderly, institutional populations, and those on the margins of society. But perhaps the most important work that needs to be done next is to define what gluten-free is and how that definition allows us to create enforceable food manufacturing standards.

If this recent and overwhelming victory is any indication of the spirit and determination of the celiac community, we may soon be asked to lobby Congress again, this time for the addition of rye, barley, and oats to the list of allergens.

American Celiac Task Force
Andrea Levario and Allison Hewitt, co-chairs, Legislative Project
www.celiaccenter.org
actf@fogworks.net

Lobbying Congress Effectively

The task force gives the following tips for effective communication with your senator or representative. First, if you don't know how to contact that person, go to www.gpo.access.gov/cdirectory/index.html or call the U.S. Capitol switchboard, (202) 224-3121, and ask for your senator or representative's office.

Ask to speak with the aide who handles the issue about which you would like to comment. Identify yourself as a constituent and tell the aide you would like to leave a brief message, such as "Please tell Senator/Representative _____ that I support/ oppose S_____/H.R._____ because _____." Always give the reasons for your position and ask for the Senator's/Representative's/Secretary's position on the bill or issue. By all means, request a written response to your phone call.

If you'd rather put your views in writing, make your petition as eloquent as you can, but don't rattle on. Be courteous, to the point, and include key information and use examples to support your position. A good rule to follow when writing to a U.S. senator or representative is one issue/one letter/one page.

Do remember a letter addressed to a senator or representative or secretary should always read "The Honorable." The salutation should say "Dear Senator _____" or "Dear Representative _____."

When writing to the secretary or chair of a committee, the salutation is always "Dear Mr. Secretary, Dear Madame Secretary, Dear Mr. Chairman, or Dear Madame Chairman."

Letters to the Speaker should begin, "Dear Mr. Speaker" or, we can only

---

Kudos

. . . .

To Alex Plotkin and Max Lapin, owners of the Philly Swirl Company, makers of Original Italian Ice Swirl, popsicle SwirlStix, Phudge & Cream Bars, and Fruit & Crème Bars for donating 25 cents off each box sold with a matching personal donation to the University of Maryland Center for Celiac Research. I know what I'm having on a hot day.
Thank them at www.phillyswirl.com.

---

hope that someday we'll need to know a letter to a female Speaker should carry the salutation, "Dear Madame Speaker."

The same guidelines and courtesies apply to e-mail.

National Foundation for Celiac Awareness

Founded in 2004 by Alice Bast, a celiac, mother, and activist, the mission of this fledgling organization funded by the National Institutes of Health is not to provide direct patient support but to advance research and raise awareness and funding for celiac disease itself. Its goals are public and physician education, widespread screening, and to improve the quality of life for children and adults and future generations affected by this autoimmune disease through grants and direct programming. With physician and public awareness as its main goal, it hopes to wipe out the many complications of untreated and undiagnosed celiac disease, among them osteoporosis, related autoimmune disorders, infertility, neurological conditions, and cancer.

To that end, the 501 (c) (3) nonprofit National Foundation for Celiac Awareness is building an influential board of directors among community and industry leaders and has attracted an expert panel from leading-edge institutions in medicine and research, among them Alessio Fasano, M.D., Center for Celiac Research, University of Maryland, Cairan P. Kelly, M.D., Harvard Medical School, and Anthony J. DiMarino, M.D., Chief of Gastroenterology and GI, and director of the Digestive Diseases Center at Thomas Jefferson University Hospital.

NFCA promotes careers in celiac research and seeks to identify and fund therapies that will lead to a cure. The board's charter is to guide the creation of funding and development, and to use its considerable fund-raising ability to launch a nationwide awareness and advocacy campaign.

Unlike many organizations that are predicated on patient support, NFCA is focusing on the fact that celiac disease is one of the most common hereditary diseases in the world and as such requires more accurate and cost-effective screening methods than those now available and in use. The vision includes a pharmaceutical cure to prevent the onset or to mediate the many manifestations of the disease, so that men and women suffering from CD and DH may lead normal lives.

NFCA works toward the day all health care professionals (not just those specializing in gastroenterology) will recognize the signs and symptoms of the clinical chameleon that is CD to enable rapid and accurate diagnosis and have the appropriate tools and materials to teach patients how to live healthy and gluten-free. NFCA will fund the first scientific journal devoted exclusively to celiac disease and will provide research money through an expert panel and formal proposal process. Findings will be communicated directly via the physician education program and the public awareness campaign.

In short, the NFCA means to shorten the now average eleven-year odyssey most patients endure before getting an accurate diagnosis and to preempt through research and awareness the debilitating, often tragic, and unnecessary repercussions of undiagnosed CD.

National Foundation for Celiac Awareness
124 South Maple Way
Ambler, PA 19002
(267) 625-5505/ fax (215) 283-2335
info@celiacawareness.org, www.celiacawareness.org

A Word about Nonprofits

The terms *nonprofit* or *not-for-profit* are bandied about not only in the celiac world but in many places in our lives. A nonprofit organization is designated a 501 (c) (3) corporation and must report its income to the IRS as such. In order to verify the nonprofit status of any organization you are considering supporting through membership and donations, go to www.guidestar.com and check its tax returns. Some associations do not have this status, which is fine, but they must fully disclose that they are "for profit."

It is also tempting to be persuaded by a banner declaring that the "profits of this or that enterprise are going to celiac research." In most cases, this is true and many companies and individuals donate a generous portion of their proceeds to good causes, but bear in mind this has become a popular marketing device for many businesses. The key word in the sentence is *profit* or, more specifically, *net profit*, which is what remains after taxes, expenses, capital improvements, overhead, salaries, etc. If nothing remains after all these matters are settled, there are no profits and thus, nothing to give to a good cause. Hollywood is famous for movies that gross in the millions but show no net profit, the substance of many a lawsuit from disgruntled actors and screenwriters whose salaries and bonuses are tied contractually to a percentage of "the net." If you're not sure about a company, ask where its profits go and more to the point, how much has already been given to celiac research.

Finally, if you want to be absolutely sure your money is going to research or to another cause of your choice, always write "For research only" on the face of your check. This way you are assured that your money is being spent in the way you intended.

How to Take No for an Answer

Some months ago, David Marc Fischer, a New York celiac who has enjoyed David Glass Ultimate Truffle Cakes for many years, wrote to the company to verify that their recipe continued to be gluten-free. The answer wasn't exactly what he expected. The correspondence is reprinted here with Mr. Fischer's permission.

> While our Ultimate Chocolate Truffle Cake recipe does not call for any gluten ingredient, the company cannot guarantee or advertise the cake as "gluten-free" because gluten is used elsewhere in the facility. Therefore we cannot give you confirmation.

Let down, but determined to give this company a reason to change its manufacturing policy, Fischer wrote back:

> Thank you for your prompt response to my inquiry about whether the Ultimate Chocolate Truffle Cake recipe would be safe for people like myself, who are on medical gluten-free diets. As someone who has enjoyed and, in a way, relied on, the cake for several years, I was disappointed to find that your company no longer feels confident about its safety, but I am grateful for your frankness.
>
> I do hope that you and the decision-makers in your company will seriously consider the benefits of producing the cake under conditions that would make it safe for people on gluten- and wheat-free diets. For most consumers, the cake, as delicious as it is, is just one of many available in assorted markets. But for the rapidly growing population of people who

must adhere to those medical diets [at this point, I would have inserted, "1 in 132 are gluten-intolerant, that's 2.2 million Americans" to give them something to chew on], the cake would be virtually unique and highly prized. I strongly suspect that the profit you would make by marketing the cake to this community would compensate for any investment you would incur in ensuring its safety. On top of that, you'd be making a lot of us very, very happy.

Thank you for considering these remarks.

This is a great letter. It's short and to the point, extremely courteous, and instead of being full of complaint, gives the recipient a solid marketing reason why the company should reconsider its manufacturing process in a way that could impact its bottom line. I have read many such letters and, frankly, most go on too long about research and symptoms. The trick is to give a business a good reason to comply. Mr. Fischer's letter does that with brevity and an upbeat tone. I'm sure he wouldn't mind if you patterned one of your own after it.

Kristin van Ogtrop, editor of *Real Simple* magazine, treasures this quote from Rabbi Paul M. Steinberg scribbled on a cocktail napkin during a wedding at which he officiated. It captures the spirit of all those who won't take no for an answer, those who support and fight for us and sometimes with each other for the greater good of all celiacs.

If you want to be happy for an hour, take a nap.
If you want to be happy for a day, go fishing.
If you want to be happy for a month, go on a honeymoon.
If you want to be happy for a year, inherit a fortune.
If you want to be happy for a lifetime, help other people.

Q: How many celiacs does it take to change a label?
A: All of us.

a puzzling condition

It is a riddle wrapped in a mystery inside an enigma.

—WINSTON CHURCHILL

In the beginning, we haven't got a clue. Our medical mystery may be solved at last, but the future is puzzling. We are handed a lifetime prescription for a diet that goes against the grain of how we have been taught to eat. We kick and scream and torture ourselves with visions of strawberry shortcake with mountains of cream. We indulge in dark moods and hungry looks at strangers in restaurants. Then, with a realization as imperceptible as sunlight across our days, we not only feel better, we *are* better. We find ourselves looking forward to seeing gluten-free friends whose faces mirror the story of our own lives, confident and strong. Suddenly, there's a bit more meat on our bones, a buttered scone in our fingers, a frothy head on cold glass of beer, a full and satisfying plate. The riddle of how we will live is solving itself. We hear our own voices ring with laughter. We are discovering no road is long in good company. A chapter has closed. We open the next with optimism, gratitude, and verve, holding other unsteady hands along the way.

And so, dear reader, it's time for some entertainment. Sharpen your pencils (and your wits) and see how much you've digested. With special thanks to Steve Zettler and Cordelia Frances Biddle, the pseudonymous Nero Blanc, author of the Berkley Prime Crime Crossword Mystery Series, I present to you *A Puzzling Condition*, the world's first gluten-free crossword puzzle.

The World's First Gluten-Free Crossword Puzzle

Across

1. Atkins or glutenous taboo
6. Impolite reach for GF samples
10. Genetically mongrel celiacs; var.
14. Strong painkiller
15. Irk
16. "Was that a crouton?"
17. Tinkyada, e.g.
18. Diari-_____
19. _____ avis
20. Corny verity?
23. Barn allergen
25. Switch positions
26. _____ and hearty
27. Most venerable
30. "Miss Muffet went that-a-_____?"
32. Celiac who's left high and dry?
33. Oats: friend or _____?
34. Home of a gluten-friendly mouse; abbr.
37. Porridge reaction
42. Picnic pest
43. Jazzy GF group?
44. It takes two celiacs to _____
45. Tax pro for GF deductions
47. A celiac's worst nightmare
48. Immed. reaction time
50. GF brew
52. Dijon donkey
53. Dangerous grains
58. Tiniest gluten particle?
59. Scottish isle
60. Yoga position
63. "Beloved" Nobelist
64. Worry, as in cross-contamination
65. Celiac honeymoon digs
66. GF flour source
67. Last word in Münster
68. Overachieve

Down

1. Celiac on the beat?
2. "It's in your head," org.
3. Beer and pretzels, e.g.
4. Firth of Clyde island
5. Tent maker
6. Aussie expert, Peter
7. Iranian coins
8. Too
9. Argument over stew thickener?
10. Celiac doc, "Hold the Mayo?"
11. Traveling gustaphobe's pantry?
12. Flourless cake
13. Deposed crumb?
21. "I'll have a pizza _____!"
22. It takes _____ cake
23. Teamster Jimmy
24. Director Woody
28. Slippery breaded fish
29. _____ Lanka
30. Beat the odds
31. "_____-Haw"
33. Brainy reaction to gluten?
34. "Discover a gluten pill? _____!"

35. 3-starrer; abbr.
36. Celiac's goal: To speak _____
38. Dreyer star catalog; abbr.
39. "Scram!"
40. Cardinals' cap letters _____
41. Org. founded in Ethiopia, 1963: Was injera served?
45. Pernicious symptom
46. Celiac support org.
47. Guy's partner
48. "I'm a celiac, also!"

49. Breadwinner or celiac named Petitpain; e.g.
50. A many-forked road?
51. Gladden
53. Purr-fect theatre?
54. Duration of diet
55. R.O.C.K. star?
56. "Read the label, or _____!"
57. Unsafe soup base
61. Shoshonean
62. Lyon GF seasoning

the resourceful celiac

Oh, I get by with a little help from my friends.

—JOHN LENNON AND PAUL MCCARTNEY

If I had to name the single most important skill any celiac must learn, it would be resourcefulness. There is an art to questioning a food or drug company, not only to get the information you need but also to educate others about the vast, untapped market of celiacs out there just dying to get their hands on a crusty gluten-free baguette.

It's also important to develop culinary vision—to look past a product's intended purpose for the one you need. I am reminded of the long-gone kosher bakery I discovered in Brooklyn when I was first diagnosed. They baked challah every Friday for Shabbat and sold wonderful sponge cakes, old-fashioned leaf cookies, macaroons, and other gluten-free treats year-round. For generations, this family survived the ups and downs of business on both sides of the Atlantic. They had perfected the art of baking with potato flour, not because it is gluten-free, but because during the severe wheat shortages of World War II, this was the only ingredient that was in plentiful supply. Their desserts were the best I'd ever tasted because they were invented for people who still had the taste of wheat in their mouths. If only a market-savvy son or daughter, seeing one celiac after another come back for more had counseled patience, had convinced their parents of a new, untapped market.

It's hard to imagine that people who outsmarted the economic repercussions of an entire world war could not make it to the millennium. I like to imagine the proprietors happily retired and on a cruise ship somewhere, tasting the ship's pastry, shaking their heads and saying, "In our sleep we could do better." The point is, companies come and go. The companies, organizations, and support group chapters listed here, as well as those gluten-free specialty businesses, bakeries, restaurants, and food manufacturers listed in previous chapters, were all up and running at press time. It is impossible to reflect the moment-by-moment moves, reversals of fortune, mergers and acquisitions, and the occasional and inevitable casualty of a changing economy. Nor am I able to guarantee addresses, phone numbers, websites, and e-mail addresses beyond this printing. It would be impossible and naive of me to try. If the previous edition is any indication, you should have this book for a good long time. I like to imagine it well-thumbed, dog-eared, and smudged with a gluten-free goodie or two, eaten in bed while you bone up on your restaurant skills, search for a gluten-free bed-and-breakfast, have a laugh or two, and resolve to try something spectacular for your next dinner party. I think it's much more important to have a comprehensive list of resources than to worry about one or two people dropping out, moving away, going out of business, or changing numbers. That's what resourcefulness really is—using what you have to find what you don't.

We've all been taught never to deface a book. In this case, I will forgive you. As the years go by, you have my permission to pencil in new companies, cookbooks, support group contacts, in the pages that follow and in each chapter. This way your celiac resources are all in one place. And if you discover something wonderful, please let me know. I'll put it in a nice clean edition for you next time.

Local Support Groups, Chapters, and Affiliates of National Organizations

These are your neighbors and friends down the block, across town, a phone call away. They know which restaurant will serve you a safe meal, where to buy gluten-free products in the area and will pool their resources to help you. The Turkish proverb has never been truer: "No road is long with good company."

Celiac Disease Foundation/Connections, cfd@celiac.org

ALABAMA

Martha Wright, Southeast Hartford, (334) 588-2156

ARIZONA

www.Phoenixceliac.com
Nina Spitzer, Phoenix,
(480) 488-0318, nina@amug.org
Diane Lake, Phoenix,
(603) 587-3885

ARKANSAS

Connie Miller,
cmillerspecial@yahoo.com

CALIFORNIA

Antelope Valley/Mojave/Inyokern
Carol Stewart, (661) 273-6952
Madeline Aday, (661) 946-5782

Burbank/Glendale/Pasadena
Nancy Shirey, (818) 558-5103
Barbara Elliott, (818) 842-1020

Central Valley
Melanie Dunlap, (559) 788-0820

Coachella Valley
Linda Borses, (760) 777-8840,
cvconnections@earthlink.net

East San Gabriel Valley
Roxanne Chapman, (909) 592-7485,
astwoareone@aol.com

Hollywood to Santa Monica
Mary Courtney, (310) 998-8487,
mary@courtney.org

Inland Empire
Kellee Shearer, (909) 242-8448,
treshearer@aol.com

High Desert/Barstow/Hisperia/Victorville
Kathleen Hemingway,
(760) 253-6952,
dkhemingway@msn.com

Manhattan Beach to Long Beach
Mimi French, (310) 372-1884
Marian White, (310) 514-3773

Northern Coast
Marie Dell'Isola, Napa,
(707) 255-4027
Leilani Smith, Sebastopol,
(707) 829-9105

Orange County Coast
Barbara Nielsen, (949) 644-4966,
barbara126@aol.com

San Fernando Valley
Linda Miller, (818) 884-8715,
lmiller3506@yahoo.com

San Francisco/Oakland
Ellen Switkes, (510) 655-0215,
Ellen.Switkes@ucop.edu

San Luis Obispo County
Betty Guthrie, Arroyo Grande
(805) 473-8495,
centralcoastceliacs@yahoo.com
Isabel Porter, (805) 929-6297

Central Coast
Dolores Kent-Olivas, Morgan Hill
(408) 778-1083,
doloreskent@msn.com

Santa Clarita Valley
Susan Singley, (661) 251-2952,
susansingley@hotmail.com
Jeanne Hammonds, (661) 298-7703

Santa Cruz
Pam Newbury, (831) 423-6904,
pknewbury@earthlink.net

South Bay
Mimi French, (310) 372-1884
Marian White, (310) 514-3773

Stanford
Kelly Rohlfs, (605) 725-4771,
kellyr@bonair.stanford.edu

Ventura County
Mary-Jean Vawter, (805) 584-6348,
maryjeanv@peoplepc.com

City of Ventura
Jo Ramsey, (805) 650-7713

LOUISIANA

Baton Rouge
Mary Mack Jeansonne,
(225) 766-8872,
e-celiacsbr@aol.com

MICHIGAN

Macomb County
Marie Girard, (586) 716-2426

NEVADA

Las Vegas
Sandi Jo Lawless, (702) 228-4128,
sidelta@aol.com
Olive Paterson, (702) 456-8202,
olivenv2@cox.net

NEW YORK

Orange County
Marisa Frederick, Celiac Kids' Club,
(845) 615-1227,
www.celiackidsclub.org

Mohawk Valley
Eleanor Wallace, (315) 736-6981,
www.csgmv.org

Syracuse/Ithaca
Ruth Wyman, (315) 463-4616

Westchester County
Chris Spreitzer, (914) 737-5291,
chris@mike-chris.spreitzer.com

NORTH DAKOTA

Lynda Nelson, P.O.Box 10052,
Fargo, ND 58106

PENNSYLVANIA

Lehigh Valley
Beverly Kistler, (610) 776-1178

SOUTH DAKOTA

Don Range, (605) 721-5429

UTAH

Logan/Ogden
Jeanine Andersen, (435) 753-9011

WASHINGTON

Seattle Area
Annette Van Dyke, (425) 377-2163

WYOMING

Jim Blick, (307) 548-6393,
scorpion5876@hotmail.com

CSA Chapters, www.csaceliacs.org

ALABAMA

Jane Hancock, (256) 837-0876,
jdshancock@aol.com

ARIZONA

Scottsdale
Donna Buls, (480) 488-8996
Jane King, Sun City, (623) 933-5160,
eliphyaleta@aol.com
Russ and Sheila Boocock, Fountain
Hills, (480) 837-1953

Tucson
Jeanette Sather, (520) 296-6809
Jeannine Faidley, (520) 298-9480
Julia Kelly, (520) 795-2923
Mary Louise Catura,
(520) 298-1038, elmarcat@juno.com
Vicki Holmes, (520) 298-2776,
vholmesaz@aol.com

ARKANSAS

Ozark Area
Leona Erskine, Gassville,
(501) 435-2415
Marilyn H. Jorgensen, Mountain
Home, (870) 492-5243
Pauline Geery, Mountain Home,
(501) 425-3818

Northwest Arkansas
Janice O. Carmichael Rogers,
(479) 636-8995,
djcarmichael@peoplepc.com

Hot Springs
Pat Detloff, (501) 922-0732,
ralpatdetloff@cox-internet.com
Rita Fordham, (501) 922-5839,
rrhsv@cox-internet.com
Edna M. Holt, (501) 922-0744

CALIFORNIA

Barstow
Kathleen J. Hemingway,
(760) 25307764,
dkhemingway@msn.com

Carlsbad
William and Helen Foreman,
(760) 931-7809,
bhforeman@webtv.net

Central Valley
Jeanne M. Morey, Stockton,
(209) 951-9608
Tim Matthies, Turlock,
(209) 632-8540,
matthies@ainet.com

Garden Grove
Cecile H. Weed, State Coordinator,
(714) 750-9543,
bcweed@earthlink.net
Diane Craig, (916) 483-8546,
dcraig101@hotmail.com

Oceanside
Glorian Beeson, (760) 721-1791,
frankbeeson@cox.net

Orange County
Barbara Strudwick, La Palma,
(714) 523-2599,
bkstrudwick@yahoo.com
Jenny View, Yorba Linda,
(714) 777-5714, jenview@cs.com

Redlands
Terri Daniels, San Bernardino,
(909) 882-4560

San Diego
Sandra Milne, San Diego
(858) 278-1413
shipmatesZ@mindspring.com

Sonoma County
Rosemary Yates, Santa Rosa
(707) 575-1848

Sacramento
Kathe Hughes, Cameron Park
(530) 672-1104

Stockton
Jeanne M. Morey, (209) 951-9608

Valinda
Patricia Q. West, (626) 337-6469,
pdqrn@aol.com

COLORADO

Colorado Springs
Steve Traini, (719) 494-8567,
celiacsteve@aol.com
Virginia Ludwig, (719) 598-6748,
ginglud@aol.com

Denver Metro
Betty Elofson, (303) 238-5145,
j-belofson@prodigy.net

Highlands Ranch
Mary Ann Peterson, (303) 683-1461,
mapetell30@aol.com

NORTHERN COLORADO

Berthoud
Bill R. Eyl,
(303) 772-3155,
billeyl@earthlink.net

Boulder
Barbara R. Sanford,
(303) 499-7259,
barbarasanford@comcast.net

Fort Collins
Phil Keller,
(970) 229-1911,
pkeller@webaccess.net
Judy Siple, Fort Collins,
(970) 493-9674, jabms@frii.net.

Grand Junction
Kathye Holland,
(970) 255-0511

Greenley
Monica Hupalo,
(970) 339-8465,
mhupalo@hotmail.com

Loveland
Dave Shaw,
(970) 669-4233, davshaw@qwest.net

CONNECTICUT

Greater New Haven
Betsey Powers, North Haven,
(203) 234-7060, betseygp@aol.com
Beverly Lombardi, Cheshire,
(203) 27209757,
bevlombardi@cox.net
Cheryl Mitchell, Wallingford,
(203) 269-5665,
alpatkel@netzero.net
Loretta Jay Stepansky, Co-Chair
Cel-Kids Network, Fairfield,
(203) 372-8721,
lorettajay@parasolservices.com

Northwest Connecticut
Carol Hoebel, Thomaston,
(860) 283-5577, kk56.ct@netzero.net
Eileen Robbins, Bristol,
(860) 583-8458
Marilyn Duffany, Thomaston,
(860) 283-8506

Sandy Hook
Eileen Gallo, (203) 426-8223,
eileen@pxmall.com

DELAWARE

William A. Locke, (804) 794-7476,
csa.region4director@comcast.net

DISTRICT OF COLUMBIA

See Maryland

FLORIDA

Pinellas County
James D. and Mary DuGranrut,
St. Petersburg (727) 522-1204,
jdug@pipeline.com
Mary Lou Thomas, Homosassa
(352) 628-9559,
mlthomas4cs@hotmail.com

Northwest Florida
Barbara Shilling, Pensacola
(850) 435-0522, bshilling@att.net

Southeast Florida
Ian and Heather Claridge,
West Palm Beach, (561) 967-8052
Norma Kagan, North Miami Beach,
(305) 945-0091,
skagnkag@prodigy.net
Rose Cruickshank, Boca Raton,
(561) 487-2377
roseforhealth@aol.com

Tampa
Janet Heitler, (813) 933-1645,
jchtbc42@tampabay.rr.com

GEORGIA

Atlanta
Nancy Wheeler, Savannah
(912) 598-8306,
ncwheelee@yahoo.com
Sam and Suzanne Shapard, Rome
(706) 234-1995,
dovedown@juno.com

Marieta
Markee Jones, (770) 992-5437,
markeej@mindspring.com

HAWAII

Kailua-Kona
Sharon Courtright, (808) 326-2380,
kona@kpmco.com

IDAHO

See Oregon

ILLINOIS

Central Illinois
Marsha Bishoff, Celiac Chapter #56,
(309) 444-7415,
marshaceliac@juno.com

Decatur
Jewel M. Barr, (217) 423-8234

Greater Chicago
Membership Voice Mail:
(847) 255-4156
Edward W. Wehling, St. Charles,
(630) 513-5125,
ewehling@ameritech.net
Ruth Smith, Barrington, (847) 381-
6106, ruthcsa@att.net

Normal
Kathryn Alexander, (309) 862-1895

Rockford
Jolyn M. Fasula, (815) 229-8804

Indiana

Martha Widener, Lafayette, (765) 447-7579, marthaw6@juno.com
Mary Moore, Crawfordville, (765) 364-9118, msmoore@tctc.com
Nancy Linneman, West Lafayette, (765) 497-0665, nancygrandma3@aol.com

Iowa

Ames
Charlotte Dougherty, (515) 296-2904
Karen Youngberg, (515) 296-2702, karenyoungberg@msn.com

Davenport
Becky Wentworth, (563) 391-2968, wentworth@netexpress.net

Waterloo
Anna Mary Cobie, (319) 235-7952, annamary@pitnet.net

Waverly
Betty Bast, (319) 352-4740, rbbast@webiowaplus.net
Gertrude Wilken, Dumont, (641) 228-1173
Kim Ovel, New Hampton, (641) 394-2379, dkjk@iowatelecom.net.

Kansas

Greater Kansas City
CSA Chapter Hotline: (913) 236-9454

Cindy Bright, Olathe, (913) 780-5258, cbright@peoplepc.com
Dean Cling, Kansas City, (816) 942-6677, dcling007@earthlink.net

Manhattan
Julia H. Griffith, (785) 537-8526

Overland Park
Wendy Percival, (913) 239-0647, wpercival4@aol.com

Topeka
Sharon Larson, (785) 379-0479, slars@kscable.com

Wichita
Beverly Eades, (316) 776-9369
Bill Dienstbach, (316) 722-1389
Marty Weeks, (316) 684-4017, martyweeks@cox.net

Kentucky

Louisville
Betty Ane Haering, (502) 969-7081, pichaering@aol.com
Harriet Langdon, Middle Town, (502) 245-8132
LaVaughn Will, (502) 425-6610, whwill@aol.com
Marilyn Reynolds, (502) 459-7643

Louisiana

Baton Rouge
Glenda Worm, (225) 751-7980, pelinc@bellsouth.net

New Orleans
Diane B. Schaefer, (504) 348-3099,
schfrpd@aol.com
Lorraine McCaslin, (504) 833-1717,
lomccaslin@aol.com

Maine

Portland
Paula J. Raleigh, Naples,
(207) 787-2279, honeybee@pivot.net
Sue E. Gefvert, Cumberland,
(207) 294-3543,
sgefverl@maine.rr.com

Maryland

Brookville
Christine Ewing, Cel-Kids Network
Liaison, (301) 570-9593,
cedesigns@comcast.net

Potomac
Juanita Ohanian,
(301) 881-4018,
jaonebel@aol.com

Westminster
Doug Rettberg,
(410) 876-3604,
rowina2@hotmail.com

Timonium
Phyllis Farmer,
(410) 560-1279, hfarmer@carr.org

Massachusetts

Boston
CSA Chapter Hotline:

(617) 262-5422 or (888) 4-CELIAC
Elise Gorseth, Waltham,
(617) 923-0172
Marjorie W. Rogers, Natick,
(508) 653-5465,
mwrogers67@aol.com
Nola Ford, Cambridge,
(617) 547-1828,
nolaford@yahoo.com

Lenox
Chaula Hopefisher, (413) 637-3641,
hopefisher@chaula.com
*Massachusetts and Rhode Island
(Children and Adults)*
Mary Arruda, West Greenwich, R.I.,
(401) 385-9175
Tanis E. Collard, Attleboro,
(508) 399-6229,
csgc@ix.netcom.com

Michigan

Traverse
Carolyn Hollenbeck,
(231) 947-9372,
jctessa7@chartermi.net
Curt Nordine, Ludington
(231) 845-7017,
dnordine@chartermi.net
Jean Sommers, Hessel
(906) 484-2099,
somrocks@cedarville.net
Linda Smith, Cadillac
(231) 775-8226, gdslws@voyager.net
Sandy Cartwright, (231) 947-8324,
scarttc@aol.com
Tom Sullivan, Grosse Pointe Woods
(313) 881-4526, msulli8400@aol.com

Lansing
Kersti Borysowicz, Michigan Capital
Celiacs/DH Chapter #43,
(517) 351-1203,
borysowi@pilot.msu.edu
Lynne Decator, (517) 485-3857,
1decator@aol.com
Sheila Verway, (517) 485-6288,
sgnoble@voyager.com

Central Michigan
Nyla Wilson, Clio, (810) 686-2539
Pat Adams, Owosso, (517) 743-3990,
pawadams4401@aol.com

Grand Rapids/West Michigan
Mitzi J. Berkhout, (616) 363-5749,
hennmitz@aol.com
Alan Fry, (616) 437-4569

Midland
Richard and Lucille King,
(989) 631-5640
Aileen Rashott, (989) 835-8747,
rashotta@chartermi.net

Newberry
Charmond Kingren, (906) 293-5742,
mkingren@hotmail.com

Steensville
Joan Carley, (269) 429-5103,
carley1@intraworldcom.net

MINNESOTA

Minneapolis/St. Paul
CSA Chapter: ncsg2002@yahoo.com
Carol Hansen, (651) 489-0645,

carolhansen@comcast.net
Judy Luger, (952) 933-1905,
judyluger@hotmail.com

Southeastern Minnesota
Coyla Sheppard, Rochester,
(507) 281-1523
Sharon McCarty, Elgin,
(507) 876-2441

MISSISSIPPI

Central Mississippi
Joy Clemmer, Madison,
(601) 856-4925
Linda Williams, Madison,
(601) 856-8846, lrw321@aol.com
Robert R. Berry Sr., Clinton,
(601) 924-0024,
rberrysr@bellsouth.net

Gulf Coast
Jane Gates Dacey, Ocean Springs,
(228) 875-2820, jgdacey@aol.com

MISSOURI

Hollister
L. June Johnson, (417) 334-0650,
georgej65672@peoplepc.com

St. Louis
Barb Berger, Chesterfield
(314) 532-3075
Barbara Ferrenbach, (314) 962-7440,
bferrenback@charter.net
Sharon Biondo, (636) 225-3947

MONTANA

R. Jean Powell, Bozeman,
(406) 586-1285

NEBRASKA

Lincoln
Jill Miller, State Coordinator,
(402) 474-6964, bjbjfam@aol.com

Midlands
Betty Wilberger, Nebraska City,
(402) 873-3620, bw54924@alltel.net
Kelly Eby, Gretna,
(402) 332-5039
Lynn Humphrey, Carroll, Iowa,
(712) 792-5866
Yvonne F. Steinback, Omaha,
(402) 455-0693,
celiac1234@aol.com

Star City
Beckee Moreland, (402) 441-9621

Western Nebraska
Mimi Frerichs, Kearney,
(308) 234-1200,
frerichs@1american.com

NEVADA

Las Vegas
Carolyn Warren, (702) 641-2542

Reno
Kathleen Frank, (775) 826) 9038,
kathleenefrank@earthlink.net

NEW HAMPSHIRE

Merrimack
Maureen Shelly, (603) 429-1228

Nashua
Carollee Hayward, (603) 889-8482,
realtyqueen@prodigy.net

NEW JERSEY

Central New Jersey
Diane Eve Paley, CSA President,
Old Bridge, (732) 679-6566,
dianecsa@aol.com
Elena Torsiello, East Windsor,
(609) 426-0292, ejtors@cs.com
Ellie Fried, Cel-Kids Network
Liaison, Short Hills, (973) 912-0253,
ejk54@hotmail.com
Melissa Daniel, East Brunswick,
(732) 545-5361

Hackettstown
Merle Morse, (908) 852-7311

Jersey Shore
Irene Kuchta, Brick, (732) 262-2378
Marie Maneri, Brick, (732) 920-3397
Joahanna Edwards, Toms River,
(732) 557-6242, jeme71@aol.com
Liz Pelly-Waldman, Cel-Kids Network
Liaison, Brielle, (732) 292-0137,
lizpelly@aol.com

Phillipsburg
Gary Powers, (908) 859-8518,
gppowers14@earthlink.net

South Jersey
Dorothea Bennet, Delran,
(856) 461-3374,
dben2300@sprynet.com
Leah Edelstein, Voorhees,
(856) 435-6785,
ledelstein@comcast.net
Lisa Martin, Turnersville,
(856) 228-0172,
csausanj@comcast.net
Patti Townsend, Collingswood,
(856) 854-5508,
tompatti@comcast.net
William Lucas, Burlington,
(609) 387-7139,
celiac9@earthlink.net

NEW MEXICO

Albuquerque
Lorraine Johnson,
(505) 298-0922
Marilyn Y. Johnson, State
Coordinator, (505) 299-5283,
marilynyj@comcast.net
Marvin E. Daniel, (505) 821-2935,
marvdaniel@earthlink.net

NEW YORK

Long Island
Catherine Curraro, Franklin Square,
(516) 437-3271
Ellen Mulligan, Hicksville, (516)
935-5109, nelle729@aol.com
James Callahan, East Meadow,
(516) 794-1654, pdfdjim@aol.com

Manhattan
Alice Chenal, (212) 755-9541
Merle Cachia, (212) 662-2464,
pjc1@columbia.edu

Rochester
Carol Becker, (585) 671-1443,
cabecker@rochester.rr.com
Norma Bartlett, (585) 436-0479

Staten Island
Lila T. Barbes, (718) 984-8547

Western New York
Cliff Hauck, Williamsville,
(716) 636-6028,
hauckc@adelphia.net
Lisa Lundy, Cheektowaga,
(716) 835-6392,
garlundy@adelphia.net
Pat Demicke, West Seneca,
(716) 675-6272,
mikedehank@aol.com

NORTH CAROLINA

Pittsboro
Ruth Thomas, (919) 542-4030

NORTH DAKOTA

Oakes
Juli Becker, (701) 742-2738

OHIO

Cleveland
Cindy Koller-Kass, (440) 248-6671,
glutenfreel@yahoo.com

Fairborn
Sandra J. Leonard, (937) 878-3221,
thebaker@sbcglobal.net

Perrysburg
Daniel R. and Linda E. Judson,
(419) 874-2519,
mrs_j314@msn.com

OKLAHOMA

Oklahoma City
Diane M. Eischen, (405) 263-7283,
mrteischen@aol.com
Heather Cline, (405) 235-1715,
hmcline@aol.com

Tulsa
Ronda Falkensten, (918) 743-3368,
cfalkensten@excite.com

OREGON

Michael Jackson, Tolovana Park,
(503) 436-9256,
mjackson@seasurf.com

PENNSYLVANIA

New Kensington
Theresa Fogle, (724) 335-4892,
tfoglel@aol.com

Philadelphia
Karen Dalrymple, (215) 757-1233

Pittsburgh
Lorraine E. Weaver, (412) 835-4983,
dweaverl@compuserve.com
Mary P. Neville, (412) 833-9507,
mpnev@aol.com

Wilkes-Barre/Scranton
Rose Marie Butera, (570) 655-0728,
rbutera@al.com

Wynnewood
Rita M. Herskovitz, (610) 642-9351,
herskovitz@email.chop.edu

RHODE ISLAND

Kathleen Thiboutot, Tiverton,
(401) 624-8888,
kathit51@hotmail.com

SOUTH CAROLINA

Gaston
Barbara Jandrisevitz,
(803) 926-8757,
bjandri@myexcel.com

Florence
Gladys Ward, (843) 662-7846,
gladward@mindspring.com

Santee
Gay Brangle, (803) 854-5002,
hankandgay@aol.com

SOUTH DAKOTA

Mitchell
Deb Pollreisz, (605) 996-4026,
craftgirl@mit.midco.net

TENNESSEE

Dickson
Sarah R. Mika, (615) 763-2934

Jackson
Joan Kay Chance, (731) 668-7468,
jkcgftn@aol.com

Memphis
Nicole Gast, (901) 377-9366,
nikkigast@yahoo.com
Sally Damron, (901) 452-5443

Nashville
Dr. Herschel Graves Jr.,
(615) 352-5442,
hagraves@comcast.net
Janet Lowery, (615) 758-2674,
janetlowery@comcast.net
Maureen Norris, (615) 591-9616,
manorris@comcast.net
Tori Ross, (615) 880-3957,
toriross@comcast.net

TEXAS

Austin
Frances Kelly, (512) 301-2224,
fkelley@austin.rr.com

Barzoria County
Cecilia McNeil, (979) 265-0819,
clmcneil@mail.esc4.com

Corpus Christi
Susan Revier, (361) 855-6810,
jandsrevier@msn.com

Eastland
Jill Hollywood, (254) 629-2200,
jillahollywood@hotmail.com

East Texas
Teresa Lux, (903) 759-7746,
tjl@internetwork.net

Houston
Janet Y. Rinehart, State Coordinator,
(281) 679-7608, txjanet@swbell.net
Gerry and Mary Lu Mase,
(713) 461-5731,
mlmase@houston.rr.com
Karen Tipton, (281) 265-7673,
karensltx@aol.com

North Richland Hills
Betty Barfield, (817) 967-2804,
betty.barfield@aa.com

San Antonio
Anne Barfield, (210) 340-0648,
annebarfield@satx.rr.com

Waco
Steve O'Connor, (254) 399-0472,
s88oconnor@aol.com

West Texas
Lois Newbold, Midland,
(915) 684-4671
Pat Gatlin, Midland, (915) 563-4847,
pgatlin@fbc-midland.org

Whitehouse
Windy Cannon, (903) 871-8213,
wlcannon@cox-internet.com

Utah

Salt Lake City
Christy Rands, (801) 637-7323
Jane Myers, (801) 268-7452,
jane.myers@mountainstarhealth.com

Vermont

St. Albans
Carol Jones, (802) 524-5156,
runnermama@peoplepc.com

Virginia

Northern Virginia
Christine Ewing, Cel-Kids Liaison,
Brookville, Maryland
(301) 570-9593,
cedesigns@comcast.net
Daniel A. DuBravec, Reston,
(703) 471-5047,
mvineyard@aol.com

Richmond
Linda Williams, (804) 27200414
Peggy Rash, (804) 262-5662
William and Deborah Locke,
(804) 794-7476,
csa.region4director@comcast.net

Tidewater Area
Penny Rogers, Virginia Beach,
(757) 424-2081,
pdrhwrbsr@aol.com
Richard and Jo Laslo, Virginia
Beach, (757) 671-9309,
dicklaslo@aol.com
Ronn Lee, Virginia Beach,
(757) 473-9817, drl48@cox.net

Washington

Jennifer Shea, Clinton,
(360) 341-8990, jshea@whidbey.com
Barbara Grow, Pasco,
(509) 545-6253,
bgrow22@charter.net

West Virginia

*Tri-State Celiac Sprue Support
Group #85*
Andrew Jones, Paintsville,
(606) 789-6457
Deborah A. Yeager, Huntington,
(304) 733-5867

Wisconsin

Antigo
Lyn Jiter, (715) 623-7254

Bloomer
Alice Zinsmaster, (715) 568-3311,
qazinzy@bloomer.net
Jenny Abernathy, (715) 568-2000

Fox Valley
Bill Morris, DePere, (920) 337-9235,
hbmorris@att.net
Mackenzie Harding, Menasha,
(920) 886-0544, kenz23@yahoo.com

Green Bay
Mary Mueller, (920) 435-4861,
cmueller@execpc.com
Pam Rourke, (920) 339-7867

LaCrosse
Mary Lou Balts, (608) 788-7398,
baltskml@centurytel.net

Madison
Aaron Avery, (608) 271-4041,
aavery77@hotmail.com
Betty Wass, (608) 233-9259
Kathleen Borner, Cottage Grove
(608) 839-3540, kborner@aol.com
Margaret Kramer, (608) 829-1554
Meghan Shannahan,
(608) 661-9848,
meshannahan@wisc.edu

Milwaukee
Beverly Lieven, (414) 354-2354,
milcs@aol.com
Jean Zachariasen, (414) 476-9017

Unity
Bertha Steinwagner, (715) 223-2075

WYOMING

Caspar
Kim Attaway, (307) 472-5889,
wyceliacassoc@alluretech.net
Laura Gossman, (307) 237-2058,
lgossman@vcn.com

Powell
Jill Smith, (307) 754-2058,
seatonjill@directairnet.com

Gluten Intolerance Group of North America, www.gluten.net

ALABAMA

Huntsville
Jeana Swaim, (256) 233-8436,
jswaim@arilion.com

ARIZONA

Phoenix
Sue Clayton, (480) 759-0199
Glutenfreegroup@glutenfreegroup
.com/Sueclayton@Cox.net

ARKANSAS

Little Rock
Anne Luther, (501) 223-3981,
aaluther@comcast.net

FLORIDA

Orlando
Mike Jones, mjones@digital.net

KENTUCKY

Benton
Rosemary Mueller,
rosemary@hcis.net

MISSOURI

Tri-Lakes Celiac Support Group
Barbara Hicks, Kimberling City,
(417) 739-2703, honedu@mchsl.com

NEVADA

Reno R.O.C.K.
Carrie Owen, (775) 857-2708,
owen4some@charter.net

NEW YORK

Buffalo
Mike Lodico, (716) 695-4302,
Glutenfree@adelphia.net,
www.buffaoceliacs.org

Syracuse
Ruth Wyman, (315) 463-4616,
jwyman@twcox.rr.com

Suffolk County
Les Doti, Kings Park,
(631) 513-9521,
ldoti@optionline.net

Westchester County
M. and C. Spreitzer, (914) 737-5291,
Ifo@westchesterceliacs.org,
www.westchesterceliacs.org

NORTH CAROLINA

Asheville
Mary Carol Koester, (828) 232-1714,
asheville@gluten.net,
www.gigofasheville.org

Piedmont
Grace Johnston, (336) 924-5326,
jimigrace@triad.rr.com

NORTH DAKOTA

Bismark
Lila Brendel, (701) 258-7800,
lybrendel@btinet.net

Fargo
Stacey Juhnke, (701) 237-4854,
redriverceliacs@gluten.net,
www.reriverceliacs.org

Oakes
Juli Becker, (701) 742-2738

OREGON

McMinnville
S. Chambers and S. Roberts,
(503) 472-0925,
schambe@linfield.edu

Portland-Vancouver
Jeanne Hufstutter, (503) 244-8224,
jeannehuff@aol.com,
www.portlancceliacs.org

Williamette Valley
Ann Grafe, (503) 982-3644,
banngrafe@worldnet.att.net

PENNSYLVANIA

Harrisburg
Linda Weller and K. Swailes,
Harrisburg (717) 520-9817,
Harrisburg@gluten.net,
www.harrisburgceliacs.org

TENNESSEE

Knoxville
Theresa Cornelius, (865) 922-8780,
tcorneli@utk.edu
Grace Collins and Jacqueline
Maxwell, (731) 402-0139,
gfcrusader@iglide.net

UTAH

American Fork
Amber Lee, (801) 763-0977
ucngig@afutah.org, www.gfutah.org

Ogden
Cheryl Archuleta, (801) 392-5093,
Cherarch@hotmail.com

VIRGINIA

Richmond
Anna Ashworth, (804) 364-3794,
agashworth@aol.com

Madelyn Smith, (804) 968-4111,
smith10900@aol.com,
www.gigofrichmond.org

WASHINGTON

Bellingham
Caroline Yorkston, (360) 676-1372,
carolinelou@yorkstonoil.com
Mary Lou Richardson,
(360) 734-4989, migarden@aol.com

Port Townsend
Adele Fosser, (360) 385-2282,
fosserha@olypen.com

Ellensburg
Delayna Breckon, (509) 933-1010,
glutenfree@elltel.net

Seattle
Earl Ley, (206) 747-1110,
earl.lev@boeing.com,
www.seattleceliacs.com

Independents, www.celiacdisease.org

The following support groups in Pennsylvania are not affiliated with any national organization, but are waiting for a single national group to emerge.

Gettysburg
Cheryl Hutchinson, (717) 642-6053,
Hutchjc@earthlink.net

Lancaster
Susan Polachak,
jpolachak@comcast.net

York
Kathie Cavanagh, (717) 428-3859,
www.celiacdisease.org

Raising Our Celiac Kids/Local R.O.C.K. Groups, www.celiackids.com

ALABAMA

Slocomb
Nichole Alexander, (334) 886-7150,
mamma_hen3@hotmailcom

ARIZONA

Gilbert
Deanna Frazee, (480) 641-8821,
deannafrazee@hotmail.com

Scottsdale
Jennifer Fabiano, (480) 905-2622,
jfabioano@cox.net

Tucson
Liz Attansio, (520) 877-9181,
lizinbox@aol.com

CALIFORNIA

Canyon County
Helaina Taylor, (661) 251-6884,
helaina@directvinternet.com

Danville
Dana Doscher, ddoscher11@aol.com

Irvine
Evelyn Tribole, Etzzzzzzzz@aol.com

Moreno Valley
Kellee Shearer, (909) 242-8448,
Treshearer@aol.com

Orange County
Carolyn Weske, (714) 771-0680,
cweske@hotmail.com

Palo Alto
Autumn Katz, (650) 328-5365,
koolcatinacan@yahoo.com

San Diego
Susan Jarrold, (619) 579-9590,
sjarrold@sdcoe.k12@.us

San Francisco
Jackie Corley, (415) 387-2969,
Jacqueline_Scott_Corley@cand
.uscourts.gov

Visalia
Shannon Williams, (559) 741-1671,
Rock_Visalia@webtv.net

COLORADO

Littleton
Randy and Kim Toltz,
(303) 470-0003,
randy@thetoltzgroup.com

CONNECTICUT

Waterford
Donna Kensel, dmkensel@aol.com

FLORIDA

Apopka
Deborah Pfeifle, (407) 880-6104,
dpfeifle@earthlink.net

Coral Springs/Palm Beach
Janna Faulhaber and Stacey Galper,
(954) 255-8855,
Staceynagel@paxson.com

Odessa
Terri Willingham,
pubmail@tampabay.rr.com

Tampa
Melissa Ransdell, (813) 265-8105,
melrans@tampabay.rr.com

ILLINOIS

Dekalb
Audrey O'Sullivan, (815) 756-2606,
Audrey08@aol.com

Springfield
Joyce Hall, Joychll@aol.com

INDIANA

Mooresville
Cindy Holder, (317) 831-9871,
Holders2@comcast.net

IOWA

Des Moines
Mary Curan,
curran621@mindspring.com

KANSAS

Overland Park
Wendy Percival, (913) 239-0647,
wpercival4@aol.com

MAINE

Portland
Nicole Richman, (207) 893-2712,
nrichmal@maine.rr.com

MICHIGAN

West Bloomfield
Gail Smoler, (248) 851-9451
GailS63@aol.com

MINNESOTA

Minneapolis/St. Paul
Lynda Benkofske, (763) 263-7679,
libenkof@ties2.net

MISSISSIPPI

Columbia
Beth Broom, sbroom@dixie-net.com

NEBRASKA

Blair
Shelly Andreasen, (402) 533-1090,
johndeerfarms@huntel.net

NEVADA

Las Vegas
Shelli Gialketsis, (702) 869-5366,
RSGINLV@aol.com

Reno
Carrie Owen, (775) 857-2708,
owen4some@charter.net

NEW JERSEY

Freehold
Sue Cavallaro, (732) 462-4660,
SusanCav@aol.com

Blairstown
Maria Benson, (808) 362-7752,
Mbenson890@aol.com

NEW YORK

Long Island
Cindy Sippin, (631) 473-5842

Rome
Rebecca Madeira, (315) 337-7671,
celiacparents@earthlink.net

NORTH CAROLINA

Raleigh
Andrea Otken-Dennis,
(919) 303-4518, adennis@ipass.net

NORTH DAKOTA

Fargo
Stacey Juhnke, (701) 237-4854,
DSJuhnke@yahoo.com

OHIO

Akron
Sue Krznaric, (330) 253-1509,
skrznaric@cs.com

Cincinnati
Beth Koenig, (513) 923-4435,
prkoenig@fuse.net

PENNSYLVANIA

Downington
Tracy Baxter, (610) 269-7300,
thebaxters@snip.net

Greenville
Fiona Garner, garner6@archgate.net

Harrisburg
Linda Weller, (717) 520-9817,
www.harrisburgceliacs.org,
harrisburg@gluten.net

Lititz
Jennifer Young, (717) 560-5739,
JenniferNYoung@hotmail.com

SOUTH CAROLINA

Lexington
Gail Fox, (803) 957-7658,
gailfox@sc.rr.com

TENNESSEE

Nashville
Janet Lowery, (615) 758-2674,
janetlowery@comcast.com

Woodlawn
Shantal Green, (931) 648-2289,
skgreen@syberwerx.net

TEXAS

Dallas/Fort Worth
Kelly LeMonds, (972) 489-9915,
klemonds@comcast.net
Dianne McConnell, (817) 849-8646,
fortworthrock@swbell.net

Houston
Janet Y. Rinehart, (281) 679-7608,
txjanet@swbell.net,
www.csaceliacs.org
Faye Sallee, (281) 496-9166,
fsallee@houston.rr.com

San Antonio
Amy Holt, (210) 481-0659,
info@rocksa.org, www.kidceliac.com

Victoria
Julie Bauknight, (361) 572-9252,
eavesfamily@coxinternet.com

UTAH

Ogden
Eileen Leatherow,
e.leatherow@attbi.com

VIRGINIA

Ashburn
Kris Domingue, (703) 724-1754,
Kdomingue@aol.com

Northern Va./Washington, D.C.
Melonie Katz, (703) 445-8305,
OneSillyYak@yahoo.com

Richmond
Carrie Martin, (804) 323-1066,
ChrisBOWHUNTER@aol.com,
www.rcssg.org

WASHINGTON

Belleview
Nick and Sue Pierson,
(425) 401-9163,
NicholasPierson@hotmail.com

Poulsbo
Tim and Dawn Simonson, (360)
779-9292, timsimonson@csi.com

WEST VIRGINIA

Karen Daniel, (304) 757-0696,
krdaniel@charter.net

WISCONSIN

Jackson
Yvonne Schwalen,
trainman280@netzero.net

Rhinelander
Cheryl Boyd, (715) 369-3735,
mboyd@charter.net

Canadian Celiac Association/
L'Association Canadienne de la Maladie Coelique, www.celiac.ca

ALBERTA

Calgary Chapter
4112 4th Street N.W.
Calgary T2K 1A2
(403) 237-0304

Edmonton Chapter
11111 Jasper Avenue, Room 5R17
Edmonton T5K OL4 (780) 482-8967

BRITISH COLUMBIA

Vancouver Chapter
1212 Broadway West, Suite 306
Vancouver V6H 3V1
(604) 736-2229,
www.vcn.bc.ca/celiac

Victoria Chapter
P.O. Box 5765, Station B
Victoria V8R 6S8
(250) 472-0141

Kamloops Chapter
116 River Road
Kamloops V2C 4P9
(250) 374-6185

Kelowna Chapter
139-595 Yates Road
Kelowna V1V 1P8
(250) 769-1935,
celiac_delowna@hotmail.com

MANITOBA

Manitoba Chapter
P.O. Box 2543
Winnipeg R3C 4B3
(204) 772-6979, www.celiac.mb.ca

NEW BRUNSWICK

Fredericton Chapter
527 Beaverbrook Court, Suite 226
Fredericton E3B 1X6
(506) 450-4357

Moncton Chapter
P.O. Box 1576
Moncton E1C 9X4

Saint John Chapter
454 Elmore Crescent
Saint John E2M 3C1
(506) 672-4454

NEWFOUNDLAND

St. John's Chapter
262 Freshwater Road
St. John's A1B 1B8

Nova Scotia/Halifax Chapter
P.O. Box 9104, Station A
Halifax B3K 5M7
(902) 464-9222,
www.ns.sympatico.ca

What Does It Take to Start a Local Chapter of a Celiac Group?

- Time. Lots and lots of time. You must be willing and able to dedicate a large block of your life to the needs of the group.
- Other questions you need to ask yourself. Honestly, now. No one's looking.
- Do you know enough about the diet yourself? Are you able to change your views as research advances our understanding of the disease?
- Are you a good listener? You must never tire of hearing newly diagnosed members' stories and be empathetic to their fears and concerns.
- How creative are you? How efficient? How dependable? How organized?
- Are you as persistent as a pit bull? Are you positive? Do you prefer the word *can* to the word *can't*?
- Does your family support your decision to support others?
- Are you worthy of another person's trust?
- And finally, look deep into your heart and answer this: What do I get out of doing this?

ONTARIO

Hamilton Chapter
P.O. Box 65580,
Dundas Postal Outlet
Dundas L9H 6Y6
(905) 572-6775

Kitchener/Waterloo Chapter
153 Frederick Street, Suite 118
Kitchener N2H 2M3

London Chapter
P.O. Box 198
Dorchester N0L 1G0
Celiaclondon@golden.net

Sudbury Chapter
P.O. Box 2794, Station A
Sudbury P3A 5J3

Ottawa Chapter
P.O. Box 39035, Billings
Ottawa K1H 1A1
(613) 786-1335,
www.celiac.ottawa.on.ca

Thunder Bay Chapter
1995 Riverdale Road, R.R. #3
Thunder Bay P7C 4V2

Toronto Chapter
Yorkdale P.O. Box 27592
Toronto M6A 3B4
(416) 781-9140

St. Catherines Chapter
Grantham P.O. Box 20193
St. Catherines L2M 7W7

Quinte Chapter
P.O. Box 20104
Belleville K8N 5V1

QUEBEC

Quebec Chapter
614-21 Lakeshore Drive
Montreal H9S 5N2

Saskatchewan/Regina Chapter
P.O. Box 1773
Regina S4P 3C6

Saskatoon Chapter
P.O. Box 8935
Saskatoon S7K 6S7

PRINCE EDWARD ISLAND

Charlottetown Chapter
P.O. Box 921
Charlottetown C1A 7N5

The Well-Read Celiac

BOOKS FOR CHILDREN AND FAMILIES

The AIA Gluten and Dairy Free Cookbook by Marilyn Le Breton and Rosemary Kessick (Jessica Kingsley Pub. 2002). AIA is the U.K.-based group, Allergy Induced Autism.

Feeding the Baby by Joachim and Christine Splichal (Ten Speed Press, 2003).

Food Allergy Field Guide: A Lifestyle Manual for Families by Theresa Willingham (Savory Palate Press, 2000).

Kid Friendly Food Allergy Cookbook by Lynn Rominger (Fair Winds Press, 2004).

Kids With Celiac Disease by Danna Korn (Woodbine House).

No More Cupcakes & Tummy Aches: A Story for Parents and Their Celiac Children to Share by Jax Peters Lowell and illustrated by Jane Kirkwood (Xlibris, 2004). Foreword by Alessio Fasano, M.D.

To order: (888) 795-4274 / www.xlibris.com.

Cookbooks

The Artful Vegan by Eric Tucker, Bruce Enloe, Amy Pearce (Ten Speed Press, 2003).

Cooking Gluten-Free, A Food Lover's Collection of Chef and Family Recipes without Gluten or Wheat by Karen Robertson (Celiac Publishing, 2003).

Cooking Without by Barbara Cousins (Thorsens, 2000).

The Gluten-Free Gourmet Series by Bette Hagman (Henry Holt, 1999): *The Gluten-Free Gourmet*, rev. ed., *More from the Gluten-Free Gourmet, The Gluten-Free Gourmet Cooks Fast and Healthy, The Gluten-Free Gourmet Makes Dessert,* and *The Gluten-Free Gourmet Bakes Bread.*

The Gluten-Free Kitchen: Over 135 Delicious Recipes for People with Gluten Intolerance by Roben Ryberg (Prima Lifestyles, 2000).

Gluten, Wheat and Dairy-Free Cookbook by Antoinette Savill (Thorsons, 2000).

Maria's Cookbook: Manioc Recipes by Sheila Thompson, www.maria-brazil.org

Rice & Risotto by Christine Ingram (Hermes House, 2003).

Risotto by Williams-Sonoma (Simon & Schuster, 2002).

Savory Baked Goods, More Than 125 Recipes for Cakes, Pies, Quick Breads, Muffins, Cookies & Other Delights by Rebecca Reilly (Simon & Schuster, 2001).

Special Diet Celebrations: No Wheat, Gluten, Dairy, or Egg by Carol Fenster (Savory Palate Press, revised 2003).

Seductions of Rice by Jeffrey Alford and Naomi Duguid (Artisan, 2003).

The Wheat-Free, Gluten-Free Cookbook Series by Connie Sarros (Contemporary Books, 2003): *Dessert Cookbook, Reduced Calorie Cookbook, Cookbook for Kids and Busy Adults,* and *Recipes for Special Diets.*

The Whole Foods Encyclopedia by Rebecca Wood (Penguin, 1999).

References

Current Bibliographies in Medicine/Celiac Disease, January 1986–March 2004 (2,382 citations currently in online databases, published by U.S. Department of Health and Human Services, Public Health Services, National Institutes of Health), National Library of Medicine, Bethesda, Maryland, www.nim.nih.gov/pubs/resources.html

Celiac Disease Nutrition Guide by Merri Lou Dobler and Tricia Thompson (American Dietetic Association). To order, (800) 977-1600, www .eatright.org/catalog

Grossman's Guide to Wine, Spirits and Beers (Scribner).

Hugh Johnson's Modern Encyclopedia of Wine (Simon & Schuster).

Larousse Gastronomique, The Encyclopedia of Food, Wine & Cookery by Prosper Montagne (Crown).

The Merck Manual of Diagnosis and Therapy (Merck).

The Physicians' Desk Reference (Medical Economics Data).

MAGAZINES AND NEWSLETTERS

Celiac Disease Foundation Newsletter, (818) 990-2354, www.celiac.org

Clan Thompson Celiac Newsletter, monthly news about research, gluten-free drugs and foods, 91 Main Street, Stoneham, ME 04231, (207) 928-3303, www.clanthompson.com

Gluten-Free Baking and More, monthly recipes from Elizabeth Barbone. (518) 279-3884, www.glutenfreebakingandmore.com

Glutenfreeda Newsletter, monthly online gluten-free cooking magazine. 4809 South Kip Lane, Spokane, WA 99224, (509) 448-9095, www. glutenfreeda.com

Gluten-Free Living, practical information presented in a straightforward style. 19A Broadway, Hawthorne, NY 10532, (847) 480-8810, www .glutenfreeliving.com

Gluten Intolerance Group Newsmagazine, (206) 246-6652, www.gluten.net

Lifeline, CSA Newsletter, (402) 558-0600, www.csaceliacs.org

Living Without, a gorgeous quarterly magazine for people with food allergies and chemical sensitivities. Recipes, resources, articles, lifestyle, and more. In health food stores, on newsstands, or by subscription, P.O. Box 2126, Northbrook, IL 60065, (847) 480-8810, www.livingwithout.com

The Long Island Spectrum (Gem Media), autism and the gluten-free diet, (516) 933-4070.

Scott Free Quarterly Newletter, monthly e-mails on research, information, and recipes from Scott Adams, www.celiac.com

Internet Message Boards, Information, Chat, Celiac Community

Always verify accuracy when getting information from the Internet.

CeliACTION Network
Celiac consumer advocacy list to share letters to drug and food manufacturers. To subscribe, send e-mail to CeliACTIONNetwork-subscribe@yahoogroups.com

Celiac Chicks Web Log
www.celiacchicks.com

Delphi Forums Archive/Listserv
www.forums.delphiforums.com/celiac

Gluten-Free Menus
Silly Yaks,
Subscribe@yahoogroups.com

Information, News, etc.
www.glutenfreeforum.com

Information/Medical
www.medscape.com
www.delpiforums.com/celiac

Information, Links, Posters
www.glutenfreecanada.com
www.glutenfreeforum.com

Kids Chat, Exchange Ideas, Coping Strategies
www.clubceliac.com

Recipes, News, Information
www.celiac.com

St. John's Celiac Listserv
To subscribe, e-mail listserv@maelstrom.stjohns.educ
To subscribe to children's list, e-mail cel-kids@maelstrom.stjohns.edu.
Archives
www.maelstrom.stjohns.edu/archives/celiac.html

Celiac and Diabetes

Diabetes, Celiac Disease and Me
www.houston.celiacs.org

Managing Diabetes and Celiac Disease . . . Together
Published by the Canadian Celiac Association
www.celiac.ca

Celiac and Sjögren's
www.dry.org

Gluten- and Casein-Free
www.gfcfdiet.com
www.aspergerssyndrome.org
www.tacanow.com
www.autistics.cc
www.tacanow.com

Kitchen Equipment

Gluten-Free Tools
Bosch mixers (not readily available
in United States), Zojirushi and Ultimate Breadman baking machines,
Zojirush rice cookers, Magic Vac
vacuum sealers, grain, seed, nut, and
spice mills.
(877) 456-7704,
www.geocities.com/glutenfreetools

Farberware Electric Rice Cooker
3- to 10-cup sizes, stainless steel,
steamer insert
(800) 233-9054,
www.esalton.com

*New York Cake and Baking
Distributors, Inc.*
56 West 22nd Street
New York, NY 10011
(212) 675-2253

Online Indian Specialty Foods—
Moong dal, chutneys, spices
www.grocerybabu.com

Panasonic Bread Machine
(800) 211-7262,
www.panasonic.com

*Salton Breadman and Toastmaster
Bread Makers*
(800) 233-9054, www.esalton.com

William-Sonoma
(800) 541-2233,
www.williams-sonoma.com

*Zojirushi Home Bakery Supreme;
Zojirushi Neuro Fuzzy Logic Rice
Cooker*
5- or 10-cup sizes, automatic keep
warm system, no-stick
(800) 733-6270, www.zojirushi.com

Home Tests, Gadgets, and Accessories

Gluten-Home Test by Elisa
Technologies
4581-L NW 6th Street
Gainesville, FL 32609
(352) 337-3029, www.elisa-tek.com

The Medic Alert Watch
Sports, fun, and children's watches
(800) 722-6955,
www.medcalalertwatch.com

York Nutritional Laboratories
Diagnos-Techs saSCAN Secretory
IgA Food Intolerance Kit
Saliva screening for egg, gluten milk,
and soy intolerance
2700 North 29th Avenue, #205,
Hollywood, FL 33020
(888) 751-3388,
www.yorkallergyusa.com

Silly Yak Shirt Company
Whimsical T-shirts and accessories
for adults and children
www.silly-yak.com

"Team Celiac" T-shirts
www.glutenfreeshirts.com

National Organizations, Information, Advocacy, Research

American Academy of Allergy,
Asthma & Immunology
611 East Wells Street
Milwaukee, WI 53202
(800) 822-2762, www.aaaai.org

American Celiac Society Dietary
Support Coalition
P.O. Box 23455
New Orleans, LA 70183
amerceliacsoc@netscape.net

American Culinary Federation
P.O. Box 3466
10 San Bartola Road
St. Augustine, FL 32085

American Dietetic Association
215 W. Jackson Blvd., Suite 800
Chicago, IL 60606
(800) 366-1655, www.ada.com

The American Gastroenterological
Association
4930 Del Ray Avenue
Bethesda, MD 20814
(301) 654-2055, www.gastro.org

American Genetic Association
P.O. Box 257
Buckeystown, MD 21717
(301) 695-9292,
www.lifesciences.asu.edu

American Health Care Association/
Nursing Home Information
1201 L Street N.W.
Washington, DC 20005
(202) 842-4444, www.ahca.org

American Medical Association
515 North State Street
Chicago, IL 60610
(312) 464-5000, www.ama-assn.org

American Society for Nutritional
Sciences
9650 Rockville Pike, Suite 4500
Bethesda, MD 20815
(301) 530-7050

Anaphylaxis Canada
416 Moore Avenue, Suite 306
Toronto, Ontario M4G1C9, Canada
(416) 785-5666,
www.anaphylaxis.org

Autism Research Institute
4182 Adams Avenue
San Diego, CA 92116
(619) 281-7165,
www.autismresearchinstitute.com

Culinary Institute of America
1946 Campus Drive
Hyde Park, NY 12538
(845) 452-9600, www.ciachef.edu

Developmental Delay Resources
4401 East West Highway, Suite 207
Bethesda, MD 20814
(301) 652-2263, www.devdelay.org

Food Allergy Network
11781 Lee Jackson Highway,
Suite 160
Fairfax, VA 22033
(800) 929-4040,
www.foodallergy.org

International Food Information
Council Foundation
1100 Connecticut Avenue NW,
Suite 430
Washington, DC 20036
www.ificinfo.health.org

International Foundation for
Functional Gastrointestinal
Disorders
P.O. Box 170864
Milwaukee, WI 53217
(888) 964-2001, www.iffgd.org

Intestinal Disease Foundation
Landmarks Building, Suite 525
100 West Station Square Drive
Pittsburgh, PA 15219
(877) 587-9606,
www.intestinalfoundation.org

Parents of Children with Food
Allergies, Inc.
118 Washington Street, Suite 10
Holliston, MA 01746
(508) 893-6977,
www.foodallergykids.org

National Adult Day Services
Association
www.helpguide.org/elder/
adult_day_services.htm

National Association of Child Care
Resources and Referral
www.nim.nih.gov/medlineplus/child
daycare.html

National Digestive Diseases
Information Clearing House
2 Information Way
Bethesda, MD 20892
(301) 654-3810, www.niddk.nih.gov

National Heartburn Alliance
www.heartburnalliance.org

National Institute of Diabetes &
Digestive & Kidney Diseases
31 Center Drive, MSC 2560
Bethesda, MD 20892
www.niddk.nih.gov

Snack Food Association
1711 King Street, Suite 1
Alexandria, VA 22314
(800) 628-1334, www.sfa.org

Society for Nutrition Education
1001 Connecticut Avenue NW,
Suite 528
Washington, DC 20036
(202) 452-8534

international dining cards

No reason to stay home because of your diet. Appearing below in English, then translated into Arabic, Chinese, Danish, Dutch, French, German, Greek, Hebrew, Italian, Japanese, Polish, Portuguese, Russian, Spanish, Swedish, Swahili, and Thai are updated gluten-free dining cards for you to photocopy, laminate for extra sturdiness on long trips, and stash extras in your luggage. Not strictly for traveling, these will also go a long way toward understanding at the ethnic restaurant right around the corner where the owners are still a bit shaky in English. People appreciate it when you try to communicate in their language, even if it's only on paper.

English Gluten-Intolerance Card

I do not speak your language.

I have celiac disease and cannot tolerate gluten.

If I eat any food, product, chemical additive, or stabilizer containing even a trace of wheat, rye, oats, barley, triticale, malt, or any derivatives of these grains, I will become ill.

I am able to eat foods containing corn and rice.

If necessary, please check with the chef to make sure my food does not contain any of the ingredients listed above and help me order a meal I can safely enjoy.

Thank you very much.

Arabic Gluten-Intolerance Card

أنا لا أتحدث لغتك.

أنا أعاني من مرض حساسية في الامعاء ولا أستطيع ان اتحمل آزوت الدقيق بأي شكل من الاشكال.

إذا تناولت اي طعام، او إنتاج، او كيماويات مضافة،او اية مادة توازن تحتوي حتى ولو على اثر بسيط من القمح، الجاودار، الشوفان، الشعير، الملت ، أو اي من المولَّدات من القمح والنباتات المذكورة، فستصبح حالتي خطرة. استطيع أن اتناول الاغذية التي تحتوي على الذرة والأرز .

ارجو منكم التحدث مع الطباخ ليتأكد من أن طعامي لا يحتوي على اي اثر من المواد المذكورة أعلاه، كما ارجو مساعدتي على طلب طعام يمكنني التمتع به بأمان. لكم شكري العميق.

Chinese Gluten-Intolerance Card

我不懂中文。

我患有腹腔病，绝对不可以食用任何形式的面筋、麸类食物。

如果我吃了含小麦、黑麦、燕麦、荞麦、大麦、小米、黑小麦、麦芽以及任何以这些谷物为原料的食物，或含化学添加剂、稳定剂的食物，我就会生病。

我可以吃玉米和大米做的食物。

如果可能的话，麻烦和厨师讲一下，我吃的食物中不能含有任何上述成分，并请选用一份我能够放心享用的饭菜。

非常感谢您的帮助！

Danish Gluten-Intolerance Card

Jeg kan ikke tale dansk.

Jeg lider af kronisk celiaki og kan ikke tåle nogen som helst form for gluten.

Hvis jeg spiser noget som helst mad, produkt, kemisk tilsætnings- eller stabiliseringsmiddel, der indeholder så meget som en anelse hvede, rug, havre, byg, tritical (hvede+rughybrid), malt eller ethvert, stof, der er afledet af disse kornsorter, bliver jeg syg.

Jeg kan spise mad, der er tilberedt med majs og ris.

Vær venlig at rådføre dig med kokken for at være sikker på, at min mad ikke indeholder nogen af de ingredienser, der står opført på ovenstående liste, og vær venlig at hjælpe mig med at bestille et måltid, som jeg kan nyde uden fare.

Mange tak!

Dutch Gluten-Intolerance Card

Ik spreek uw taal niet.

Ik lijd aan coeliakie (glutenovergevoeligheid) en kan geen enkele vorm van gluten tolereren.

Als ik een (voedsel) product, chemisch additief of stabiliseer-stof eet die zelfs een minuscule hoeveelheid tarwe, rogge, haver, gerst, triticaal, mout of een van deze graansoorten afgeleide stof bevat, dan word ik ziek.

Ik kan voedsel eten dat maïs en rijst bevat.

Spreekt u a.u.b. met de kok om zeker te zijn dat mijn maaltijd geen van de hierboven vermelde bestanddelen bevat en help me iets te bestellen waarvan ik veilig kan genieten.

Met oprechte dank!

French Gluten-Intolerance Card

Je ne parle pas votre langue.

J'ai une maladie intestinale. Je ne peux pas tolerer gluten en beaucoup des formes.

Si je mange n'importe quelle genre de nourriture, produit, additife chemique ou stabilisateur, contenant même une trace de blé, seigle, avoine, orge, triticale, malte ou les extraits de ses graines, je tomberai malade.

Je peux manger de la nourriture à baser de maïs et riz. Veillez si'il vous plaît averter le chef cuisinier d'être sur que ma nourriture ne contienne pas les engrais que je viens de mentioner et de m'aider à choisir un repas que je pourrai savourer sans inquiétude.

Merci beaucoup.

German Gluten-Intolerance Card

Ich spreche Ihre Sprache nicht.

Ich habe eine Krankheit. Ich vertrage keine Gluten in irgendeiner Form.

Wenn ich Speisen, Erzeugnisse, Zusaetze oder Stabilisatoren esse, die auch nur eine Spur von Weizen, Roggen, Hafer, Buchweizen, Gerste, Hirse, Malz, Gertreideessig oder Derivate dieser Getreidearten enthalten, werde ich krank.

Koennen Sie bitte dem Küchenchef meine Probleme erklaeren so dass meine Speise keine der oben genannten Bestandteile enthaelt, und ich waere Ihnen dankbar, wenn Sie mir helfen koennten, ein Gericht zu bestellen, dass ich gefahrlos essen darf.

Herzlichen Dank!

Greek Gluten-Intolerance Card

Δεν μιλάω τη γλώσσα σας.
Υποφέρω από την ασθένεια κοιλιοκάκη και δεν
μπορώ να ανεχθώ τη γλουτένη υπό οποιαδήποτε
μορφή.
Εάν φάω οποιαδήποτε τροφή, προϊόν, χημικό
πρόσθετο, ή σταθεροποιητή που περιέχει ακόμη και
ίχνος σίτου, σίκαλης, βρώμης, κριθαριού,
χειμερινού σιτηρού triticale, βύνη ή οποιοδήποτε
παράγωγο αυτών των δημητριακών, θα
αρρωστήσω.
Μπορώ να φάω τροφές που περιέχουν καλαμπόκι
και ρύζι.
Σας παρακαλώ ρωτήστε το μάγειρα για να
σιγουρευτείτε ότι το φαγητό μου δεν περιέχει
κανένα από τα συστατικά που δίνονται παραπάνω
και βοηθήστε με να παραγγείλω ένα γεύμα που θα
μπορέσω να απολαύσω με ασφάλεια.
Ευχαριστώ πολύ!

Hebrew Gluten-Intolerance Card

כרטיס אלרגיה מ "גלוטן"

אני לא מדבר את השפה שלכם
יש לי מחלת "מליאק".
אם אני אוכל מאכל כלשהו, מוצר, תוספת כימית או
מיצב שיש בו אפילו טיפה: חיטה, שיפוך, שיבולת שועל,
חיטה מוסלמית, שעורת דותך, "טריטיקאל", חמץ של
גרעין, לתת או כל מוצר שנגזר מהנ"ל, אני אחלה.

אני יכול לאכול כל דבר שעשוי מתירס ואורז.
אם יש צורך, אנא תבדוק עם הטבח כדי לאשר שבאוכל
שלי אין אף רכיב/דבר מהמרכיבים הנ"ל ובבקשה תעזור
לי להזמין משהו שאוכל אאהנה עם בטחון.
תודה רבה.

Italian Gluten-Intolerance Card

Non parlo Italiano.

Sono affetta dal marbo Celiaco, e nontolleroglutine in alcuna forma.

Se mangio del cibo contenente prodotti o solo trace di grano, avena, segala, orzo, crusca, malto e germogli di questi cereali, me sento molto male.

Posso peró mangiare cibi che contengano riso e granturco.

Laprego di consultargi con il cuoco per assicurarsi che il mio cibo non contenga nessuno dei prodotti sopra elencati, e mi aiuti a ordinare un bon pasto.

Grazie.

Japanese Gluten-Intolerance Card

　日本語を話せませんが、私はセーリアック病という腸の持病があり、グルテンを含む食物はどのような形でも受け付けません。
　たとえ極く微量でも小麦、ライ麦、オート麦、大麦、ライ小麦、麦芽、そしてこれら穀物から派生するものを含む食物、製品、化学調味料、安定剤を食べると病気になります。
　米とトウモロコシを材料とする食物は食べられます。
　そこでお願いですが、シェフに伺って私の食事に上に挙げた材料が入っていないか確かめて頂きたいのです。そして安全に食べられる食事を選べるようお手伝いをお願いします。
　どうぞよろしく。

Polish Gluten-Intolerance Card

Nie władam Pana/Pani językiem.

Choruję na celiaklię (zaburzenie wchłaniania z jelit), mój organizm nie toleruje glutenu.

Jeżeli zjem jakiekolwiek pożywienie, środki konserwujące czy wyrób zawierający nawet śladowe ilości pszenicy, żyta, owsa, gryki, jęczmienia (pęczka, kasza perłowa), prosa, octu zbożowego, słodu czy jakichkolwiek pochodnych tych zbóż, rozchoruję się.

Mogę za to jeść pożywienie zawierające kukurydzę lub ryż.

Proszę pomóc mi wybrać posiłek, który nie zagrażałby mojemu zdrowiu, jak również, jeżeli jest to konieczne, proszę upewnić się u szefa kuchni, że moje jedzenie nie zawiera żadnego z powyższych składników.

Bardzo dziękuję.

Portuguese Gluten-Intolerance Card

Eu não falo a sua língua.

Tenho a doença celíaca e não consigo tolerar nenhuma forma de glúten.

Se comer qualquer alimento, produto, aditivo químico ou estabilizador que contenha o menor vestígio de trigo, centeio, aveia, cevada, tritical, malte ou qualquer derivado destes cereais, fico muito doente.

Posso comer alimentos que contenham milho e arroz.

Por favor, confirme com o chefe de cozinha que a minha comida não contém nenhum dos ingredientes indicados acima e ajude-me a pedir uma refeição que eu possa saborear em segurança.

Os meus agradecimentos!

Russian Gluten-Intolerance Card

Я не говорю по-русски.
У меня глютеиновая болезнь, и я не переношу глютен, в каком бы-то ни было виде.
Мне станет плохо, если я съем любую еду, продукт питания, химическую добавку или стабилизатор, содержащие пусть даже незначительное количество пшеницы, ржи, овса, ячменя, тритикале, солода или любых производных от этих зерен.
Мне можно есть продукты, в которых содержится кукуруза и рис.
Убедительно прошу Вас обратиться к повару и проверить, не содержит ли моя пища какого-либо из ингредиентов, перечисленных выше, и помочь мне заказать еду, которая была бы для меня безопасной.
Большое Вам спасибо!

Spanish Gluten-Intolerance Card

No hablo su idioma.

Suffro de una infermidad celiaca. No puedo tolerar gluten in ninguna forma.

Si como un alimento o producto, aditivo quimico o establizador que contenga trigo, avena, cebada, tricale, malta o ninguno de los derivados de estos granos m'enferman.

Puedo comer cualquier alimento que contenga maiz y arroz.

Si es posible, por favor informe el cocinero para asegurarse que mi comida no contenga ningun ingrediente de los especificados anteriormente y ayudeme a ordenar una comida que pueda disfrutar.

Muchas gracias.

Swahili Gluten-Intolerance Card

Nina ugongwa unayoitwa 'celiac,' na sifai kula chakula che chote chenye asili ya ngano au aina nyingine ya nafaka.

Nikila chakula chenye ngano, shayiri, unga wa porridgie na kadhalika, hata kama ni kidogo, nitakuwa mgongwa sana.

Naweza kula chakula chenye mahindi na mchele.

Tafadhali hakikisha kwa mpishi wenu kwamba chakula changu hakina vitu vilivyotajwa. Nisaidie kuagiza chakula kizuri kwa usalama wangu.

Asanta sana.

Swedish Gluten-Intolerance Card

Jag talar inte ert språk.

Jag har celiaki och tål inte gluten i någon form.

Om jag äter någon mat, produkt, kemisk tillsats eller konsistensgivare som innehåller bara den minsta aning av vete, råg, havre, korn, rågvete, malt eller något derivat av dessa sädesslag blir jag sjuk.

Jag kan äta mat som innehåller majs och ris.

Var snäll och tala med köksmästaren för att vara säker på att min mat inte innehåller någon av ovannämnda ingredienser och hjälp mig beställa en måltid som jag kan njuta av utan risk.

Tack så mycket för hjälpen!

Thai Gluten-Intolerance Card

ฉันพูดภาษาของคุณไม่เป็น
ฉันเป็นโรคในช่องท้อง จึงไม่สามารถรับประทานโปรตีน
ข้าว (Gluten) ได้ ทั้งนี้ไม่ว่าจะเป็นในรูปแบบใดก็ตาม
ถ้าหากว่าฉันได้รับประทานอาหารใดๆ ผลิตภัณฑ์ใดๆ สาร
เคมีต่อเติมใดๆ หรือสารกันการเปลี่ยนแปลงใดๆ ที่
ประกอบด้วยข้าวสาลี, ข้าวไรย์, ข้าวโอ๊ต, ข้าวบาร์เลย์, ข้าว
พันธุ์ผสมทรีทีเคล, มอลต์ หรือสิ่งใดที่ผลิตจากเมล็ดข้าว
ชนิดดังกล่าวมานี้ ทั้งนี้ไม่ว่าปริมาณจะน้อยก็ตาม ฉันจะ
เกิดป่วยอย่างหนัก
ฉันยังสามารถรับประทานอาหารที่ประกอบด้วยขาวโพดหรือ
ข้าวได้
กรุณาถามพ่อครัวดูก่อน เพื่อให้แน่นอนว่า อาหารที่ฉันจะ
รับประทานจะไม่มีส่วนประกอบใดๆ ที่ได้ระบุข้างต้นนี้
และช่วยฉันสั่งอาหารที่ฉันสามารถกินอย่างเอร็ดอร่อยและ
ปลอดภัยได้
ขอขอบพระคุณ

answers to the world's first gluten-free crossword puzzle

(The puzzle can be found on pages 448–449)

¹C	²A	³R	⁴B	⁵O	■	⁶G	⁷R	⁸A	⁹B	■	¹⁰M	¹¹U	¹²T ¹³S
¹⁴O	P	I	U	M	■	¹⁵R	I	L	E	■	¹⁶U	H	O H
¹⁷P	A	S	T	A	■	¹⁸E	A	S	E	■	¹⁹R	A	R A
■	²⁰K	E	R	N	E	L	²¹O	F	²²T	R	U	T	H
²³H	²⁴A	Y	■	²⁵O	N	S	■	²⁶H	A	L	E	■	
²⁷O	L	D	²⁸E ²⁹S	T	■	³⁰W ³¹H	E	Y	■				
³²F	L	I	E	R	■	³³F	O	E	■	³⁴F ³⁵L ³⁶A			
³⁷F	E	E	L	I	³⁸N ³⁹G	O	N	E	S	⁴⁰O ⁴¹A	T	S	
⁴²A	N	T	■	⁴³G	I	G	■	⁴⁴T	A	N	G	O	
■	⁴⁵A ⁴⁶C	C	T	■		⁴⁷G	L	U	T	E	N		
⁴⁸M ⁴⁹I	N	S	■	⁵⁰T ⁵¹E	A	■	⁵²A	N	E				
⁵³C	E	R	⁵⁴E ⁵⁵A	L	K	I	L	L	E	⁵⁶R ⁵⁷S	■		
⁵⁸A	T	O	M	■	⁵⁹I	O	N	A	■	⁶⁰L	O	T	⁶¹U ⁶²S
⁶³T	O	N	I	■	⁶⁴F	R	E	T	■	⁶⁵S	U	I	T E
⁶⁶S	O	Y	A	■	⁶⁷E	N	D	E	■	⁶⁸E	X	C	E L

sources

1. The Brave New Celiac

Can I Use Oats? Gluten-Intolerance Group Web site, www.gluten.net.

Celiac Disease, What Happens, Symptoms, Cause, Diagnoses and Treatment, Celiac Disease Foundation, www.celiac.org.

"Celiac Facts and Stats," University of Chicago Celiac Disease Program, *Living Without,* Summer 2003.

"Facts and Figures 2003," *Chicago Celiac Disease Program Newsletter.*

"Consumer Group Petitions FDA to Require "Diarrhea" Notice on Foods that Contain Sorbitol," Center for Science in the Public Interest, Press Release, September 1999.

Gluten-Free Diet, Mayo Clinic Patient and Health Education Center, Rochester, MN.

The Gluten-Free Diet, Gluten Intolerance Group Web site, www.gluten.net.

Gluten-Free Diet, Shelly Case, R.D., Centax Books, revised ed., 2002.

"Gluten-Free Guidelines," *Manual of Clinical Dietetics,* 6th ed., 2000.

"Gluten-Restricted, Gliadin-Free Diet," American Dietetic Association, *Manual of Clinical Dietetics.*

Grains and Glossary, CSA/USA Library of Resource Materials.

The History of Celiac Disease and of Its Diagnostic Practices, Stefano Guandalini, M.D. and Michelle Melin-Rogovin, University of Chicago Celiac Disease Program.

"Know the Facts," Amy Ratner, *Gluten-Free Living,* September–October 2001.

Merck Manual of Diagnosis and Therapy, 16th ed. (Merck).

"Oats and the Gluten-Free Diet," *Journal of the American Dietetic Association* 103, March 2003.

On the Celiac Condition: A Handbook for Celiac Patients and Their Families, CSA/USA.

"Presentation on Celiac Disease and the Gluten-Free Diet," Emily Rubin, R.D., Thomas Jefferson Hospital Digestive Diseases Institute, Philadelphia, September 2003.

"Prevalence of Celiac Disease in At-Risk and Not-At-Risk Groups in the United States, A Large Multi-Center Study," Fasano et al., *Archives of Internal Medicine* 163, February 2003.

"Questionable Foods and the Gluten-Free Diet," Tricia Thompson, R.D. *Journal of the American Dietetic Association* 100, April 2000.

"Quick Start Guide for a Gluten-Free Diet," Celiac Disease Foundation and Gluten Intolerance Group, *Living Without*, Fall 2002.

"The Range of Celiac Symptoms," Mary Courtney, *Celiac Disease Foundation Newsletter* 6–3, Summer 1993.

Vegetarian Gluten-Free and Gluten-Containing Foods, Vegetarian Society, www.vegsoc.org/info/gluten.html.

"Wheat Starch, Gliadin and the Gluten-Free Diet," Tricia Thompson, R.D., *Journal of the American Dietetic Association* 101, December 2004.

3. *Thinking Like a Celiac*

"Celiac Disease and the Military," Capt. John Himberger, U.S. Air Force, Family Nurse Practitioner, *Lifeline*, CSA, Summer 2003.

Facts and Fallacies about Digestive Diseases, National Digestive Diseases Information Clearinghouse Web site, digestive.niddk.hih.gov.

Family Protection Program, Federal Emergency Management Agency, Washington, D.C.

Healing with Whole Foods, Oriental Traditions and Modern Nutrition, Paul Pitchford (North Atlantic Books, 1993).

"Foods that Pack a Wallop," *Time*, January 2002.

"If You Can't Eat Bread, Drink Only the Wine," Rabbi Marc Gellman and Msgr. Thomas Hartman, *Newsday*, May 22, 2004.

Information Bulletin, The Canada Revenue Agency.

"More on the Communion Issue," *Houston Celiac-Sprue Support Group Newsletter*, September 2000.

Nutritional Supplements, U.S. Internal Revenue Service Pamplet #502.

"Science Article Raises Possibility of Pill to Block Gluten," Stefano Guandalini, M.D., *University of Chicago Celiac Disease Program Newsletter*, Winter 2002.

"Stomach Trouble," Michelle Andrews, *Self*, February 2004.

"The Structural Basis for Gluten Intolerance in Celiac Disease," Lu Shan, Chaitan Khosla et al. *Science*, September 27, 2002.

"Target Celiac Disease," Bon Harder, *Science News* 163, June 21, 2003.

"Gluten Response in Children with Celiac Disease," F. Koning and W. Vader, *Gastroenterology 122*, June 2002.

13. *Sex and the Celiac*

"Non-Malignant Complications of Coeliac Disease," G. K. T. Holmes, Department of Medicine, Derbyshire Royal Infirmary, Derby, UK, *Acta Paediatric Supplement* 412, 1996.

"Coeliac Disease and Unfavorable Outcome of Pregnancy," P. Martinelli et al., University of Naples Federico II, *Gut*, March 2000.

"Infertility and Ceoliac Disease" by P. Collin et al., Department of Medicine, University of Tampere, Finland, *Gut* (1996).

"Coeliac Disease in the Father Affects the Newborn," J. F. Ludvigsson, and, J. Ludvigsson, Obrero Medical Centre Hospital and Linkoping University, Sweden, *Gut* (2001).

"Coeliac Disease," by Peter H.R. Green, Bana Jabri, *The Lancet* (August 2003).

"Physician Awareness in Celiac Disease, A Survey of Complications Involving Fertility, Pregnancy, and Lactation" and "A National Survey of Infertility in Women with Untreated Celiac Disease," fielded by Joseph B. Palascak, M.D., Monica B. Awsare, M.D., Emily Rubin, R.D., Alice Bast, Anthony J. DiMarino, M.D.

"Fertility and Pregnancy in Women with CD," by Michelle Melin-Rogivin, *Celiac Disease Foundation Newsletter,* Fall 2002.

"Pregnancy and the Celiac," by Gloria Scarparo, R.D., *CSA Lifeline*, Fall 2003.

Letters to the Editor, *Gut* 49 (2001); by K. K. Hozyasz, Pediatric Department, National Research Institute of Mother and Child, Warsaw, Poland.

"Undiagnosed Coeliac Disease Does Not Appear to Be Associated with Unfavorable Outcome of Pregnancy," *Gut* 53 (2004); by L. Greco et al., University of Naples Federico II, Italy.

"All About Eating for Two," by Judith Levine Willis, *FDA Consumer* (April 1990).

"Lactation Reduces Breast Cancer Risk in Shandong Province, China," by Zheng et al., *American Journal of Epidemiology*, December 15, 2000.

American Academy of Pediatrics, *Breastfeeding Policy Statement: Breast Feeding and the Use of Human Milk.*

"Nutrition and Dental Decay in Infants," by W. J. Loesche, *American Journal of Clinical Nutrition,* February 1985.

"Breast-Feeding Best Bet for Babies," by R. D. Williams, U.S. Food and Drug Administration statement.

"The Nine Months of Living Anxiously," by Alex Kuczynski, *New York Times*, May 23, 2004.

"Foods to Avoid during Pregnancy and Eating for Two," American Pregnancy Association, www.americanpregnancy.org.

15. *The Doctor Will See You Now*

"Ask the Doctor," by Michelle Pietzak, M.D., *Celiac Disease Foundation Newsletter*, Winter 2003.

"Doctor Discipline," by Josh Goldstein, *Philadelphia Inquirer*, November 16, 2003.

"The Iceberg Cometh: Establishing the Prevalence of Celiac Disease in the United States and Finland," Daniel S. Kamin, Glenn T. Furuta, *Gastroenterology,* January 2004.

"Is Intestinal Biopsy Always Needed for Diagnosis of Celiac Disease?" by R. Scoglio, et al., *American Journal of Gastroenterology,* June 2003.

The Merck Manual of Diagnosis and Therapy, 16th ed. (Merck).

Mosby's Medical Dictionary, 6th ed., Harcourt Health Sciences (2002).

"Perfect Health, Other Than the Quintuple Bypass," by Jay Neugeboren, *New York Times*, April 2, 2004.

"Small-Bowel Endoscopy," by T. Roscht, *Endoscopy*, November 2002.

"Strong Medicine," by Joanne Kaufman, *New York Magazine,* December 2, 2002.

"Ten Diseases Doctors Miss," by Alice Lesch Kelly, *Prevention*, February 2004.

"Wash Those Hands," by Christine Gorman, *Time,* March 29, 2004.

16. *The Seven-Year Itch & Other Associated Conditions*

"The Celiac/Autoimmune Thyroid Connection," *Digestive Diseases and Sciences* 45, February 2000.

"Celiac Disease and the Skin," by John J. Zone, M.D., presentation at symposium, Celiac Disease Center, Columbia University, New York, November 2, 2002.

"Common Associated Medical Conditions—Established and Emerging," by Dr. Edward Hoffenberg, M.D., *CDF Newsletter*, Winter 2001.

"Dermatitis Herpetiformus, Skin Disorders," www.nutramed.com.

"Detecting Celiac Disease in Your Patients," by Harold T. Pruessner, M.D., *American Academy of Family Physicians*, March 1998.

"Endocrinological Disorders and Celiac Disease," by Pekka Collin et al., *Endocrine Reviews*, August 2002.

"Focus on Vitamin D: A Need That Doesn't Change with the Seasons" and "Shining a Light on the Health Benefits of Vitamin D," by Claudia Dreifus, *New York Times,* January 28, 2003.

"Immunity Challenged," by Angelina Sciolla, *Philadelphia Magazine,* March–April 2004.

"Non-Hodgkin's Lymphoma and Lymphoma," The Lymphoma Research Foundation, www.lymphoma.org.

"Risk of Malignancy in Patients with Celiac Disease," by Peter H. R. Green, M.D., et al., *American Journal of Medicine* 115, 2003.

"SIGEP Study Group for Autoimmune Disorders in Celiac Disease," by A. Ventura et al., *Gastroenterology* 117, August 1999.

"Was JFK the Victim of An Undiagnosed Disease Common to the Irish?" by Peter H. R. Green, M.D., History News Network, November 2002.

"What Diabetes Is," National Diabetes Information Clearinghouse, www.diabetes.niddk.nih.gov.

"The Widening Spectrum of Celiac Disese," by Joseph A. Murray, M.D., *American Journal of Clinical Nutrition* 69, 1999.

17. Rx for Health

"Help Yourself to Gluten-Free Medication," by Sr. Jeanne Patricia Crowe, Pharm. D., R.Ph., *Greater Philadelphia Celiac Sprue Support Group Newsletter,* August 2002.

"Celiac Sprue: A Guide through the Medicine Cabinet," by Marcia Milazzo, Medford, N.J., 2004.

"A Practical Guide to Contemporary Pharmacy Practice" (School of Pharmacy, 2nd edition, 2004).

"Clearing Up Cosmetic Confusion," *Celiac Disease Foundation Newsletter,* Summer 2001.

19. How Many Celiacs Does It Take to Change a Label?

"Alice's Story" by Alice Bast, *Greater Philadelphia Celiac Sprue Support Group Newsletter,* March 2003.

American Celiac Task Force Web site, www.celiaccenter.org/taskforce.asp.

Canadian Celiac Association Web site, www.celiac.ca.

CSA Web site, www.csaceliacs.org.

Celiac Disease Foundation Web site, www.celiac.org.

Gluten Intolerance Group Web site, www.gluten.net.

Letter to David Glass Ultimate Chocolate Truffle Cake, by permission of David Marc Fischer.

Minor Use and Minor Species Animal Health Act, 108th Congress, 2nd Session, H.R.S. 741.

National Foundation for Celiac Awareness Web site, www.celiacfoundation.org.

acknowledgments

One never accomplishes a task like this alone.

For their suggestions, insightful review and careful reading of the medical sections of this book, I am indebted to the following experts: Frederick B. Vivino, M.D., F.A.C.R., Chief, Division of Rheumatology, University of Pennsylvania Medical Center, Director, PENN Sjögren's Syndrome Center; Serge Jabbour, M.D., F.A.C.P., F.A.C.E., Clinical Assistant Professor of Medicine, Division of Endocrinology, Diabetes and Metabolic Diseases, Thomas Jefferson University Hospital; Kays Kaidbey, M.D., Professor of Dermatology, Ret., University of Pennsylvania; Alessio Fasano, M.D., University of Maryland; John Zone, M.D., Professor of Dermatology, University of Utah; and Anthony J. DiMarino, M.D., Chief, Division of the Digestive Diseases Center at Thomas Jefferson University Hospital.

A special thanks to Jay DiMarino for his kind words and excellent foreword and to Dr. Michelle Pietzak for her important introduction to the subject of pediatric celiac disease—and for dropping everything to do it. Passion, optimism, and empathy are gifts these dedicated physicians give us.

I shall always be indebted to Dr. Joseph Murray of the Mayo Clinic for all he has done for me, both personally and professionally.

For sharing the latest American Dietetic Association information on the gluten-free diet, as well as research on infertility and problems of pregnancy among undiagnosed celiacs, I thank Emily Rubin, R.D., of Thomas Jefferson

University Hospital Celiac Center, and Alice Bast, founder of the National Foundation for Celiac Awareness.

So, too, am I grateful to Elaine Monarch, Diane Eve Paley, Mary Schluckebier, Janet Rinehart, Jeannie Gee, Cynthia Kupper, and Danna Korn, for their support, friendship, many kindnesses, and good, good work.

I salute publisher Peggy Wagener for her essential *Living Without* magazine and for giving me a forum for my "slightly eccentric" views. You are a gluten-free goddess.

My appreciation to "Gluten-Free Lee" Tobin and Karen Shoenholtz of Whole Foods Market for their enthusiastic participation in this project, and especially for *The "No More Tummy Aches" Cupcake*. Birthdays will be much brighter because of these good people.

Many thanks to Beth Hillson, celebrity chef, celiac activist, and pal. Your generosity is boundless. And so, too, I am grateful to Johnny Alamilla, Rick Bayless, Rebecca Bunting, Barbara Cassidy, Betty Lou Davis, Workeye Ephrem, Bobby Flay, Joe Garrera, Bette Hagman, Nigella Lawson, Aimee Olexy, Shola Olunoyo, Cristina Pirello, Sarah Pluta, Rebecca Reilly, Connie Sarros, Bryan Sikora, and Bill Wavrin of Miraval Spa for their glorious gifts of food. At the end of the day, this is what celiac disease is really about. Eating well is the best revenge.

For putting his dagger down and deadline aside to help me plot the world's first gluten-free crossword puzzle (a murderously difficult procedure), I thank my good friend Steve Zettler, who with his wife and writing partner, Cordelia Frances Biddle, is the mayhem-meister behind the wildly popular Crossword Puzzle Mystery Series from Berkley Prime Crime.

There are good and true friends and kind strangers who rallied, read, encouraged, cooked, copied, downloaded, Googled, sent kisses, cookies, prayers, food, flowers, tested recipes, strategized, answered technical questions, cooked my pasta, served gluten-free rolls, nudged busy doctors, chefs, and other well-known personages, helped me keep body and soul together, and otherwise cheered me on—Betty Lou Davis, Joan Milarsky, Phyllis Moffo, Jack Cassidy, Tom Smitley, Susan Kaidbey, George Ritchie, Cordelia Biddle, Regina DiMartino, Toni O'Donnell, Kathy Lowry, Pam King, Bernadette Brescia, Andrew Marconi, Anne Eiswerth, Dr. Leonard Molczan, Adam Bere, Fiona Kingdon, Judy and Yigal Ron, chef Oscar Reyes and Nikki Gross of Fitzwater Café, and Keeli Manning. For his first-rate translations and good Lebanese coffee, Issam Masri of Al-Warak, Inc.

I am grateful to my agent Wendy Sherman for her steady and wise council, and I am blessed to have worked with editor Lisa Considine. Her unflagging enthusiasm and keen instinct nudged me toward a better book than the one I had in mind. Without Danny Reid, where would anybody be? Or without Holt's ongoing belief in a celiac market?

I shall never fully repay Jane Kirkwood for her fierce grace and lifelong friendship.

On these pages and in our hearts, Phyllis Brogden is here in so many ways.
And John, always—friend, partner, guiding light, love.

recipe acknowledgments and permissions

Chicken Crepes, Blondies, General Tso's Chicken, Gluten-Free Matzoh, Pad Thai by permission of Beth Hillson and the Gluten-Free Pantry.

Quinoa Potato Gratin with Ancho Chili Cream by permission of Johnny Alamilla and Alma Restaurant.

Classic Cheese Soufflé and Dark Chocolate Soufflé by permission of Shola Olunoyo and the Studio Kitchen.

Roasted Vegetable Lasagna, "No More Tummy Aches" Cupcakes, and Gluten-Free Fruit Cake by permission of Lee Tobin and Whole Foods Market.

Warm Ricotta Mousse by permission of Betty Lou Davis.

Saffron Risotto Cakes with Shrimp, Chili Oil, and Chive Oil by permission of Bobby Flay and Bolo Restaurant.

Spring Vegetable Paella and Rice Pudding from *Everything You Wanted to Know about Whole Foods but Were Afraid to Ask* by Christina Pirello (HP Books, 2004); and Miso Soup from *Cooking the Whole Foods Way* by Christina Pirello (HP Books, 1997) reprinted by permission of Christina Pirello.

Roasted Chili Polenta with Shiitake Tomatillo Sauce by permission of Bill Wavrin, Miraval Spa.

Goat Cheese Cake with Nut Crust and Lemon Curd, Chickpea Socca, and Savory Parmesan Crisps by permission of Bryan Sikora and Aimee Olexy, Django, Philadelphia.

Apple Pie, Chicken Pot Pie, Red Pepper Lobster Quiche and Native Corn Bread from the forthcoming *Sumptuous and Savory without Gluten or Wheat* by permission of Rebecca Bunting.

Quesadillas Asadas from *Rick Bayless's Mexican Kitchen* (Scribner, 1996) reprinted by permission of Rick Bayless.

Pakoras with Sweet and Spicy Chutney and Cucumber Raita by Sara J. Pluta reprinted by permission of *Living Without* magazine, www.livingwithout.com.

Ghenet Ethiopian Injera by permission of Yeworkwhoha "Workeye" Ephrem of Ghenet Restaurant, SoHo, New York, New York.

A Twice-Baked Teething Biscuit and Hamantashen by permission of Joe Garrera.

Cornmeal Porridge with Dried Fruit courtesy *Gourmet*, © 1991 by Condé Nast Publications, Inc.

Face Paint, Bubbles, and Play Dough from *Wheat-Free, Gluten-Free Cookbook for Kids and Busy Adults* (Contemporary Books, 2003) reprinted by permission of Connie Sarros.

Bath Tub Paint reprinted by permission of Elaine Monarch, *Celiac Disease Foundation Newsletter,* Spring 2003.

Give Thanks Gluten-Free Gravy, Cassidy Family Sweet Potato Casserole, and Count-Your-Blessings Cheesecake by permission of Barbara Cassidy.

Classic Gluten-Free Bread Stuffing with Crisp Sage Dressing from *Gluten-Free Baking: More Than 125 Recipes for Delectable Sweet and Savory Baked Goods, Pies, Quick Breads, Muffins, and Other Delights* (Simon & Schuster, 2001) by permission of Rebecca Reilly.

Gluten-Free Sponge Cake from the *Wheat-Free, Gluten-Free Desert Cookbook* (Contemporary Books, 2003) reprinted by permission of Connie Sarros.

A Proper Christmas Trifle from *Nigella Lawson: How to Eat, The Pleasure and Principles of Good Food* (John Wiley & Sons, 2002) by permission of Nigella Lawson.

index

General Index

Bob's Red Mill, 110
Boca Burger, 78
Bocuse, Paul, 135
Bolo, 131
Bonefish Grill, 183–84
bone(s), xviii, 3, 5, 56, 57, 372–75; density
   scan, 56, 355, 373
Bone Suckin' Sauce, 110
Bonne Bell company, 404
books, 475–77
Boozler, Elaine, 156
Boston Market, 184
Bouchard Family Farms, 110
bowel movements, 67
Boy Meets Grill (Flay), 131
brain cells, 58
brain fog, 4, 383, 401
Brazilian food, 198, 205, 227–28
breads: best, 102, 104–5; Ethiopian, 227;
   Indian, 234; restaurant terms for, 177;
   shopping for, 81; stocking in pantry, 22;
   yes and no, 9
Breadshop's Natural Foods, 111
breadsticks, favorite, 102
breast-feeding, 293, 300–301, 307–8
Brescia, Bernadette, 403
brewer's yeast, 275
Bristol Myers Squibb, 393
broccoli, 58, 59
Brogden, Phyllis, 414, 430
Brown, Dan and Michelle, 216
brownies, 102, 133
Bruno King of Ravioli, 211
bubbles, 335, 337
buckwheat, 12, 23
Bufferin, 399
Bumblebar, 107, 111
BUN levels, 376
Bunny Hop Café, 83
Bunting, Rebecca, 47, 122, 124–29, 418–19
Burger King, 190–91
Burt's Bees, 404
Bush, George W., 440
Butte Creek Mill Cornmeal, 111

Café Baldo, 211
Café Pescara, 212
caffeine, 268, 298, 320
cake: anti-cheating strategies, 257; best,
   101–2, 106; Malaysian, 223
Cala Luna Resort, 216
calcium, 5, 57, 296, 298, 355, 372–74
Campbell Soup Company, 118
Camp Celiac, 339, 435

Camp Kanata, 339
Camp Stealth, 339
Canada, 49–50, 94–95, 205, 212, 438–39
Canadian Celiac Association (CCA), 25, 49,
   438–39; local chapters, 473–75
Canadian Food Inspection Agency, 439
cancer, 308, 309
candy, 14, 324–28
canned goods, 79
Canyon Ranch, 214
Cape Verde, 226
caramel coloring, 18, 392
carbohydrates, 57, 268; intolerance, 14
Caribbean food, 228–29
Carrabba's Italian Grill, 184–85
Carvel, 118, 191
Casabe Rainforest Crackers, 111
Casa du Spaghetti, 212
Case, Shelly, 432
casein allergy, 14
Cassidy family, 419
caterer, 153–54, 283
Catholics, 16, 278, 279
Cause You're Special, 105, 111
Cavanaugh, Kathie, 431–32
caviar, 27–28
CDF Connections, 434
Cecilia's Gluten-Free Grocery, 95
Cedar House Bed & Breakfast, 217
Cedarlane Natural Foods, 111
Celebrex, 394
Celiac Awareness Month, 431
Celiac Chicks web site, 91, 282
celiac disease: adjusting attitude to, 26–41;
   American with Disabilities Act and, 281;
   associated conditions and, 368–86; bad
   news about, 8–9; biopsy for, 354; blood
   tests for, 353–54; breast-feeding and,
   300–301; chances of family having,
   xxi–xxii, 3–4; children and, 303–41;
   college and, 281; crossword puzzle on,
   447–49, 501; defined, 306–7; diagnosis
   of, xviii, xxii, xxv, 3–9, 65, 369; diagnosis
   of children with, 306–9; discovering you
   have, 3–9; doctor on children and,
   306–10; doctors and medical issues and,
   345–67; drug companies and, 393;
   emergency preparedness and, 50–52;
   enablers and, 286; fertility problems and,
   293–94; follow-up care for, xviii–xvix;
   food labeling bill and, 440–41; GI Bill of
   Rights and doctors, 347; good news
   about, 4–8; growing awareness of,
   xxii–xxiv; hygiene and, 292–93; internet

about the author

JAX PETERS LOWELL has been a diagnosed celiac—and gluten-free—since 1981. A lifestyle expert, advocate, and contributing editor to *Living Without* magazine, Lowell lives in Philadelphia in a converted bread factory with her husband and several cartons of rice pasta. She is the author of a novel, *Mothers.*